Clinical Trials

A Practical Guide to Design,
Analysis, and Reporting

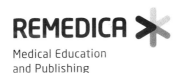

REMEDICA
Medical Education
and Publishing

£ 30.00

Also available from Remedica:
The Clinical Research Survival Guide
Handbook of Clinical Trials
Responsible Research: A Guide for Coordinators

Published by Remedica
Commonwealth House, 1 New Oxford Street, London WC1A 1NU, UK
Civic Opera Building, 20 North Wacker Drive, Suite 1642, Chicago, IL 60606, USA

info@remedicabooks.com
www.remedicabooks.com
Tel: +44 20 7759 2999
Fax: +44 20 7759 2951

Publisher: Andrew Ward
In-house editors: Catherine Harris, Carolyn Dunn, and Anuradha Choudhury
Design and artwork: AS&K Skylight Creative Services

First published 2006
Reprinted 2007

Printed in Spain

Remedica is a member of the AS&K Media Partnership.

ISBN-10: 1 901346 72 2
ISBN-13: 978 1 901346 72 5
British Library Cataloguing-in-Publication Data
A catalogue record for this book is available from the British Library.

Clinical Trials

A Practical Guide to Design, Analysis, and Reporting

Duolao Wang and Ameet Bakhai, Editors

Duolao Wang, PhD
Senior Statistician
Medical Statistics Unit
London School of Hygiene & Tropical Medicine
London, UK

Ameet Bakhai, MBBS, MRCP
Consultant Cardiologist
Barnet General & Royal Free Hospitals
AMORE Studies Group
London, UK

Author Biographies

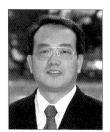

Duolao Wang, BSc, MSc, PhD

Dr Duolao Wang is a senior lecturer at the world renowned London School of Hygiene and Tropical Medicine, London, UK. He has more than 10 years of experience in clinical trials, and provides educational and consulting services to pharmaceutical companies, physicians, and contract research organizations. He has published extensively on medical and epidemiological research as well as statistical methodology in peer-reviewed journals, and has taught several hundreds of postgraduate students.

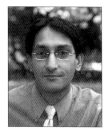

Ameet Bakhai, MBBS, MRCP

Dr Ameet Bakhai is a consultant cardiologist and physician at Barnet General & Royal Free Hospitals, London, UK. He has worked in clinical trials for 7 years, directing coronary intervention trials and leading collaborative Health Technology Assessments commissioned for groups such as the UK National Institute for Clinical Excellence. He has over 50 publications and gained statistical, trial, and economic evaluation expertise at the Harvard Clinical Research Institute, MA, USA. He is also a director of the Asha Medical Outcomes Research and Economic (AMORE) studies group.

Contributors

Radivoj Arezina, MD, MSc
Research Director
Richmond Pharmacology
St George's Hospital Medical School
London, UK

Ameet Bakhai, MBBS, MRCP
Consultant Cardiologist
Barnet General & Royal
Free Hospitals
AMORE Studies Group
London, UK

Amit Chhabra, MD, MPH
Research Associate
Harvard Clinical Research Institute
Boston, Massachusetts, USA

Tim Clayton, BSc, MSc
Senior Lecturer
Medical Statistics Unit
London School of Hygiene
& Tropical Medicine
London, UK

Felicity Clemens, BSc, MSc
Lecturer
Medical Statistics Unit
London School of Hygiene
& Tropical Medicine
London, UK

**Maurille Feudjo-Tepie,
BSc, MSc, PhD**
Senior Data Analyst
GlaxoSmithKline
Middlesex, UK

**Marcus Flather, BSc, MBBS,
FRCP**
Director
Clinical Trials & Evaluation Unit
Royal Brompton Hospital
London, UK

Zoe Fox, BSc, MSc
Statistician
Department of Primary Care
& Population Sciences
Royal Free & University College
Medical School
London, UK
Copenhagen HIV Programme (CHIP)
Hvidovre University Hospital
Copenhagen, Demark

Christopher Frost, MA, Dipstat
Reader
Medical Statistics Unit
London School of Hygiene
& Tropical Medicine
London, UK

Ashima Gupta, MD
Clinical Research Fellow
Barnet General Hospital
London, UK

Joseph Kim, BSc, MPH, PhD
Lecturer
Medical Statistics Unit
London School of Hygiene
& Tropical Medicine
London, UK

Stephen L Kopecky, MD
Associate Professor
Division of Cardiovascular Diseases
Mayo Clinic
Rochester, Minnesota, USA

Belinda Lees, BSc, PhD
Senior Research Coordinator
Clinical Trials & Evaluation Unit
Royal Brompton Hospital
London, UK

Ulrike Lorch, MD, MFPM, FRCA
Medical Director
Richmond Pharmacology
St George's Hospital Medical School
London, UK

James F Lymp, BSc, PhD
Research Scientist
Child Health Institute
University of Washington
Seattle, Washington, USA

Umair Mallick, MD
Associate Director
Clinical Trials Centre
Royal Free & University College
Medical School
London, UK

Sam Miller, BA, MSc
Senior Statistician
GlaxoSmithKline
Harlow, UK

Colin Neate, BSc, MSc
Senior Statistician
GlaxoSmithKline
Harlow, UK

Dorothea Nitsch, MD, MSc
Research Fellow
Medical Statistics Unit
London School of Hygiene
& Tropical Medicine
London, UK

Sonia Patel, BSc, MSc
Researcher
Clinical Trials & Evaluation Unit
Royal Brompton Hospital
London, UK

Craig Ritchie, MB, ChB,
MRC Psych, MSc
Director
Clinical Trials Centre
Royal Free & University College
Medical School
London, UK

Jaymin Shah, MD
Associate Director
Brigham & Women's Hospital
Angiographic Core Laboratory
Boston, Massachusetts, USA

Fiona Steele, BSc, MSc, PhD
Reader
Graduate School of Education
University of Bristol
Bristol, UK

Rajini Sudhir, MD, MRCP
Cardiologist
Barnet General Hospital
London, UK

Anil K Taneja, BSc, MBBS,
MRCP, MSc
Senior Research Fellow
Clinical Trials & Evaluation Unit
Royal Brompton Hospital
London, UK

Ann Truesdale, BSc
Trials Advisor
Medical Statistics Unit
London School of Hygiene
& Tropical Medicine
London, UK

Claudio Verzilli, BSc, PhD
Research Associate
Department of Epidemiology
& Public Health
Imperial College
London, UK

Duolao Wang, BSc, MSc, PhD
Senior Lecturer
Medical Statistics Unit
London School of Hygiene
& Tropical Medicine
London, UK

Hilary C Watt, BA, MA, MSc
Lecturer
Medical Statistics Unit
London School of Hygiene
& Tropical Medicine
London, UK

Hong Yan, MD, MSc
Professor
Medical Statistics Unit
Xi'an Jiaotong University
Xi'an, China

Wenyang Zhang, BSc, MSc, PhD
Senior Lecturer
Institute of Mathematics & Statistics
University of Kent at Canterbury
Kent, UK

Preface

Randomized controlled trials are rightly seen as the key means by which new treatments and interventions are evaluated for their safety and efficacy. There are now more randomized trials being undertaken and published than ever before – they provide the cornerstone of evidence-based medicine in current practice.

Hence, more and more people from a broad range of professional backgrounds need to understand the essentials of clinical trials as regards their design, statistical analysis, and reporting. This book is an admirable venture, in that it covers this whole field at a level of methodological detail that gives a good working knowledge of the subject. At the same time, it avoids undue technicalities or jargon so that even those with little or no previous knowledge of statistics, study design, or reporting practices will be able to follow all of the material presented.

The book's structure, with 38 chapters grouped into five broad sections, helps the reader to focus on one specific topic at a time, and should also make it a useful text to accompany taught courses in clinical trials.

The book represents a well-balanced account of clinical issues and statistical methods, which are clearly explained and illustrated with relevant examples throughout. The book also contains over 300 references, facilitating a more in-depth pursuit of each topic if desired. Overall, I think this book is an excellent contribution, which I recommend as a rewarding read for anyone interested in clinical trials and their methods.

Professor Stuart Pocock, PhD
Medical Statistics Unit
London School of Hygiene & Tropical Medicine

Acknowledgments

We are greatly indebted to Professor Stuart Pocock for his encouragement, support, and advice on the construction of this book. We also appreciate the useful comments and discussions about parts of the book with Professor Stephen Evans and Dr Marcus Flather, both experienced and renowned clinical trial specialists in their own rights.

We would also like to thank all our wonderful and professional contributors for their diligence and hard work in producing various chapters. We are deeply grateful to our editors Catherine Harris, Carolyn Dunn, Philip Shaw, and Andrew Ward for their efforts in bringing this book into publication, which they did so professionally and without stress.

Finally and most importantly for us - we are personally indebted to our wonderful respective partners Yali and Varsha, and our children (Emma, Tom, Anisha, and Asha), for their support, enthusiasm, and tolerance, without which this book would have never been completed. We have stolen many precious moments from them, making this work as much theirs as ours. Thank you to all of our family and friends.

Contents

Introduction

The inspiration...

Over 7 years ago, while working on design and analyses of projects conducted at the Clinical Trials and Evaluation Unit at the Royal Brompton Hospital, London, a young clinician and statistician began what was to become a long journey together into clinical trials. We were fortunate to meet Andrew Ward, Publisher from Remedica, along the way, and our journey culminated in the creation of this book – initially starting with short 500-word articles explaining concepts such as P-values and confidence intervals, and concluding in 5,000 word articles explaining multicenter studies and meta-analyses.

Along the way, we have published more than 30 peer-reviewed and invited papers with others, continually building our writing style to be able to appeal to clinicians, statisticians, and trial workers alike. This book is therefore unique in that it quickly demystifies and brings the language of clinical trials within reach of all.

The audience...

This book describes and explains the issues that occur during all stages of clinical trials, covering design, analysis, and reporting of clinical trials, with an emphasis on open, practical, and effective communication. The material is therefore ideal for those involved in designing, conducting, analyzing, evaluating, interpreting, or publishing clinical trials – including physicians, medical students, clinical and medical researchers, study co-ordinators, project managers, medical writers, data managers, pharmaceutical scientists, statisticians, medical economists, medical analysts, and those working in the health services who have to evaluate such material.

The material...

Our book consists of 38 chapters in five sections: fundamentals of trial design, alternative trial designs, basics of statistical analysis, special trial issues in data analysis, and reporting of trials. The chapters can be read consecutively or individually, with Chapter 1 providing an overview and some reading guidelines. To hold interest, the chapters are scattered with numerous practical examples of concepts and illustrations relating to trials, and there are even chapters enabling one to become a polished trial sceptic. The chapters on tables and figures are essential for those submitting their reports for regulatory approval or for publication, and the statistical chapters provide step-by-step guidance on which tests to use.

The clincher...

More importantly, most chapters can be read in 30 minutes – essential for commuters, those who like to read during lectures or lunch breaks, and those who might need to fall asleep on a book. Even more appealing is that the 5 hours it often takes to cross the Atlantic give you enough time to land as a smarter conference delegate after digesting key sections of this book.

Duolao Wang
Ameet Bakhai
Editors

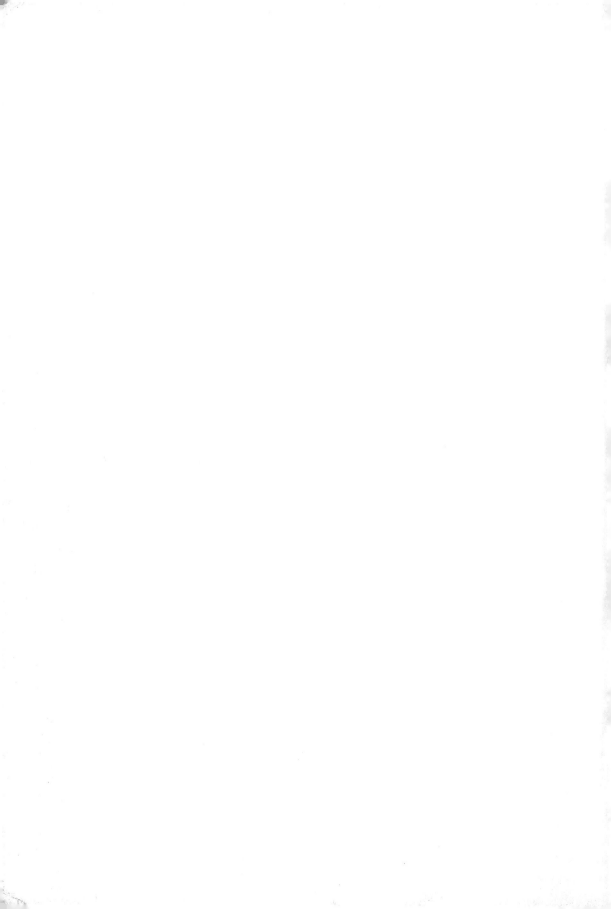

Part I

Fundamentals of Trial Design

Chapter 1

Randomized Clinical Trials

Duolao Wang, Dorothea Nitsch,
and Ameet Bakhai

Randomized clinical trials are scientific investigations that examine and evaluate the safety and efficacy of new drugs or therapeutic procedures using human subjects. The results that these studies generate are considered to be the most valued data in the era of evidence-based medicine. Understanding the principles behind clinical trials enables an appreciation of the validity and reliability of their results. In this chapter, we describe key principles and aspects of clinical trial design, analysis, and reporting. We also discuss factors that might lead to a biased study result, using a contemporary clinical trial to illustrate key concepts. Throughout, the reader is referred to later chapters that offer more detailed discussions.

What is a randomized clinical trial?

A clinical trial evaluates the effect of a new drug (or device or procedure) on human volunteers. These trials can be used to evaluate the safety of a new drug in healthy human volunteers, or to assess treatment benefits in patients with a specific disease. Clinical trials can compare a new drug against existing drugs or against dummy medications (placebo) or they may not have a comparison arm (see **Chapter 2**). A large proportion of clinical trials are sponsored by pharmaceutical or biotechnology companies who are developing the new drug, but some studies using older drugs in new disease areas are funded by health-related government agencies, or through charitable grants.

In a randomized clinical trial, patients and trial personnel are deliberately kept unaware of which patient is on the new drug. This minimizes bias in the later evaluation so that the initial blind random allocation of patients to one or other treatment group is preserved throughout the trial. Clinical trials must be designed in an ethical manner so that patients are not denied the benefit of usual treatments. Patients must give their voluntary consent that they appreciate the purpose of the trial. Several key guidelines regarding the ethics, conduct, and reporting of clinical trials have been constructed to ensure that a patient's rights and safety are not compromised by participating in clinical trials [1–3].

Are there different types of clinical trials?

Clinical trials vary depending on who is conducting the trial. Pharmaceutical companies typically conduct trials involving new drugs or established drugs in disease areas where their drug may gain a new license. Device manufacturers use trials to prove the safety and efficacy of their new device.

Clinical trials conducted by clinical investigators unrelated to pharmaceutical companies might have other aims. They might use established or older drugs in new disease areas, often without commercial support, given that older drugs are unlikely to generate much profit. Clinical investigators might also:

- look at the best way to give or withdraw drugs
- investigate the best duration of treatment to maximize outcome
- assess the benefits of prevention with vaccination or screening programs

Thus, different types of trials are needed to cover these needs; these can be classified under the following headings.

Phases

The pharmaceutical industry has adopted a specific trial classification based on the four clinical phases of development of a particular drug (Phases I–IV) [4–7]. In *Phase I*, manufacturers usually test the effects of a new drug in healthy volunteers or patients unresponsive to usual therapies. They look at how the drug is handled in the human body (pharmacokinetics/pharmacodynamics), particularly with respect to the immediate short-term safety of higher doses. Clinical trials in *Phase II* examine dose–response curves in patients and what benefits might be seen in a small group of patients with a particular disease.

In *Phase III*, a new drug is tested in a controlled fashion in a large patient population against a placebo or standard therapy. This is a key phase, where a drug will either make or break its reputation with respect to safety and efficacy before marketing begins. A positive study in Phase III is often known as a *landmark* study for a drug, through which it might gain a license to be prescribed for a specific disease.

A study in *Phase IV* is often called a *postmarketing* study as the drug has already been granted regulatory approval/license. These studies are crucial for gathering additional safety information from a larger group of patients in order to understand the long-term safety of the drug and appreciate drug interactions.

Trial design

Trials can be further classified by design. This classification is more descriptive in terms of how patients are randomized to treatment. The most common design is the parallel-group trial [4,5]. Patients are randomized to the new treatment or to the standard treatment and followed-up to determine the effect of each treatment in parallel groups. Other trial designs include, amongst others, crossover trials, factorial trials, and cluster randomized trials.

Crossover trials randomize patients to different sequences of treatments, but all patients eventually get all treatments in varying order, ie, the patient is his/her own control (see **Chapter 10**) [8,9]. *Factorial* trials assign patients to more than one treatment-comparison group. These are randomized in one trial at the same time, ie, while drug A is being tested against placebo, patients are re-randomized to drug B or placebo, making four possible treatment combinations in total (see **Chapter 11**). *Cluster randomized* trials are performed when larger groups (eg, patients of a single practitioner or hospital) are randomized instead of individual patients (see **Chapter 15**).

Number of centers

Clinical trials can also be classified as *single-center* or *multicenter* studies according to the number of sites involved. While single-center studies are mainly used for

Phase I and II studies, multicenter studies can be carried out at any stage of clinical development (see **Chapter 16**). Multicenter studies are necessary for two major reasons:

- to evaluate a new medication or procedure more efficiently in terms of accruing sufficient subjects over a shorter period of time
- to provide a better basis for the subsequent generalization of the trial's findings, ie, the effects of the treatment are evaluated in many types of centers

Other classifications

Trials can also be described as superiority studies, equivalence studies, or noninferiority studies in terms of what the study was designed to prove. A *superiority* study aims to show that a new drug is more effective than the comparative treatment (placebo or current best treatment) [4]. Most clinical trials belong to this category. On the other hand, an *equivalence* study is designed to prove that two drugs have the same clinical benefit. Hence, the trial should demonstrate that the effect of the new drug differs from the effect of the current treatment by a margin that is clinically unimportant (see **Chapters 12** and **13**). A *noninferiority* study aims to show that the effect of a new treatment cannot be said to be significantly weaker than that of the current treatment (see **Chapter 14**). In the latter two trials the new treatment might still turn out to be more effective than the comparative treatment, but this is not the prior assumption of the trials.

Clinical trials can also be classified by whether the trial is the first to compare a specific treatment (*exploratory*) or is a further trial trying to confirm a previous observation (*confirmatory*) [10]. An exploratory study might also seek to identify key issues rather than to confirm or challenge existing results regarding the treatment effect. For example, it might look at the impact of a new drug in a specific subset of patients who have additional diseases to the main disease of interest, such as diabetic patients with heart disease. On occasions, a study can have both confirmatory and exploratory aspects. For instance, in a confirmatory trial evaluating a specific treatment, the data can also be used to explore further hypotheses, ie, subgroup effects that have to be confirmed by later research.

Why might clinical trial results not represent the true difference?

In a clinical trial, the observed treatment effect regarding the safety and efficacy of a new drug may represent the 'true' difference between the new drug and the comparative treatment or it may not. This is to say that if the trial were to be repeated with all the available patients in the world then the outcome would either be the same as the trial (a true result) or different (making the trial result a chance event, or an erroneous false result). Understanding the possible sources of erroneous results is critical in the appreciation of clinical trials. Reasons for erroneous results fall into three main categories.

- Firstly, the trial may have been biased in some predictable fashion.
- Secondly, it could have been contaminated (confounded) by an unpredictable factor.
- Thirdly, the result might simply have occurred by random chance.

Bias/systematic errors

Bias can influence a trial by the occurrence of systematic errors that are associated with the design, conduct, analysis, and reporting of the results of a clinical trial. Bias can also make the trial-derived estimate of a treatment effect deviate from its true value (see **Chapter 6**) [4,5,11]. The most common types of bias in clinical trials are those related to subject selection and outcome measurement. For example, if the investigator is aware of which treatment a patient is receiving, it could affect the way that he/she collects information on the outcome during the trial, or he/she might recruit patients in a way that could favor the new treatment, resulting in a selection bias.

In addition, exclusion of subjects from statistical analysis because of noncompliance or missing data (see **Chapter 30**) could bias an estimate of the true benefit of a treatment, particularly if more patients were removed from analysis in one group than the other (see **Chapter 22**) [12]. Much of the advanced design strategies seek to reduce these systematic errors.

Confounding

Confounding represents the distortion of the true relationship between treatment and outcome by another factor, eg, the severity of disease (see **Chapter 26**). Confounding occurs when an extra factor is associated with both the outcome of interest and treatment group assignment. Confounding can both obscure an existing treatment difference and create an apparent difference that does not exist.

If we divided patients into treatment groups based on inherent differences (such as mean age) at the start of a trial then we would be very likely to find the benefit of the new treatment to be influenced by those pre-existing differences. For example, if we assign only smokers to treatment A, only nonsmokers to treatment B, and then assess which treatment protects better against cardiovascular disease, we might find that treatment B performs better – but the benefit may be due to the lack of smoking in this group. The effect of treatment B on cardiovascular disease development would therefore be confounded by smoking.

Randomization in conjunction with a large sample size is the most effective way to restrict such confounding, by evenly distributing both known and unknown confounding factors between treatment groups. If, before the study begins, we know which factors may confound the trial then we can use randomization techniques that force a balance of these factors (*stratified randomization*) (see **Chapter 7**). In the analysis stage of a trial, we might be able to restrict confounding using special statistical techniques such as *stratified analysis* and *regression analysis* (see **Chapter 24**).

Random error

Even if a trial has an ideal design and is conducted to minimize bias and confounding, the observed treatment effect could still be due to random error or chance [4,5]. The random error can result from sampling, biologic, or measurement variation in outcome variables. Since the patients in a clinical trial are only a sample of all possible available patients, the sample might yet show a chance false result compared to the overall population. This is known as a *sampling error*. Sampling errors can be reduced by choosing a very large group of patients or by using special analytic techniques that combine the results of several smaller studies, called a meta-analysis (see **Chapter 38**). Other causes of random error are described elsewhere [5].

Statistical analyses deal with random error by providing an estimate of how likely the measured treatment effect reflects the true effect (see **Chapters 18–21**). Statistical testing or inference involves an assessment of the probability of obtaining the observed treatment difference (or more extreme difference for an outcome), assuming that there is no difference between treatments. This probability is often called the *P*-value or false-positive rate. If the *P*-value is less than a specified critical value (eg, 5%), the observed difference is considered to be statistically significant. The smaller the *P*-value, the stronger the evidence is for a true difference between treatments. On the other hand, if the *P*-value is greater than the specified critical value then the observed difference is regarded as not statistically significant, and is considered to be potentially due to random error or chance. The traditional statistical threshold is a *P*-value of 0.05 (or 5%), which means that we only accept a result when the likelihood of the conclusion being wrong is less than 1 in 20, ie, we conclude that only one out of a hypothetical 20 trials will show a treatment difference when in truth there is none.

Statistical estimates summarize the treatment differences for an outcome in the form of point estimates (eg, means or proportions) and measures of precision (eg, confidence intervals [CIs]) (see **Chapters 18–21**). A 95% CI for a treatment difference means that the range presented for the treatment effect is 95% likely to contain (when calculated in 95 out of 100 hypothetical trials assessing the same treatment effect) the true value of the treatment difference, ie, the value we would obtain if we were to use the entire available patient population.

Finally, testing several different hypotheses with the same trial (eg, comparing treatments with respect to different outcomes or for several smaller subpopulations within the trial population) will increase the chance of observing a statistically significant difference purely due to chance (see **Chapter 29**). Even looking at the difference between treatments at many time points (interim analyses) throughout the length of the trial could lead to a spurious result due to multiple testing (see **Chapter 28**) [13]. Therefore, the aim should always be to plan a trial in such a way that the occurrence of any such errors is minimal (see **Chapter 31**). For the reader it is also important to be able to appraise the trial publication or report, to spot potential for such errors (see **Chapter 37**).

The CHARM program: an example of a randomized clinical trial

To design and analyze a clinical trial, one needs to ask several questions. For example:

- What are the objectives and endpoints of the study?
- What patient population or disease is the drug meant to treat?
- What criteria should be used to select patients eligible for the study?
- How large should the sample size be so that the study will have enough power to detect a clinically significant benefit?
- How sure can we be about the observed treatment benefits and that they will reflect a genuine treatment difference with minimal influence of systematic errors, confounding, or chance?

We will use the CHARM (Candesartan in Heart failure – Assessment of Reduction in Mortality and morbidity) trials to illustrate some of the main points that have to be considered in trial design, analysis, and reporting [14–17]. Patients with chronic heart failure (CHF) are at high risk of cardiovascular death and recurrent hospital admissions. The CHARM program consisted of three independent, but parallel, trials comparing the angiotensin receptor blocker candesartan to placebo in terms of mortality and morbidity among patients with CHF. The three patient populations enrolled (all with heart failure) were distinct but complementary, so that the effects of candesartan could be evaluated across a broad spectrum of patients with heart failure.

Objectives and endpoints

A clinical trial should have clear objectives that are measured by endpoints (see **Chapters 3** and **4**). The main objective of the CHARM program was to determine whether the use of candesartan could reduce mortality and morbidity in a broad population of patients with symptomatic heart failure. To test these hypotheses, the primary endpoint was defined as the time from randomization to death from any cause in the total CHARM population [14]. In each component trial, the primary endpoint was the time to the first occurrence of cardiovascular death or emergency hospitalization for the management of CHF (accordingly, the primary analysis of each component trial was based on this endpoint) [15–17].

It was ethically acceptable to perform this trial since there was not enough evidence to support the use of candesartan in patients with CHF prior to this study. The objectives and the endpoints were clearly stated in advance, and conclusions with respect to the effect of candesartan were based on these prespecified objectives and endpoints.

Study design

CHARM was a multicenter study consisting of three separate, two-arm, randomized, double-blinded, placebo-controlled subtrials into which patients were allocated depending on their left ventricular ejection fraction (strength of their heart function) and background use of angiotensin-converting enzyme (ACE) inhibitors at presentation [14–17]. Patients who had preserved left ventricular function (left ventricular ejection fraction ≥40%) were randomly allocated to either candesartan or placebo in the 'CHARM-Preserved' trial. Patients who had left ventricular ejection fraction <40% were split into a further two trials, depending on whether they had a known intolerance of ACE inhibitors ('CHARM-Alternative' trial) or were already on an ACE inhibitor ('CHARM-Added' trial). They were then randomized to candesartan versus placebo.

As demonstrated in the CHARM study, it is crucial to randomize patients to minimize systematic bias or confounding at the start of the study (see **Chapters 7** and **8**). In order to later have valid estimates of the effect of candesartan in one of these distinct patient populations with heart failure (preserved function, with or without intolerance to ACE inhibitors) it was necessary to split patients into these groups at the design stage.

Patient population

It should be noted that the results of a clinical trial can only be generalized to patients who are similar to the study participants (see **Chapter 5**). The CHARM investigators' aim was to assess candesartan in a broad spectrum of patients. Hence, the CHARM study population consisted of symptomatic heart failure patients (New York Heart Association class II–IV) aged ≥18 years, except those with recent major events or a very poor prognosis (such as patients with myocardial infarction, stroke, or open heart surgery in the previous 4 weeks, and any noncardiac disease judged likely to limit 2-year survival) [14–17]. Due to the principle of not harming patients, the study also excluded patients who presented with contraindications to treatment with candesartan. All patients gave their written informed consent before being enrolled.

Sample size calculation

The sample size calculation was used to minimize random error (see **Chapter 9**). We call this process *power* calculation. The study needed sufficient 'power' to be able to say something definitive about the effect of the treatment (relating to the primary endpoints) so it was important to include a sufficient number of patients.

A variety of rules exist on how to calculate the sample size for any given trial [18,19]. These are based on statistical models that take account of the recruitment of patients into the trial and the type of statistical test to be used. Different formulas are used depending on the trial design – conventional parallel-arm trials, cluster randomized trials, factorial trials, and crossover trials – as well as on the type of endpoint chosen, such as continuous outcomes (eg, average difference in blood pressure after treatment), binary outcomes (eg, disease-related event), and time-to-event or survival outcomes (eg, time to death) (see **Chapter 17**).

In the CHARM program, the overall study was designed to address the question of all-cause mortality [14]. The investigators assumed an annual overall mortality in the placebo group of 8%. On that basis, the program of investigation had >85% power to detect a 14% reduction in mortality at a significance level of 0.05, based on the log-rank test [14]. Each component trial independently estimated its respective sample size based on the anticipated event rate for the combined outcome of cardiovascular death or admission to hospital for CHF [15–17].

Conduct of the trial

The CHARM component trials recruited patients from 618 sites in 26 countries, with use of uniform procedures and management, and coordination via a single central unit [14]. Between March 1999 and March 2001, 7,599 patients were randomly assigned in a double-blind fashion to candesartan or matching placebo, stratified by site and component trial, with randomization provided through telephone to the central unit. The initial dose used was either 4 or 8 mg of the study drug. The dose was increased or decreased in response to the patient's clinical status, and algorithms were provided as guidelines for the management of hypotension or kidney dysfunction.

After the titration, visits were scheduled every 4 months, with a minimum planned duration of 2 years. Discontinuations because of patients' preferences or physicians' decisions were recorded, and these patients were followed-up for outcomes if possible. All deaths and first CHF hospital admissions were adjudicated by an endpoint committee (see **Chapter 3**). Neither doctors nor patients were able to deduce which treatment was given before ('allocation concealment') or during the course of the trial ('blinding') (see **Chapter 8**).

Interim monitoring

In the CHARM program, the assignment code of randomly assigned patients was held at an independent statistical center and an independent data and safety monitoring board (DSMB) was established to oversee the safety of patients enrolled in the trial and to monitor trial progress [20]. It had access to all data through the independent statistical center. Predefined stopping rules for efficacy or safety concentrated on mortality from the overall trial program (see **Chapter 31**) [13].

A pharmaceutical company that has heavily invested in a trial has a considerable interest in ensuring that the conduct of the trial does not jeopardize the likelihood of a positive outcome of the trial, eg, that the drug of interest is safe and efficacious. The use of an independent statistical center and a DSMB makes the whole process more transparent as these groups have patient safety as their primary concern. At predefined time points the existing data are therefore analyzed by the independent statistical center and the results are discussed with the DSMB.

The DSMB has to make sure that the new drug that patients are taking is not harmful. If, during the course of the trial, such evidence is found then the trial has to stop (*stopping for safety*). This idea can also be turned around: if there is major evidence for a beneficial effect of the new treatment before the planned end of the trial then the trial also has to stop. This is called *stopping for efficacy* because there is evidence of conclusive benefit of the treatment. Monitoring trial results is ethically challenging and has to balance individual ethics with the long-term interest in obtaining sufficient data [21].

Final data analysis

Intention-to-treat analysis means that outcomes of patients who were randomized but who subsequently discontinued or changed treatment are taken into account as if they had finished the trial (see **Chapter 22**). This is a pragmatic realization of the view that at the time of treatment start we will never be sure whether a patient will continue with that treatment. Hence, the intention-to-treat analysis reflects the general policy of using/prescribing the treatment in a given situation (ie, inclusion criteria).

All analyses in the CHARM program were done by intention-to-treat, and *P*-values were two-sided (see **Chapter 18**). All time-to-event endpoints were analyzed with the log-rank test, stratified by three substudies and displayed on Kaplan–Meier plots by treatment. The estimated hazard ratio from the Cox proportional hazards model was used to assess the size of treatment effect (candesartan against placebo) (see **Chapter 21**). In addition, a covariate-adjusted

Cox regression model was fitted with the prespecified 33 baseline covariates to adjust the hazard ratio for other factors that might affect prognosis (see **Chapters 24** and **25**). Prespecified subgroup analyses were done, each using a test for heterogeneity to assess for possible interactions between treatment and selected baseline variables (see **Chapters 23** and **27**). These elements will be discussed in more detail in later chapters.

Statistical analyses are usually prespecified in the trial protocol and should be performed as planned to ensure credibility and to deal with the issue of multiple testing (see **Chapter 29**) [22]. The principal statistical test for the primary endpoint analysis that was prespecified in the sample size calculation should be applied [4,5]. This means that it is imperative to plan a trial with care and to use current evidence that is as rigorous as possible in order to avoid as much bias as possible at the planning stage. Subgroup analysis can be performed, but it has to be recognized that a significant effect seen in a subgroup is not definitive evidence of a differential effect within subgroups of patients, unless the trial was powered initially to assess this (see **Chapter 23**) [22].

CHARM was designed and powered to assess separately the effects of candesartan on cardiovascular death or CHF hospitalization in different populations of patients with heart disease (CHARM-Preserved, -Added, -Alternative). In contrast, it was not designed to assess whether there was a differential effect of candesartan in diabetic participants compared to other patients with heart failure.

Trial reporting

The eventual results of the CHARM program were published in four reports [14–17], which followed the CONSORT (Consolidated Standards of Reporting Trials) statement and guidelines of reporting (see **Chapter 32**) [2,3]. A trial profile was provided to describe the flow of participants through each stage of the randomized controlled trial (enrollment, randomization, treatment allocation, follow-up, and analysis of a clinical trial) (see **Chapter 33**). The baseline characteristics of patients (including demographic information, heart disease risk factors, medical history, and medical treatment) were displayed in an appropriate format for each component trial as well as the overall program (see **Chapter 34**). These tables showed that the subtrials and the overall trial were comparable in terms of the patients' characteristics, making the estimates of unadjusted hazard ratio reliable.

The results with respect to the prespecified primary endpoints and relevant secondary endpoints were provided in appropriate tables and figures (see **Chapters 35** and **36**). For example, the main results were: 7,599 patients were followed for at least 2 years with a median follow-up time of 37.7 months. During the study, 886 patients (23%) in the candesartan group and 945 (25%) in the placebo group (as predicted, 8% annual mortality) died from any cause (unadjusted hazard ratio 0.91 [95% CI 0.83, 1.00], $P = 0.055$), with fewer cardiovascular deaths (691 [18%] vs 769 [20%], unadjusted hazard ratio 0.88 [0.79, 0.97], $P = 0.012$) in the candesartan group. It was concluded that treatment of a broad spectrum of patients with symptomatic heart failure with candesartan resulted in a marginally significant reduction in deaths, notably because of a significant 12% hazard reduction in cardiovascular deaths [14]. Results on the effects of candesartan on cardiovascular death or CHF hospitalization in different populations of patients with heart disease (CHARM-Preserved, -Added, and -Alternative) were reported in three separate articles [13–17].

Conclusion

Randomized clinical trials are a major investment in terms of patient and personnel involvement, and the funding needed to undertake the trial for the progress of medical care. We have provided a short overview on the various types of clinical trials, and the main types of errors that can arise and can seriously compromise our ability to draw valid conclusions from clinical trials.

Many of the concepts mentioned in this chapter deal with minimizing bias and maximizing precision. An appropriate design requires a clear definition of the primary and secondary hypotheses in terms of measured outcomes and an explicit definition of the study population in order to avoid systematic errors. Statistical analyses deal with random errors due to sampling or random variation in the outcome variables. Interpretation of these statistical measures of treatment effect and comparisons should consider the potential contribution of bias or confounding. Finally, it is ethically imperative that a trial is conducted and monitored in such a way as to minimize harm to patients, while looking to answer the initial questions posed by the trial of whether the new treatment is better, worse, or similar to the comparison group.

References

1.	World Medical Association Declaration of Helsinki. Ethical Principles for Medical Research Involving Human Subjects. Available from: www.wma.net/e/policy/b3.htm. Accessed May 6, 2005.
2.	Altman DG, Schulz KF, Moher D, et al. The revised CONSORT statement for reporting randomized trials: explanation and elaboration. *Ann Intern Med* 2001;**134**:663–94.
3.	Moher D, Schulz KF, Altman DG. The CONSORT statement: revised recommendations for improving the quality of reports of parallel-group randomized clinical trials. *Lancet* 2001;**357**:1191–4.

4. Pocock SJ. *Clinical Trials: A Practical Approach.* New York: John Wiley & Sons, 1983.

5. Chow SC, Liu JP. *Design and Analysis of Clinical Trials: Concept and Methodologies*. New York: John Wiley & Sons, 1998.

6. Friedman LM, Furberg CD, Demets D. *Fundamentals of Clinical Trials*, 3rd edition. New York: Springer-Verlag, 1998.

7. Matthews JNS. *An Introduction to Randomized Controlled Clinical Trials*. London: Arnold, 2000.

8. Senn S. *Cross-over Trials in Clinical Research*, 2nd edition. Chichester: John Wiley & Sons, 2002.

9. Jones B, Kenward MG. *Design and Analysis of Cross-over Trials*, 2nd edition. London: Chapman and Hall/CRC, 2003.

10. Day S. *Dictionary of Clinical Trials*. Chichester: John Wiley & Sons, 1999.

11. Jadad AR. *Randomized Controlled Trials: a User's Guide*. London: BMJ Books, 1998.

12. Everitt BS, Pickles A. *Statistical Aspects of the Design and Analysis of Clinical Trials*. London: Imperial College Press, 1999.

13. Jennison C, Turnbull BW. *Group Sequential Methods with Applications to Clinical Trials*. New York: Chapman & Hall/CRC, 2000.

14. Pfeffer MA, Swedberg K, Granger CB, et al.; CHARM Investigators and Committees. Effects of candesartan on mortality and morbidity in patients with chronic heart failure: the CHARM-Overall programme. *Lancet* 2003;**362**:759–66.

15. McMurray JJ, Ostergren J, Swedberg K, et al. Effects of candesartan in patients with chronic heart failure and reduced left-ventricular systolic function taking angiotensin-converting-enzyme inhibitors: the CHARM-Added trial. *Lancet* 2003;**362**:767–71.

16. Granger CB, McMurray JJ, Yusuf S, et al. Effects of candesartan in patients with chronic heart failure and reduced left-ventricular systolic function intolerant to angiotensin-converting-enzyme inhibitors: the CHARM-Alternative trial. *Lancet* 2003;**362**:772–6.

17. Yusuf S, Pfeffer MA, Swedberg K, et al. Effects of candesartan in patients with chronic heart failure and preserved left-ventricular ejection fraction: the CHARM-Preserved Trial. *Lancet* 2003;**362**:777–81.

18. Kirkwood B, Sterne J. *Essential Medical Statistics*, 2nd edition. Oxford: Blackwell Publishing, 2003.

19. Machin D, Campbell MJ, Payers PM, et al. *Statistical Tables for the Design of Clinical Studies*, 2nd edition. Oxford: Blackwell Science, 1997.

20. Pocock SJ. A major trial needs three statisticians: why, how and who? *Stat Med* 2004;**23**:1535–9.

21. Pocock SJ. When to stop a clinical trial. *BMJ* 1992;**305**:235–40.

22. Food and Drug Administration, Section 5.8 of the International Conference on Harmonization: Guidance on Statistical Principles for Clinical Trials. Available from: http://www.fda.gov/cber/gdlns/ichclinical.pdf. Accessed March 31, 2005.

Chapter 2

Uncontrolled Trials

Joseph Kim, Dorothea Nitsch, Duolao Wang, and Ameet Bakhai

Uncontrolled clinical trials are defined as clinical studies where new treatments are studied in the absence of a control group. As a result, these studies provide less information on the therapy than controlled trials. Nonetheless, uncontrolled trials play an integral part in the evaluation of novel therapies, particularly in the early stages of clinical research where they are used to help justify and plan large-scale clinical trials. In this chapter, we review the merits and limitations of uncontrolled trials, and describe their potential usefulness in clinical research.

Introduction

Clinical trials form the basis for evidence-based medicine. The primary aim of most clinical trials is to provide an unbiased evaluation of the merits of using one or more treatment options for a given disease or condition of interest. Ideally, clinical trials should be performed in a way that isolates the effect of treatment on the study outcome and provides results that are free from study bias. A common approach by which to achieve this aim is through randomization, whereby patients are assigned to a treatment group by random selection. When performed appropriately using a sufficiently large sample size of patients, random treatment allocation ensures that many of the potential forms of bias are balanced out evenly between treated and untreated groups. For example, unknown factors that lead to favoring one treatment over the other for selected patients at baseline can be prevented through a randomized study design [1]. However, it is not always possible or necessary to have a randomized approach since the objective of the trial may not be to evaluate the treatment effect against a control. In such situations we undertake uncontrolled trials.

Uncontrolled clinical trials are a subset of a class of studies referred to as *nonrandomized* trials, since a comparison group is not utilized. Hence, uncontrolled trials attempt to evaluate the effect of a treatment in a group of patients who are all offered the same investigational treatment.

Rationale for performing an uncontrolled trial

Whether a control group is needed in a clinical trial ultimately depends on the goals of the investigator. There are two settings where uncontrolled trials can be particularly advantageous. These are when the goal of the study is to:

- determine the pharmacokinetic properties of a novel drug (eg, through a Phase I or Phase II clinical trial)
- generate new hypotheses for further research (eg, through a case study or case series study)

Phase I trials
In the early stages of clinical research, a control group might not be desirable since the pharmacokinetic and safety profiles of a novel drug have not been established. After gathering sufficient data from initial preclinical studies through *in vitro* studies or through animal models, an investigator might wish to proceed to the first stage (or 'phase') of clinical investigations. This is known as a *Phase I* clinical trial.

The primary aims of a Phase I trial might be to:

- determine how well the investigational drug can be tolerated in humans
- find the maximum-tolerated dose in humans

Secondary aims might be to:

- study the drug's clinical pharmacology on human patient volunteers who were typically nonresponsive to conventional therapy
- study the drug's toxicity on human volunteers

Example

An example of a Phase I trial is illustrated by Bomgaars et al., who conducted a study to determine the maximum-tolerated dose, dose-limiting toxicities, and pharmacokinetics of intrathecal liposomal cytarabine in children with advanced meningeal malignancies [2]. The investigators enrolled 18 patients, who were given cytarabine either through an indwelling cerebral ventricular access device or via lumbar puncture. The initial dose was 25 mg, but this was subsequently escalated to 35 mg, and then to 50 mg.

The authors found that headache due to arachnoiditis was dose limiting in two of eight patients on the 50 mg dose, despite concomitant treatment with dexamethasone. They also found that eight of the 14 patients assessable for response demonstrated evidence of benefit (manifest as no further disease progress or disease remission). Based on these results, the authors suggested that the maximum-tolerated and recommended optimal dose of liposomal cytarabine was 35 mg, if given together with dexamethasone twice daily.

Phase II trials

The primary aims of a *Phase II* clinical trial are:

- initial assessment of a drug's therapeutic effects
- initial assessment of a drug's consequent adverse effects

Phase II trials are usually performed across multiple study centers, and might even include a control group and, possibly, randomization. If treated patients show an adequate response to treatment, the drug will be further evaluated in a large-scale *Phase III* (randomized) clinical trial.

Example

Smit et al. performed an uncontrolled Phase II study of bexarotene, a novel synthetic retinoid for the treatment of psoriasis [3]. Fifty patients with moderate to severe plaque-type psoriasis were treated with bexarotene at sequential increasing doses (0.5–3.0 mg/kg/day) administered for 12–24 weeks. Overall response rates (≥50% improvement from baseline) were noted for: psoriasis area and severity index (in 22% of patients); plaque elevation (52% of patients); and physician's global assessment of disease (36% of patients).

In addition, the authors found no serious adverse events related to the bexarotene therapy; mild adverse events included hypertriglyceridemia and decreased thyroxine levels. Based on these results, the authors suggested that bexarotene was safe and warranted further investigation through Phase III clinical trials.

Advantages of uncontrolled trials

Uncontrolled trials are often conducted to provide justification for the potential health risks and economic costs associated with undertaking a large-scale randomized clinical trial. The absence of a control group is both a strength and weakness of uncontrolled trials; though less informative than controlled trials, uncontrolled trials are faster, more convenient, and less expensive to perform. Moreover, in the absence of complete information about the pharmacokinetics and safety profile of an untested drug, uncontrolled trials limit the number of subjects exposed to a potentially harmful new treatment.

Uncontrolled trials can be used to generate hypotheses to be answered in future large-scale controlled trials. They can involve as few as one patient, in which case the trial is referred to as a *case study*. An example of a case study is shown by Farid and Bulto, who studied the effect of buspirone on obsessional compulsive disorder in a man who failed all existing therapy, including psychosurgery [4]. The authors presented his positive response to the recommended dose of buspirone and its effect on the severity of his obsessive compulsive symptoms.

When a case study is conducted over a series of patients, it is usually published as a *case series study*. Soderstrom et al. performed such a study to evaluate the effect of olanzapine (5–20 mg/day) on six extremely aggressive teenage boys with neuropsychiatric disorders [5]. All but one of the subjects responded within 1 week of therapy. The subjects described a markedly increased sense of wellbeing during the olanzapine treatment. The authors concluded that the therapeutic benefit observed in four of the boys outweighed the relatively mild side-effects of weight gain and sedation.

Another advantage of uncontrolled trials is that, in certain situations, uncontrolled trials might be the only study design allowable given a set of ethical considerations. For example, it is unlikely that patients who experienced a cardiac arrest would be randomized to resuscitation versus no intervention to evaluate the efficacy of resuscitation, since untreated patients would certainly die. Similarly, if the new treatment involved a surgical procedure involving general anesthetic it might be unethical to perform a 'sham' operation given the risk of the anesthesia.

Limitations of uncontrolled trials

A major limitation of uncontrolled trials is the absence of a randomly selected comparison group, making these trials unsuitable for fully evaluating the efficacy of a new drug. For instance, uncontrolled trials would be inappropriate for evaluating whether a particular cholesterol-lowering drug reduces the risk of coronary events since it would require studying a comparable untreated group (eg, a placebo control group). The use of a control group would ensure that the lowering of cholesterol is attributable to the drug itself and not to some other cause, such as changes in diet and exercise patterns.

Investigator bias

Another limitation is that, compared with controlled trials, the results of uncontrolled trials are more likely to lead to enthusiastic results in favor of the treatment. This specific form of study bias is known as *investigator bias* [6]. For example, suppose that an investigator wishes to conduct a new clinical trial in search of a promising new therapy. However, desire for the drug's success drives the investigator to unconsciously recruit a healthy group of individuals into the study. These individuals are likely to do well simply from being in the trial itself (ie, through a placebo effect), biasing the results in favor of therapy. Had the investigator chosen to include a control group in the study, it is likely that the results of the study would not have shown an advantage

In general, uncontrolled trials are more likely to lead to positive results compared to trials using appropriately selected controls [6]. For instance, case series and observational studies have found corticosteroids to be beneficial in patients with head trauma. However, a randomized clinical trial was terminated early because patients randomized to corticosteroids experienced a significantly greater risk of death compared to patients in the placebo group [7]. Thus, it is possible that over-interpretation of the results of uncontrolled trials prior to the publication of the randomized clinical trial led to numerous excess deaths resulting from inappropriate steroid prescription [8]. This example illustrates that over-interpreting the results of uncontrolled trials can have significant adverse public health consequences.

Table 1. Advantages and limitations of uncontrolled trials.

Advantages	Limitations
Used to generate hypotheses and can provide justification for a large-scale clinical trial	Susceptible to investigator bias because there is no randomly selected group for comparison
Can assess pharmacokinetic properties of a novel drug	Susceptible to over-interpretation
Might be the only study design available due to ethical considerations, such as a surgical procedure	Much less informative than any other studies that have a concurrent nonrandomized control group

Historical controls

Researchers sometimes use results from case series to create *historical controls*, where the results from more recent case series are compared against those of previous reports. For example, Torres et al. assessed the efficacy of immunosuppressive treatment in patients with kidney disease (idiopathic membranous nephropathy) [9]. The authors observed that patients diagnosed before changes in treatment policy eventually progressed to end-stage renal failure, whereas those who were diagnosed after these changes had a better outcome. The authors hypothesized that this policy change resulted from the publication of a small trial that reported some efficacy of immunosuppression [10].

However, the use of historical controls is limited. In this case, it remains uncertain as to whether the effect of treatment policy on end-stage renal failure was attributable entirely to the policy change alone. For example, the observed difference in outcome could have been a result of differences in diagnostic criteria between treated and historical controls and changes in patient profiles, rather than due to the changes in treatment policy. Such problems related to using historical controls have been well-described in epidemiology, particularly with respect to changes in disease coding or definitions over time [11].

Conclusion

Uncontrolled clinical trials have a specific role in clinical research, such as in the pharmacological evaluation of novel therapies and providing justification for performing a large-scale clinical trial. In particular, uncontrolled studies might be preferred over controlled trials in certain situations where a controlled trial is neither logistically feasible nor ethically justifiable (see **Table 1**). However, care should be taken when interpreting the results of uncontrolled trials – the absence of both a control group and a randomization process can artificially enhance the validity of these clinical studies.

References

1. Greenland S. Randomization, statistics, and causal inference. *Epidemiology* 1990;**1**:421–9.

2. Bomgaars L, Geyer JR, Franklin J, et al. Phase I trial of intrathecal liposomal cytarabine in children with neoplastic meningitis. *J Clin Oncol* 2004;**22**:3916–21.

3. Smit JV, Franssen ME, de Jong EM, et al. A phase II multicenter clinical trial of systemic bexarotene in psoriasis. *J Am Acad Dermatol* 2004;**51**:249–56.

4. Farid BT, Bulto M. Buspirone in obsessional compulsive disorder. A prospective case study. *Pharmacopsychiatry* 1994;**27**:207–9.

5. Soderstrom H, Rastam M, Gillberg C. A clinical case series of six extremely aggressive youths treated with olanzapine. *Eur Child Adolesc Psychiatry* 2002;**11**:138–41.

6. Pocock SJ. *Clinical Trials: A Practical Approach*. New York: John Wiley & Sons, 1983.

7. Roberts I, Yates D, Sandercock P, et al. Effect of intravenous corticosteroids on death within 14 days in 10,008 adults with clinically significant head injury (MRC CRASH trial): randomised placebo-controlled trial. *Lancet* 2004;364:1321–8.

8. Sauerland S, Maegele M. A CRASH landing in severe head injury. *Lancet* 2004;**364**:1291–2.

9. Torres A, Dominguez-Gil B, Carreno A, et al. Conservative versus immunosuppressive treatment of patients with idiopathic membranous nephropathy. *Kidney Int* 2002;**61**:219–27.

10. Ponticelli C, Zucchelli P, Passerini P, et al. A randomized trial of methylprednisolone and chlorambucil in idiopathic membranous nephropathy. *N Engl J Med* 1989;**320**:8–13.

11. Guevara RE, Butler JC, Marston BJ, et al. Accuracy of ICD-9-CM codes in detecting community-acquired pneumococcal pneumonia for incidence and vaccine efficacy studies. *Am J Epidemiol* 1999;**149**:282–9.

Chapter 3

Protocol Development

Umair Mallick, Radivoj Arezina, Craig Ritchie, and Duolao Wang

Once a clinical question has been postulated, the first step in the conception of a clinical trial to answer that question is to develop a trial protocol. A well-designed protocol reflects the scientific and methodologic integrity of a trial. Protocol development has evolved in a complex way over the last 20 years to reflect the care and attention given to undertaking clinical experiments with human volunteers, reflecting the high standards of safety and ethics involved as well as the complex statistical issues. In this chapter, we describe in some detail the various aspects covered in a trial protocol. This section is particularly relevant to those involved in setting up, evaluating, or coordinating a trial, or those wanting an insight into the design of a trial protocol.

Introduction

The trial protocol is a formal document that specifies how a clinical trial is to be conducted (**Table 1**). It describes the objective(s), design, methodology, statistical considerations, and administrative structure of the trial [1]. We can also regard the protocol as a scientific, administrative, and organizational project guideline that may be the basis of a contractual relationship between an investigator and a trial sponsor [1]. Well-designed protocols are important for conducting clinical trials safely and in a cost-effective manner. Different trial protocols will retain very similar key components. However, adaptations may be necessary for each trial's particular circumstances.

In scientific research, the first step is to set up a hypothesis, and then to construct an appropriate study design to test that hypothesis. In clinical trials, the hypothesis is usually related to one form of therapeutic intervention that is expected to be superior or equal to another in terms of specific outcomes.

Once this hypothesis is developed, the study's aims, design, methodology, statistical methods, and analyses should be formulated. The protocol should clearly address issues related to the study's conduct, set up, organization, monitoring, administrative responsibilities, publication policy, and timelines, in appropriate sections. Trial guidelines and regulatory requirements, such as the International Conference on Harmonisation guidelines for Good Clinical Practice (ICH–GCP) [1], the Declaration of Helsinki [2], the EU Clinical Trials Directive (EUCTD) [3], and the US Food and Drug Administration (FDA) Regulations Relating to Good Clinical Practice and Clinical Trials [4], should be followed as appropriate.

Protocol writing in a clinical trial

Protocol writing is a joint effort that typically involves a lead investigator (who is an expert clinician and researcher), along with his/her co-investigators, a clinical scientist(s), and an expert medical statistician who is familiar (ideally) with the subject matter. A group of experienced and renowned experts is chosen to peer review the document; their consultations and opinions are sought as appropriate.

Most common problems in protocol writing – such as incompleteness, ambiguity, and inconsistency – reflect an inefficient writing process [5]. Studies have shown that protocol development is a collaborative scientific writing process, the aim of which is to achieve consensus within a group of interdisciplinary clinical trial experts [6,7]. Important characteristics of a good quality protocol are summarized in **Table 2**.

Table 1. Questions addressed by a protocol.

- What is the clinical question being asked by the trial?
- How should it be answered, in compliance with the standard ethical and regulatory requirements?
- What analyses should be performed in order to produce meaningful results?
- How will the results be presented?

Table 2. Qualities of a good protocol.

- Clear, comprehensive, easy to navigate, and unambiguous
- Designed in accordance with the current principles of Good Clinical Practice and other regulatory requirements
- Gives a sound scientific background of the trial
- Clearly identifies the benefits and risks of being recruited into the trial
- Plainly describes trial methodology and practicalities
- Ensures that the rights, safety, and well-being of trial participants are not unduly compromised
- Gives enough relevant information to make the trial and its results reproducible
- Indicates all features that assure the quality of every aspect of the trial

Regular review by the peers and trial organizers is essential during the protocol development process. All materials and documentation should be kept, including protocol versions, meeting minutes, and correspondence discussing protocol-related issues. The final, comprehensive document should elicit a systematic approach to the development of a clinical trial, which is acceptable on scientific, organizational, and ethical grounds.

Implications of guidelines in the development of trial protocol

ICH–GCP [1] has set standards for clinical trials that fall under the UK Medicines for Human Use (Clinical Trials) Regulations 2004 (SI2004/1031) [8], EUCTD [3], and FDA Regulations Relating to Good Clinical Practice and Clinical Trials [4]. Most clinical trials (excepting nonintervention trials) involving a medicinal product(s) in human subjects are encompassed by the EUCTD and FDA regulations, and the protocol should therefore meet the standards required by ICH–GCP. Once the protocol is completed according to the given standards, it is reviewed by the local research ethics committee or institutional review board. Other key agencies – such as the Medicines and Healthcare Products Regulatory Agency (MHRA) in the UK or the FDA in the US – may also be asked to comment on a trial design.

Key components of a trial protocol

The trial protocol is a comprehensive document and the core structure of the protocol should be adapted according to the type of trial. ICH–GCP can be used as a reference document when developing a protocol for pharmaceutical clinical trials (Phase I to Phase IV) involving a pharmaceutical substance (the investigational medicinal product [IMP]) [1]. Most institutions and pharmaceutical companies use a standard set of rules to define the main protocol outline, structure, format, and naming/numbering methods for their trials. In this section, we briefly describe the main components of a typical protocol.

Protocol information page

The front page gives the:

- trial title
- trial identification number
- protocol version number
- date prepared

The descriptive title of the protocol should be kept as short as possible, but at the same time it should reflect the design, type of population, and aim of the trial. ICH–GCP suggests that the title of a pharmaceutical trial should additionally include the medicinal product(s), the nature of the treatment (eg, treatment, prophylaxis, diagnosis, radiosensitizer), any comparator(s) and/or placebo(s), indication, and setting (outpatient or inpatient) [1]. The key investigational site, investigator, and sponsor should also be detailed on the title page.

Table of contents

A table of contents is a useful tool that allows easy navigation through the protocol. The table of contents may vary according to the design of the clinical trial. **Table 3** gives an example table of contents for a typical protocol.

Definition of abbreviations

All abbreviations used in the protocol should be defined in a separate section. These should be accepted international medical or scientific abbreviations.

Table 3. Illustration of a table of contents in a protocol.

Component	Details
Protocol information page	Study title, trial ID number, version, list of appendices, definition of abbreviations and terms
Study summary or synopsis	A summary of one or two pages in a table format
Trial flow chart	Describing flow of the trial
Introduction	Trial background and rationale
Study objectives	Primary and secondary objectives
Investigational plan	*Overall study design and plan* Trial design, study population (inclusion criteria, exclusion criteria), randomization, blinding, premature discontinuation criteria, record of study participants, study medication (description and labeling, storage, administration, dosing strategies, accountability, over-dosage, occupational safety) *Study conduct* Study schedule, study flow chart, written informed consent, participant numbering, screening entry, treatment phase (visit numbers), early withdrawal, concomitant medication, blood and urine sampling, processing of samples *Safety and efficacy evaluations* Safety assessments, efficacy evaluations, unscheduled visits *Recording safety information* Adverse events (glossary, adverse drug reactions, serious adverse events, reporting of overdose, pregnancy, breaking of study blinding by the investigator) *Participant completion and discontinuation* Premature withdrawal of participants from the study, procedure for handling withdrawals
Statistical issues	Primary and secondary endpoints, sample size calculations, intention-to-treat population, per-protocol population, efficacy population, safety population, handling of dropouts and missing data, efficacy analyses (primary, secondary, tertiary), safety analysis, pharmacokinetic and pharmacodynamic analysis, adjusted analysis, subgroup analysis, statistical methods for various analyses
Ethics	Participant information sheet and informed consent, ethics approvals
Regulatory requirements, administrative issues, and monitoring	Regulatory requirements, protocol amendments, curriculum vitae, investigators, administrative structures, investigator's statement, trial monitoring (safety monitoring, quality control, auditing and inspecting), case report form, archiving of records, final reports, study documentation and publication of study results, financial agreement, termination of the study, study discontinuation by the sponsor and by the clinical investigator, insurance policy
References	Listing of references to justify the study rationale
List of appendices	Informed consent form, Declaration of Helsinki, notable values for laboratories and/or vital signs, investigator's statement, etc.

Trial summary or synopsis

A synopsis should provide the key aspects of the protocol in no more than two pages, and can be prepared in a table format. The main components of the protocol summary include:

- full title
- principal investigator
- planned study dates
- objectives
- study design
- study population
- treatments
- procedures
- sample size
- outcome measures
- statistical methods

Flow chart

A flow chart is a schematic diagram that summarizes trial design, procedures, and stages. It emphasizes the timing of enrolment procedures, study visits, study interventions, and follow-up assessments.

Background and rationale of the trial

The background section is built on experience gained from previous research. It describes the test treatment, including an outline of what is known about the effects of the treatment from previous research, and gives a rationale for the current research study. The main aim of the study background is to give the reader the knowledge they require to understand the questions or hypothesis of the study.

A systematic review of the study topic should be performed beforehand. This is an effective way to summarize the relevant available data. The basic structure of the background section should include (in this order):

1. known research on the topic
2. what is unknown about the topic
3. the study question or hypothesis

In clinical trials that involve an IMP, various aspects of the treatment and the disease should be elaborated on. These include existing epidemiological data regarding the disease (along with references to the literature), possible existing caveats in available therapies, and potential benefits that can be achieved through this trial.

Table 4. Information that should be given in trials using an intervention related to a drug treatment.

• Type of drug	• Dosage regimen	• Randomization
• Blinding methods	• Drug initiation and duration	• Drug supply
• Labeling and packaging	• Storage of trial drugs	• Drug accountability
• Treatment safety	• Occupational safety	• Over-dosage
• Concomitant medications	• Discontinuation criteria	• Return instructions

ICH–GCP specifically requires information referring to pharmacological and clinical data regarding the IMP, in particular from nonclinical studies and other clinical trials, to justify use of the IMP in a trial [1]. In such trials, a description and justification of route, dosage, dosage regimen, and treatment period is a vital part of the protocol. Please refer to the later section on trial documentation (p. 34) for further details.

Study objectives

Research objectives describe the information the investigator aims to obtain from the study. Each specific aim should be a precisely worded definition of a stated question or hypothesis to be tested. The protocol must distinguish between prospective (*a priori*) research hypotheses and ones that have been based on knowledge of the data (retrospective).

- When the effect of an intervention is investigated in a specific group of patients, the aim of the study should be stated as a *question* – eg, "What is the effect of aspirin on mortality in patients with myocardial infarction?"
- When the study is investigating the believed effect of an intervention in a specific group of patients, the aim of the study should be stated as a *hypothesis* – eg, "Aspirin is associated with a reduction of mortality in patients with myocardial infarction."

Each trial must have a primary question (*primary hypothesis*) as well as secondary questions (*secondary hypotheses*) if needed.

Investigational plan for the trial, study conduct, and safety issues

This section is one of the most important components of the trial protocol. Various subsections should give detailed descriptions of the trial, design, study population (eligibility criteria), issues related to practical aspects of an intervention, and drug safety issues in the clinical trial (**Table 4**).

In double-blind studies, procedures on how to unblind must be stated. A separate section with adverse event-related identification, reporting, and management is mandatory in drug trials.

Practicalities of the trial in terms of assessments and periods (screening entry, treatment phase, patient visit numbers), blood and urine sampling, or other investigations, measurements, or assessments are most appropriately given in a table format. In addition to study efficacy and safety variables, data quality-related issues should also be given in this section. Participant completion and discontinuation information, such as premature withdrawal of a participant from the trial, along with appropriate procedures for handling withdrawals, also constitute an important part. ICH-GCP requires that stopping rules or discontinuation criteria, accountability procedures, randomization codes maintenance, and breakage criteria, along with other details, should be specifically mentioned in this section of the protocol.

Trial design

The choice of trial design (eg, parallel-group trial, cross-over trial, factorial trial, cluster randomized trial) largely depends upon the research question that is being asked. The design specification should be able to reflect the:

- type of treatment and number of treatments
- method of randomization
- type of blinding
- type of study question
- study medication

For example, in randomized clinical trials, while describing the study design, the type of treatment (active or placebo) received by population groups should be described, as well as the type of blinding (unblinded, single blinded, double blinded). A statement relating to superiority, inferiority, and noninferiority between the treatment groups should be given.

Eligibility criteria

In a clinical trial, the eligibility criteria aim to define the study population. The study population is a subset of the population with the medical condition in which the intervention is to be tested. Eligibility criteria are related to patients' safety and the anticipated intervention effect. The eligibility criteria will have a significant impact on the generalizability of the study results, as well as on recruitment rates of the study; using eligibility criteria that are too restrictive can lead to difficulty in recruiting sufficient patients.

Eligibility criteria are categorized into two groups: *inclusion* criteria and *exclusion* criteria. Appropriate justifications should be given for the use of certain inclusion and exclusion criteria. Any contraindications to continuing in the study should be stated, together with criteria and procedures for participant withdrawal from the study.

Randomization

Randomization is a process that allocates participants to the intervention or control group by chance. The trial protocol should include the randomization procedures, including important issues that must be considered in the randomization process. These include the allocation ratio, types of randomization, and mechanisms of randomization.

Enrolment process

A section on the enrolment process should explain how the patients will be identified, screened, and consented into the trial. It must be emphasized that consent procedures will be followed and written consent forms signed before patients are enrolled into the trial. Screening procedures must be specified, including investigations performed in the individual patient in order to determine whether they meet the eligibility criteria.

Procedures, treatments, and follow-up

The type and duration of treatment or follow-up should be specified, along with dose regimens, etc., and an indication of who will perform the work, specifying requirements that must be met in order to be an investigator in the trial. Details of any tests (eg, blood or urine samples) or procedures to be performed, together with their timing, must be given. Criteria for modification of the treatment schedule should also be described. Length of follow-up of the study and timing of follow-up visits should be included.

Outcome measures or endpoints

An *outcome measure* or *endpoint* is a direct or indirect measurement of a clinical effect in a clinical trial, required to be able to make an effective claim regarding the intervention under investigation. The goal of a clinical trial is to assess the effect of treatment on these outcome measures with as few biases as possible. A *primary* endpoint is used to address the primary objective of a study, whereas a *secondary* endpoint is related to the secondary objective. A clear definition of each outcome measure must be stated (eg, death or cardiovascular death in a cardiovascular drug trial).

Sample size

A clinical trial should have enough statistical power to detect clinically important differences between the treatment groups. Thus, estimation of the sample size with provision of the expected treatment effect, level of significance, and power are absolutely critical to the success of the trial. The sample size is usually estimated to test the primary hypothesis of no difference between the therapies to be tested.

Statistical issues

In this section, the statistical analysis plan is described; this is based on the study design, objectives, and outcomes (primary and secondary) The type of statistical analyses and their justification for use should be given, as appropriate – eg, the type of analysis (such as intention-to-treat or per-protocol analysis) should be stated. The selection of the statistical methods will depend on the type of outcome measure variables and the study design.

The protocol should specify how to deal with dropouts and missing data. If an adjusted analysis is planned, the protocol should specify the covariates to be included in the adjusted analysis. Similarly, subgroup analyses should be defined *a priori* on the basis of known biological mechanisms or in response to the findings of previous studies.

Ethics

Ethical considerations should be taken into account from the beginning of the protocol design, addressing issues related to participants' rights, confidentiality, and safety, as well as treatment efficacy issues for trials that evaluate the therapeutic effects of an IMP.

The main objective of this section is to establish that the study design conforms with ICH–GCP [1], the Declaration of Helsinki [2], and local ethical and legal requirements. All research involving human participants must receive favorable approval from the local research ethics committee or institutional review board before its start. Before patients can be included in the study, they must read a patient information letter and sign a written informed consent form.

Regulatory requirements and administrative considerations

The development and sale of drugs and devices for human use is supervised by government-appointed regulatory authorities, such as the MHRA in the UK and the FDA in the US. These authorities ensure that the products or devices are safe and effective, and that all aspects of development, manufacturing, and clinical investigation conform to agreed quality standards. The application to government authorities for regulatory issues of the trial must be stated in the protocol. Furthermore, protocol amendments from previous versions and details of the trial documentation, investigators, administrative structures, the investigator's statement, financial agreement, and issues related to trial discontinuation by the sponsor and by the clinical investigator should all be given.

Trial monitoring

Trial monitoring describes a systematic and independent examination of trial-related activities, documents, and safety data to ensure that the trial is conducted in accordance with the protocol and standard operating procedures, and regulatory requirements [1]. If applicable, the monitoring plan for the trial should be given in detail. In clinical trials, data monitoring is performed for clinical safety issues as well as for source data verification in order to comply with ICH–GCP; the former is usually undertaken by the data and safety monitoring board. A protocol must state the procedures for completing the case record form (CRF) and source data verification, auditing and inspection, and record keeping and archiving of data collected and any relevant study material. Hoax patient recruitment is one of many reasons for trial monitoring.

Publication policy

The publication policy should state the need for clinical investigators to retain the right to present and publish the results of their study. An indication of the type of journal that will be targeted for publication of the main study manuscript should be specified at the start of a study. Issues related to data confidentiality, copyright, and authorship should be briefly incorporated in the trial protocol.

Study timetable

A study timetable is given at the end of the protocol document. This should include a summary of the steps and timing from study start-up to production of the final clinical report. This section may vary according to the type of clinical trial. In general, the timetable includes timelines for:

* completion of protocol
* completion of CRF and other study documentation
* submission for ethical approval (central or local ethical)
* database development and trial registration
* center selection
* initial study negotiations (feasibility, budget, etc.)
* investigator meetings
* site initiation meetings
* enrolment period (screening and treatment)
* site monitoring visits
* completion of follow-up
* interim and final data analyses
* final report preparation
* submission of the study manuscript to a journal
* presentation of study results at scientific meetings

References

References should be used where required. The design of a study protocol requires an evidence-based approach. This should justify the study rationale and background, and will also be relevant for preclinical and clinical information given in the 'investigators' brochure'. A reference list must be included at the end of the protocol, before any appendices, relating to rationale and statistical methods.

Case record form and trial documentation

The CRF is a printed or electronic document designed to capture a required record of data and other information for each patient during a clinical trial, as defined by the clinical protocol. In a protocol, the type of CRF (paper or electronic) and the method for transmitting data from the CRF to the coordination center (eg, mail, fax, electronic) for data management and analyses should be specified.

The investigators' brochure is a compilation of clinical and nonclinical data on the IMP(s) relevant to the study of the product in human participants. This document can be an integrated part of the protocol or prepared as a separate document to provide researchers with information to help them understand the rationale and comply with the protocol. Its main aim is to support clinical management of the participants in a clinical trial.

If any protocol amendments exist, these should be integrated into the protocol or provided in separate appendices. Any other appendices (eg, flow charts, assessments, measurements) should accompany the protocol as appropriate. Documents such as the participant information sheet, consent form, and information letter to participants' physicians are normally provided to the study investigators separately from the protocol.

Trial committees

The study organization will depend on the complexity and size of the trial. The following committees are usually set up for most Phase III trials and described in the protocol if relevant.

Executive committee

The executive committee is responsible and accountable for [9]:

- proper design and conduct of a trial
- ethical and professional standards of a trial
- ensuring that the results of clinical trials and scientific endeavors are arrived at in the most economical manner possible
- considering and implementing any recommendations from the data and safety monitoring board (see below)

Steering committee

The steering committee is responsible for [9]:

- guiding the overall conduct of the trial
- ensuring that the trial protocol meets the highest scientific standards
- protecting the rights and well-being of trial participants

In some trials, only a steering committee is set up, taking the responsibilities of both the executive committee and the steering committee.

Data and safety monitoring board or committee

The independent data and safety monitoring board will regularly review interim data from the trial and can recommend that the trial stop early for one of the following reasons [10]:

- The trial shows a large number of serious adverse events in one of the treatment groups.
- The trial shows a greater than expected benefit early into the trial.
- It becomes clear that a statistically significant difference by the end of the trial is improbable (futility rule).
- Logistical or data-quality problems are so severe that correction is not feasible.

Clinical event review committee

The independent clinical event review committee, or endpoint committee, reviews major clinical events (usually primary endpoints) that occur during the trial, and adjudicates or codes them into categories for later analyses.

Conclusion

Writing a protocol for a clinical trial is a complex, intellectual, and creative task, which is fulfilled by a team of researchers and experts in various areas of research including scientific, medical, statistical, ethical, regulatory, and administrative fields. The protocol is a document that carefully synchronizes knowledge in these areas in accordance with the scientific core of a clinical trial and various quality and regulatory recommendations.

In recent years, the development of guidelines has tremendously helped to develop standards for protocol writing in clinical research. This, in turn, has improved the methodology, conduct, and quality of clinical trials, with an ever-increasing ethical emphasis for all participants in the trial. Lastly, such protocols have become publications in their own right, allowing for peer review and feedback on trial assumptions at an early stage in the conduct of a trial.

References

1. International Conference on Harmonisation. E6: Good Clinical Practice: Consolidated Guidelines. Available from: www.ich.org/UrlGrpServer.jser?@_ID=276&@_TEMPLATE=254. Accessed May 6, 2005.

2. World Medical Association Declaration of Helsinki. Ethical Principles for Medical Research Involving Human Subjects. Available from: www.wma.net/e/policy/b3.htm. Accessed May 6, 2005.

3. Directive 2001/20/EC of the European Parliament and of the Council of 4 April 2001 on the approximation of the laws, regulations and administrative provisions of the Member States relating to the implementation of good clinical practice in the conduct of clinical trials on medicinal products for human use. *Official Journal of the European Union* 2001;**121**:34.

4. FDA Regulations Relating to Good Clinical Practice and Clinical Trials. Available from: www.fda.gov/oc/gcp/regulations.html. Accessed May 6, 2005.

5. Musen MA, Rohn JA, Fagan LM, et al. Knowledge engineering for a clinical trial advice system: uncovering errors in protocol specification. *Bull Cancer* 1987;**74**:291–6.

6. Gennari JH, Weng C, McDonald D, et al. An ethnographic study of collaborative clinical trial protocol writing. *Medinfo* 2004;**11**:1461–5.

7. van der Lei J. What is in a protocol? An Invitational Workshop: Towards Representations for Sharable Guidelines, March 3–4, 2000. Position Paper. Available from: www.glif.org/workshop/position_stmt/vanderLei.pdf. Accessed May 6, 2005.

8. The Medicines for Human Use (Clinical Trials) Regulations 2004. Statutory Instrument 2004 No. 1031. Available from: www.legislation.hmso.gov.uk/si/si2004/20041031.htm. Accessed May 6, 2005.

9. Day S. *Dictionary of Clinical Trials*. Chichester: John Wiley & Sons, 1999.

10. DeMets DL, Furberg CD, Friedman L, editors. *Data Monitoring in Clinical Trials: A Case Studies Approach*. New York: Springer Verlag, 2006.

Chapter 4

Endpoints

Ameet Bakhai, Amit Chhabra, and Duolao Wang

"The greatest challenge to any thinker is stating the problem in a way that will allow a solution," said Bertrand Russell (1872–1970). This maxim holds as strongly for clinical trials as for any quest in life. While the first clinical trials asked questions about events such as the rate of death or recurrence of infection, researchers are now interested in more sophisticated clinical trial endpoints for measuring combined outcomes (eg, avoiding death or hospitalization, or disease-specific outcomes such as asthma exacerbations or heart attacks). Researchers are also becoming more interested in economic outcomes for evaluating whether clinically effective treatments are also cost-effective. Surrogate endpoints are also used in trials that are related to disease-specific outcomes; eg, cholesterol level is a surrogate endpoint related to the risk of heart attacks. In this chapter, we discuss the types of endpoints that can be used in clinical trials.

What is a clinical trial endpoint?

A clinical trial endpoint is defined as a measure that allows us to decide whether the null hypothesis of a clinical trial should be accepted or rejected. In a clinical trial, the null hypothesis states that there is no statistically significant difference between two treatments or strategies being compared with respect to the endpoint measure chosen. An endpoint can be composed of a single outcome measure – such as death due to the disease – or a combination of outcome measures, such as death or hospitalization due to the disease.

Clinical trial endpoints can be classified as *primary* or *secondary* endpoints. Primary endpoints measure outcomes that will answer the primary (or most important) question being asked by a trial, such as whether a new treatment is better at preventing disease-related death than the standard therapy. In this case, the primary endpoint would be based on the occurrence of disease-related deaths during the duration of the trial. The size of a trial is determined by the power needed to detect a difference in this primary endpoint.

Secondary endpoints ask other relevant questions about the same study; for example, whether there is also a reduction in disease measures other than death, or whether the new treatment reduces the overall cost of treating patients. Occasionally, secondary endpoints are as important as the primary endpoint, in which case they are considered to be co-primary endpoints. When secondary endpoints are also important then the trial must be sufficiently powered to detect a difference in both endpoints, and expert statistical and design advice might be needed.

What are the main types of endpoints?

An endpoint may be based on [1]:

- a binary clinical outcome indicating whether an event –
  such as death from any cause – has occurred
- death from a disease-specific cause (eg, a fatal stroke for a trial
  comparing blood pressure treatments)
- the occurrence of disease signs or symptoms
- the relief of symptoms
- quality of life while disease is active
- the use of healthcare resources (eg, the number of hospital admissions)

Ideally, a trial should have a single endpoint based on just one outcome measure. However, as the art of trial design has evolved, most large trials have a primary (composite) endpoint consisting of multiple outcome measures.

An endpoint can also be the time taken for an event to occur. For such an endpoint, the events of interest for which a time is to be recorded – such as stroke or heart attack – must be predefined. Trial endpoints can also be a quantitative measurement of a biochemical or socioeconomic parameter such as cholesterol level or quality-of-life score. Therefore, there are a number of different outcomes – which can be evaluated both individually and in combination – on which the primary endpoint of a trial can be based.

How are clinical endpoints chosen?

When choosing endpoints for a clinical trial, it is important to ensure that they:

- are clinically meaningful and related to the disease process
- answer the main question of the trial
- are practical so that they can be assessed in all subjects in the same way
- occur frequently enough for the study to have adequate statistical power

If the endpoint to be measured consists of more than one outcome, then these outcomes should be easily differentiable from each other so that the events may be quantified independently. For example, in a cancer treatment trial, good outcomes to choose would be the primary tumor size and the number of new tumor metastases.

Why is death or time to death not always the best endpoint to measure?

Although death is the ultimate clinical endpoint and probably the best yardstick to judge treatments by, it may not be the best endpoint to measure in all studies for the following reasons:

- Death may be a rare event within the timeframe of the trial.
- Following all patients until a significant difference is seen in the number of deaths or the time to death may take many years of follow-up, so substantial resources may be required.
- Death may result from causes other than the disease being treated (eg, deaths due to car accidents, assuming that the disease process does not impair driving ability).

One rare example where all patients died in the timeframe of the study and, therefore, where time to death was the primary outcome measured, was a study in Zambia where patients with HIV were given fluconazole for proven cryptococcal meningitis [2]. In this case it was feasible to follow all patients to death because the disease is rapidly fatal, even with treatment. Therefore, the endpoint of this trial was the mean time to death for each treatment group, and the results showed that patients given fluconazole lived an average of 9 days longer than those who were not.

Composite endpoints

While some guidelines – such as the guidance on trial design in the International Conference on Harmonisation guidelines for Good Clinical Practice – prefer a primary endpoint based on a single outcome that will be defined before the study begins, many studies include multiple outcomes as part of a composite endpoint. Exploratory clinical investigations or early-phase studies are more likely to have multiple outcomes, with some of these being developed during the study. An example of a clinical trial with a composite endpoint of multiple outcomes is the CURE (Clopidogrel in Unstable Angina to Prevent Recurrent Events) study [3]. This study looked at the effects of clopidogrel in patients with acute coronary syndromes without ST-segment elevation. In this trial, the primary endpoint was a composite of the following clinical outcomes:

- death from cardiovascular causes
- stroke
- nonfatal myocardial infarction (heart attacks)

The second primary endpoint was the composite of the outcomes forming the first primary endpoint plus refractory ischemia (angina unresponsive to medical therapies).

When multiple outcomes can be experienced by any of the patients it is often best to present both the total number of outcomes per patient and hierarchical counts of outcomes. In the latter, only one outcome can be counted for each patient, and it is usually the most serious outcome that is recorded. The rules for the hierarchy of outcomes are usually established in advance of the trial, with a fatal outcome taking precedence over a nonfatal one.

Another way of combining outcomes would be to compare the number of recurrences of identical outcomes, such as the number of seizures experienced by patients with epilepsy during a follow-up period.

Advantages of using composite endpoints

There are two main advantages of using a composite endpoint. An endpoint with multiple outcomes means that more outcome events will be observed in total. Since the number of patients needed in the trial decreases as the number of events occurring in the control group increases, a composite endpoint allows us to evaluate a new treatment by using a smaller number of patients in the trial. For example, if the expected 1-year rate of events (death alone) is 1%, a sample size of 21,832 subjects will be required to show a 40% reduction in death (a type I error rate = 0.05 with 90% power). (For an explanation of how to determine the sample size for a clinical trial, see **Chapter 9**.) If, on the other hand, we look at the combined outcome of death or heart attack, which may be expected to occur at an annual rate of 10%, then this study would require a sample size of 2,028 subjects to capture a 40% reduction. This does, of course, assume that both the rate of deaths and the rate of heart attacks are expected to be reduced equally by 40%, which may not always be the case, and so this needs to be factored into the sample size calculation.

The other advantage of combining several outcomes is that a more comprehensive evaluation of a treatment can be given across more than just one category of outcome. For example, for a study on colon carcinoma, the outcome variables could be any of the following categories [4]:

- clinical (eg, symptoms of constipation)
- pathologic (eg, histologic evaluation from colon biopsy)
- visual (eg, endoscopic evaluation of tumor size)
- biochemical (eg, laboratory evaluation of tumor markers or signs of liver damage due to secondary tumors)

If the trial is adequately sized, the action of the treatment can then be assessed on each and every outcome.

Limitations of composite endpoints

In a composite endpoint of multiple outcomes we make the assumption that avoiding any one outcome has an equal importance as avoiding any other outcome. However, this is rarely the case. For example, in the case of colon carcinoma, avoiding constipation might not be as important as shrinking the tumor mass or delaying death – although, from a patient's point of view, avoiding constipation might be critical since constipation might lead to the need for a surgical solution if not resolved by drugs.

The second assumption made when using composite endpoints is that all individual outcome measures are related to the disease process and are equally meaningful. This is not always the case. Many trials, for example, consider rehospitalization or escalation of treatment usage to be outcome measures. However, it is possible for such outcomes to occur for reasons that are somewhat independent of the disease process itself, such as initial poor compliance with treatment requiring higher doses of therapy as a corrective measure. The occurrence of these measures may therefore not correlate strongly with the disease process, but their absence might be a strong indicator of treatment effect. This is a fairly complex matter and requires further discussion and debate. For now, bodies such as the US Food and Drug Administration (FDA) prefer clinically meaningful outcomes such as disease-specific death rates.

An additional limitation of composite endpoints is that they can also give inconsistent results, with certain outcomes improving and others worsening, making overall interpretation of the study difficult. Whether the outcomes chosen are clinical, biochemical, pharmacologic, pathologic, physiologic, or other, their relative importance should be determined prior to data collection, during the design of the trial.

Surrogate endpoints

As we have discussed, it is not always practical or feasible to base endpoints on 'true' clinical outcomes that, like death, might only occur after some time. Therefore, to be able to assess potential treatment effects, alternative measures are needed. One solution that has recently been attracting interest is *surrogate* endpoints. Temple defines a surrogate endpoint in a clinical trial as a laboratory measurement or physical sign used as a substitute for a clinically meaningful endpoint that measures directly how a patient feels, functions, or survives [1]. Changes induced by a therapy on a surrogate endpoint are expected to reflect changes in a clinically meaningful outcome measure [5].

A potential surrogate endpoint should be chosen based on strong biological rationale. Commonly used surrogate endpoints include [6]:

- pharmacokinetic measurements, such as concentration–time curves for a drug or its active metabolites in the bloodstream
- *in vitro* measurements, such as the mean concentration of an antibiotic agent required to inhibit growth of a bacterial culture
- radiological appearance, such as increased shadowing seen on a chest X-ray film of a patient with smoking-related lung disease that is related to a patient's breathing capacity

- a change in the levels of disease markers, such as a change in blood pressure as a predictor of a future occurrence of a stroke or kidney disease
- the macroscopic appearance of tissues, such as the endoscopic visualization of an area of erosion in the stomach that is considered by gastroenterologists to be the precursor of stomach bleeds

Advantages of surrogate endpoints

Like a composite endpoint, use of a surrogate endpoint can reduce the sample size needed for a study and thereby the duration and cost of performing a clinical trial. Surrogate endpoints are particularly useful when conducting Phase II screening trials to identify whether a new intervention has an effect, since a change is often seen in a surrogate endpoint long before an adverse event occurs. If there is sufficient change, it might then be justifiable to proceed to a large definitive trial with clinically meaningful outcomes.

Limitations of surrogate endpoints

It is important to realize that surrogate endpoints are only useful if they are a good predictor of a clinical outcome. If this relationship is not clearly defined, surrogate endpoints can be misleading. One classic example is the following case of three particular antiarrhythmic treatments.

Example

Three drugs (encainide, flecainide, and moricizine) were found to reduce arrhythmias and received FDA approval for use in patients with life-threatening or severely symptomatic arrhythmias. This was based on the assumption that if irregularities in heart rhythm were reduced, there should be lower numbers of cardiac deaths from disturbances of heart rhythm. More than 200,000 patients per year took these drugs in the US. However, it was subsequently shown in the CAST (Cardiac Arrhythmia Suppression Trial) study of 2,309 subjects that rates of death were higher in patients taking these drugs compared to those on placebo [7–9].

Health-economic endpoints

Economic endpoints are becoming increasingly important for new treatments. The Medical Research Council in the UK believes that clinical trial reports should always be accompanied by economic evaluations [10]. The growing number of economic analyses being submitted to medical journals led to the then editor of the *BMJ* announcing a policy that stated that economic results from clinical trials would now always have to be submitted with their respective clinical results, or they would not be accepted [10]. Therefore, assessments of health economics and technology, which are done to compare the quality of life of patients in different treatment groups or the costs of care of new treatments (which are usually more expensive than standard treatments), have become increasingly relevant in the approval and reimbursement of new therapies.

There are two main measures of health economics: quality-adjusted life-years (QALYs) gained – a measurement of the duration of an individual's life, taking into account the well-being that they experience during that time [11] – and cost. These measures can also be combined to give a cost-effectiveness ratio, which is the cost of gaining an extra year of life or a benefit in the quality of life for the patient. The most robust cost-effectiveness studies are conducted alongside clinical trials, and these collect resource-use costs for all subjects from each center.

Advantages of health-economic endpoints

While other treatment-specific endpoints such as sight-years gained, symptom-free time, and cases of disease prevented can also be used [12], they cannot easily be compared directly. Since the primary economic question is how to get the most benefit from health expenditure, a US panel on cost-effectiveness has recommended using a QALY analysis where possible in order to be able to make comparisons across diseases [13,14]. By calculating the cost per QALY gained for different treatments, healthcare providers can compare where best to invest their limited resources.

One of the interesting differences between clinical trial reports and cost analyses is that, often, trial reports focus only on the worst or first event that a patient experiences, while cost analyses aim to calculate the cost of all events experienced by each patient.

Limitations of health-economic endpoints

Estimating health-economic endpoints alongside clinical trials is a relatively recent concept and, therefore, is only as good as the experience of the economic investigators. The data captured for an economic analysis might not even be used if the treatment is both more expensive and less effective than standard care. Many assumptions often need to be made in an economic analysis, making the data less robust. Economic analyses might not be easily transferable across countries since the cost of care can be very different internationally, and clinical results are dependent on local practice patterns and the availability of facilities.

Certain disease states affect the patient only briefly and might not have a long-term impact if they are not fatal. For example, a collapsed lung might not kill a patient, so the negative impact on the patient's quality of life is only brief and therefore the cost-effectiveness of treating the condition would be unfavorable.

However, treatment can be given almost immediately, few physicians would withhold treatment for this condition, and few patients would wish to remain untreated. This shows that economic analyses are not necessarily valuable in isolation. For this reason, other economic endpoints are being reviewed, such as the amount that patients would be willing to pay to avoid such an event.

Conclusion

As trial designs evolve, endpoints are becoming more complex. There are often both primary and secondary endpoints in a trial. Endpoints may consist of more than one clinical outcome and can also include biochemical outcomes. Surrogate endpoints are particularly useful for early-stage trials, once it has been established that the surrogate marker is strongly related to the clinical outcome for the disease process. Economic outcomes are becoming more important and are now more frequently evaluated. Given all these choices, it is wise to appreciate the strengths and limitations of each type of endpoint at an early stage of study design.

References

1. Temple RJ. A regulatory authority's opinion about surrogate endpoints. In: Nimmo WS, Tucker GT, editors. *Clinical Measurement in Drug Evaluation*. New York: John Wiley & Sons, 1995:3–22.
2. Mwaba P, Mwansa J, Chintu C, et al. Clinical presentation, natural history, and cumulative death rates of 230 adults with primary cryptococcal meningitis in Zambian AIDS patients treated under local conditions. *Postgrad Med J* 2001;**77**:769–73.
3. Yusuf S, Zhao F, Mehta SR, et al. Effects of clopidogrel in addition to aspirin in patients with acute coronary syndromes without ST-segment elevation. *N Engl J Med* 2001;**345**:494–502.
4. Spilker B. *Guide to Clinical Trials*. New York: Raven Press, 1991.
5. Fleming TR, DeMets DL. Surrogate end points in clinical trials: are we being misled? *Ann Intern Med* 1996;**125**:605–13.
6. Greenhalgh T. How to read a paper. Papers that report drug trials. *BMJ* 1997;**315**:480–3.
7. Preliminary report: Effect of encainide and flecainide on mortality in a randomized trial of arrhythmia suppression after myocardial infarction. The Cardiac Arrhythmia Suppression Trial (CAST) Investigators. *N Engl J Med* 1989;**321**:406–12.
8. Echt DS, Liebson PR, Mitchell LB, et al. Mortality and morbidity in patients receiving encainide, flecainide or placebo. The Cardiac Arrhythmia Suppression Trial. *N Engl J Med* 1991;**324**:781–8.
9. Effect of the antiarrhythmic agent moricizine on survival after myocardial infarction. The Cardiac Arrhythmia Suppression Trial II Investigators. *N Engl J Med* 1992;**327**:227–33.
10. Smith R. New *BMJ* policy on economic evaluations. *BMJ* 2002;**325**:1124.
11. Patrick DL, Erickson P. *Health Status and Health Policy. Quality of Life in Health Care Evaluation and Resource Allocation*. New York: Oxford University Press, 1993.
12. Ramsey SD, McIntosh M, Sullivan SD. Design issues for conducting cost-effectiveness analyses alongside clinical trials. *Annu Rev Public Health* 2001;**22**:129–41.

13. Garber AM, Phelps CE. Economic foundations of cost-effective analysis.
    J Health Econ 1997;**16**:1–31.
14. Gold MR, Siegel JE, Russell LB, et al. *Cost-Effectiveness in Health and Medicine*.
    New York: Oxford University Press, 1996:72–3.

Chapter 5

Patient Selection

Belinda Lees, Dorothea Nitsch, Duolao Wang, and Ameet Bakhai

When designing a clinical trial, the objective is to select a sample of patients with the disease or condition under investigation. Consideration should be given to the source of the patients, the investigators who are going to recruit them, disease status, and any ethical issues surrounding participation. A set of carefully defined eligibility criteria is essential. This should ensure that the study findings have 'external validity' or, in other words, are generalizable for the treatment of future patients with the same disease or condition. In this chapter, we discuss some of the important issues to consider when selecting patients for clinical trials.

Introduction

The aim of a clinical trial is to investigate the efficacy of an intervention in patients with a particular disease or condition. When performing a trial, it is impossible to enroll every patient with the particular disease or condition – instead, a sample of patients is selected that represents the population of interest. It is therefore essential that the selected sample truly reflects the population it represents, and that the eligibility criteria are not so restrictive that they hamper recruitment or limit the generalizability of the findings. Essentially, the findings from the trial should have relevance to patients in future clinical practice, ie, the study should have *external validity* or *generalizability*. In order to ensure generalizability, it is essential to have an understanding of the disease and its current treatment options. However, eligibility criteria also serve the function of choosing a sample who can tolerate being in a trial and those in whom there are less co-morbidities that might dilute the effect of the intervention. Also, for clinical safety it is worthwhile selecting a sample who are less likely to have adverse effects (not the elderly or those on multiple co-therapies).

Example

During the planning of the CHARM (Candesartan in Heart failure – Assessment of Reduction in Mortality and morbidity) trial, it was already known that angiotensin-converting enzyme (ACE) inhibitors are beneficial to patients with severe heart failure. Since the pharmacological targets of candesartan and ACE inhibitors are related, it seemed unethical to stop ACE inhibitor treatment in patients already receiving this medication unless they were experiencing negative, drug-related side-effects. However, at the same time, it seemed valid to include a group comprising patients with less severe heart failure who were not receiving ACE inhibitors, since candesartan was expected to have some effects in patients with preserved heart function. Therefore, the CHARM program consisted of three trial subpopulations [1] These subpopulations contained patients with:

- severe heart failure on ACE inhibitor therapy (CHARM-Added)
- severe heart failure who had ceased previous ACE inhibitor therapy due to side-effects (CHARM-Alternative)
- heart failure despite preserved heart function (CHARM-Preserved)

In this way, any benefit of candesartan could be demonstrated to be broadly generalizable to patients with heart failure, whilst ensuring that useful comparison groups for other specific situations were chosen.

General considerations

Source of patients

One of the first considerations when designing a clinical trial is to establish where the patients will be recruited from. The sample size and the clinical outcomes to be measured will need to be balanced against practical considerations. For studies that involve a large number of very detailed observations, it may only be practical to enroll a small number of patients.

Phase I and II pharmaceutical studies usually involve small numbers of patients and are therefore frequently performed in specialist centers (eg, asthma laboratories in hospitals with dedicated research units). Phase III studies, however, typically require larger numbers of patients. Enrolment for these studies might be conducted, for example, through a primary care physician's surgery, although the extent of patient evaluation might be restricted as a consequence.

When researchers select centers to be used to recruit patients, there is often a tendency to concentrate on 'centers of excellence'. This is because the investigators at these centers are often experienced in clinical trials or experts in the disease area. It is important to bear in mind, however, that patients at 'centers of excellence' can be highly selected, with different patterns of referral from more general centers. It is also possible that more difficult or complex cases are handled more skillfully, and therefore efficacy and safety might be overstated; this is often seen in surgical studies, where there is usually a learning curve associated with new surgical techniques.

Investigators and centers

In order for recruitment to be successful, it is important that patient selection is performed at centers with enthusiastic investigators who are convinced of the scientific importance of the trial. Investigators must have an understanding of what is required for the trial so that they can clearly communicate this information to potential participants.

Investigators also need to have access to the facilities and equipment that are required to perform the trial-related tests and measurements (eg, echocardiography measurements in a study of heart valves). Patient selection can be compromised if investigators are performing competing studies; it will certainly be compromised if the investigators do not have enough dedicated research staff to screen patients and perform the trial-related procedures.

When estimating the likely number of patients to be selected for a trial at a particular center, the investigator often relies on guesswork based on the number of previous patients with the condition. A more useful method is to request that investigators complete a screening log, prior to the start of the study, of all patients who present with the condition within a predetermined timeframe, and to record whether each patient is eligible for the study.

Recruitment will often not be possible at a single center due to its limited capacity and resources; there might also be an insufficient number of patients presenting with the disease, resulting in the center failing to recruit the required numbers within the allotted timeframe. It is important to recruit patients for a study in as short a timeframe as possible in order to maintain enthusiasm for the study. One way of improving recruitment centers is to enroll more centers; however, this is not the most economical way to conduct a trial, given the resources needed to train new centers.

Eligibility criteria

In order to reduce bias and variability in a clinical trial, and therefore increase the power of the study, it is essential to have well-developed eligibility criteria. However, these criteria must not be too restrictive as this will result in a smaller patient population – there could be difficulties with patient recruitment, and whilst the patient population would be more homogeneous, the generalizability of the findings would be reduced in the non-trial setting.

A key aspect of eligibility criteria is to define patients with the disease or condition under investigation. The disease state must be established using standardized criteria. Although some diseases are more difficult to define, it should not be left to subjective clinical assessment as this makes it hard to relate the study findings to other patients with the condition. In these cases, it might be sensible to use more than one definition for the disease criteria.

Eligibility criteria are usually based on:

- patient characteristics
- diagnostic test results
- disease duration
- disease severity

Patients must meet all of the inclusion criteria and none of the exclusion criteria. A general rule is to have one or two inclusion criteria and several exclusion criteria. In the CHARM trial, for example, the investigators stated two inclusion criteria and multiple exclusion criteria (see **Table 1**) [1]. The aim was to include as

Table 1. CHARM (Candesartan in Heart failure – Assessment of Reduction in Mortality and morbidity) eligibility criteria [1].

Inclusion	Age ≥18 years
	Symptomatic heart failure (NYHA class II–IV for at least 4 weeks' duration)
Exclusion	Serum creatinine ≥265 µmol/L
	Serum potassium ≥5.5 mmol/L
	Known bilateral renal artery stenosis
	Symptomatic hypotension
	Women of childbearing potential who are not using adequate contraception
	Critical aortic or mitral stenosis
	Myocardial infarction
	Stroke
	Open heart surgery in previous 4 weeks
	Use of angiotensin receptor blocker in previous 2 weeks
	Any noncardiac disease limiting 2-year survival

NYHA = New York Heart Association.

many patients with the disease as possible (in this example, patients with heart failure), but to exclude those with co-morbidities that might affect outcome (in this example, stroke, severe aortic, or mitral stenosis) and those in whom safety may be compromised (in this example, existing severe renal impairment as candesartan can worsen renal function in certain circumstances).

If particular tests or measurements are to be performed as part of the eligibility criteria, it is essential to ensure that the results of these investigations are available prior to randomization of the patient into the study. Stratification or minimization techniques can be employed at the randomization stage to ensure balance between groups in important variables that may affect outcome; therefore, it is important to ensure that these data are available in a timely fashion. For example, in a study of cystic fibrosis, patients were stratified by their breathing capacity (as measured by forced expiratory volume in 1 second) and their atopy status, so it was essential that the results of the lung function and skin prick tests were available at randomization.

Disease status

Some diseases are subject to seasonal factors that affect the timing of patient selection (eg, immunotherapy studies of hay fever). Other diseases are subject to variability, and repeated measurements are often required to confirm diagnosis in these conditions (eg, repeat blood pressure measurements for the diagnosis of hypertension). It is important to select patients who are ill enough to improve with the intervention, but some patients might be too ill to participate in the study.

It might also be necessary to consider what effect previous treatments might have or to actually withdraw a treatment (washout period) before starting the treatment under investigation. Depending on the length of time a drug stays in the body, a specific washout period may need to be defined. For example in CHARM, a period of 2 weeks for drugs similar to candesartan was specified [1].

Selecting patients who have not been treated previously is a common requirement, as previous therapies can mask or reduce the effect of the treatment under investigation. However, in some chronic diseases (eg, asthma) this will be impractical. With other studies, withholding treatment can be unethical (eg, in Alzheimer's disease or cancer). In these studies, unequal numbers are often allocated to the treatment and control arms (eg, in a 2:1 ratio) to move quickly and to gain patient experience with the new drug [2].

Ethical issues

As mentioned previously, it is important not to make the eligibility criteria too stringent, otherwise there may be difficulty in enrolling sufficient patients – a balance needs to be achieved between scientific and practical issues. For example, individuals aged >65 years are frequently excluded from clinical trials because they are more likely to be taking concomitant medications and might be less responsive to treatment, more affected by side-effects, and/or more difficult to evaluate. However, if the treatment or intervention under investigation is intended to be used in clinical practice by individuals in this age group then they should be included.

Special consideration should be given to children or neonates as they can respond to medications differently to adults. A report by the EU revealed that >50% of medicines used in children have not have been adequately studied in this age group [3]; consequently, the EU is developing legislation that will require data on children to form part of the authorization application for medicines that are to be used in children.

There are other ethical issues to consider when selecting patients for study inclusion. For example: repeat visits or tests might be onerous for patients; tests can be painful or uncomfortable; the study might require the patient to take time off from work or school; and the study will often require patients to wait in hospital for tests or for the study drug to be issued from the pharmacy.

A fundamental consideration in patient selection is to enroll patients who are likely to comply with the study procedures. Patients must be willing to participate, and it is essential to take the time to discuss the risks and benefits of the study, to explain to the patient what is expected from them, and for them to have the opportunity to ask questions. Where possible, it is suggested that patients discuss the study with their family, friends, or primary care physician. Generally, patients must provide written informed consent to be enrolled in the study [4], except for in emergency situations where intended or verbal assent is allowed. Ensuring the patient is adequately informed will minimize dropout rates (patients who choose not to complete the trial) (see **Chapter 9**).

Reasons why eligible patients are not selected

Eligible patients might not be selected to enter a trial because of administrative reasons. For example:

- The patient is unavailable during the screening process.
- Study personnel are unavailable to screen the patient.
- The study drug or intervention is unavailable (eg, if the drug has exceeded its shelf life or if the pharmacist is unavailable to formulate an infusion).
- The study procedure is unavailable (eg, faulty echocardiography instrument).
- The patient may not be able to attend follow-up visits.

These reasons can usually be avoided by careful planning and organization. If large numbers of patients are being excluded due to a particular eligibility criterion, it is worth considering making small changes to the criteria. This can make a large difference to recruitment without necessarily affecting outcome or generalizability. Any changes to the eligibility criteria must, of course, be submitted as a protocol amendment for ethical review before being implemented.

Conclusion

When designing a clinical trial, careful consideration must be given not only to the source of patients and the investigators who are going to select the patients, but also to the disease under consideration and any ethical issues regarding patient participation. A specific set of eligibility criteria should be used to define the patient population under study. These eligibility criteria should ensure that the patients included in the study are representative of patients with a particular disease or condition. This will ensure that the study findings can be applied to treat future patients in clinical practice.

References

1. Pfeffer MA, Swedberg K, Granger CB, et al.; CHARM Investigators and Committees. Effects of candesartan on mortality and morbidity in patients with chronic heart failure: the CHARM-Overall programme. *Lancet* 2003;**362**:759–66.

2. Chow SC, Liu P. *Design and Analysis of Clinical Trials: Concepts and Methodologies*. New York: John Wiley & Sons, 1998:94–103.

3. European Union. Proposal for a Regulation of the European Parliament and of the Council on Medicinal Products for Paediatric Use and Amending Regulation (EEC) No 1768/92, Directive 2001/83/EC and Regulation (EC) No 726/2004. September 29, 2004. Available from: http://pharmacos.eudra.org/F2/Paediatrics/docs/_2004_09/EN.pdf. Accessed February 23, 2005.

4. World Medical Association Declaration of Helsinki. Ethical Principles for Medical Research Involving Human Subjects. Available from: www.wma.net/e/policy/b3.htm. Accessed May 6, 2005.

Chapter 6

Source and Control of Bias

Radivoj Arezina and Duolao Wang

The aim of a randomized controlled trial is to provide unbiased evaluation of the efficacy and safety of a medicinal product or a therapeutic procedure. Unfortunately, the treatment effect estimates generated in a study are rarely free of all bias. This is due to a number of biases or errors that occur during a study from conception, through conduct, to completion of the trial, and even beyond the end of the trial when communicating trial results. These contributing factors can be classified into three categories: bias, confounding, and random error. In this chapter, we provide an overview of the ways in which bias can enter at different stages of a clinical trial and review ways of minimizing bias in clinical research.

What is bias in clinical research?

Bias is an "opinion or feeling that favors one side in an argument or one item in a group or series; predisposition; prejudice" [1]. In clinical research, bias is defined as systematic distortion of the estimated intervention effect away from the truth, caused by inadequacies in the design, conduct, or analysis of a trial [2], or in the publication of its results. In other words, in a biased trial, the results observed reflect other factors in addition to (or, in extreme cases, instead of) the effect of the tested therapeutic procedure alone.

The list of potential biases in research is long [3]. A correspondingly large proportion of the effort and skill in clinical research goes into avoiding bias. It is commonly accepted that it is impossible to completely eliminate the possibility of bias. However, it is also recognized that bias can be reduced with, among other things, careful planning and prudent study design. Although bias is typically introduced into a trial inadvertently, due consideration should be given to this problem since it can invalidate research: the mere suggestion that bias is present is often sufficient to cause the validity of a trial to be questioned. The main types of bias and ways of reducing such unwanted influences on the study outcome are listed in **Table 1** and described below.

Selection bias

Selection bias occurs if a systematic difference exists in the way in which study subjects are enrolled (accepted or rejected) into a trial or in the way that treatments are assigned to those enrolled, which in turn has an effect on the trial conclusions. For example, a trial investigator might have reason to believe that diabetic patients are less likely to respond to a new blood-pressure-lowering drug and, consequently, tend to include them in the group receiving the established (control) drug. If the investigator's assumption proves to be correct, the results will show an exaggerated treatment difference and the trial conclusions will favor the new treatment more than they should.

Prevention of this type of bias depends, to a great extent, on how adequate the treatment allocation is. This is the main reason for the use of randomization methods in clinical trials. When randomization is employed properly, all study subjects are given the same chance of being assigned to each of the study treatments. Moreover, the treatment allocation in such a trial cannot be influenced by the investigator. Examples of good methods of treatment randomization include computer-generated codes, random number tables, and even the toss of a coin. Inadequate methods of randomization include alternate assignment and assignment

Table 1. Summary of the most common types of bias in clinical trials and methods of bias control.

Type of bias	Method of bias control
Selection bias	Randomized treatment assignment Concealment of treatment assignment
Bias in study management	Standardized study procedures Standard equipment Training and certification of research personnel
Observer ascertainment bias	Blinding or masking
Bias introduced by exclusions after randomization	Intention-to-treat analysis Worst-case scenario analysis
Publication bias	Prospective registration of clinical trials Publication of 'negative' trials

by odd/even date of birth or hospital number. However, it should be noted that, even when carried out properly, simple randomization does not guarantee the elimination of selection bias – it only reduces the possibility of this unwanted effect.

To further help minimize selection bias, stratification of randomization is used. This involves patients first being classified into subgroups, or 'strata', by one or more characteristics that may influence treatment response, such as age or severity of disease. Patients within each stratum are then randomized separately to ensure that, based on the stratification characteristics, the patients are well-balanced across the treatment groups.

With respect to randomization, there are two processes of equal importance:

- creation of a random treatment assignment code
- concealment of that code until treatment allocation occurs

Some investigators working in clinical research appreciate the code-generating process of randomization but then disregard concealment. Without satisfactory concealment, even the best, most unpredictable randomization codes may be undermined. Chalmers et al. reported manifold overestimation of treatment effect in trials without adequate concealment of treatment allocation [4]. By using proper concealment procedures, such as keeping individual treatment codes in sealed opaque envelopes and making them accessible only to authorized personnel, those who are admitting volunteers into a study are protected from knowing the treatment allocation that will be used.

Selection bias can also be introduced if a highly selected group is enrolled into a trial (eg, in order to ease the demands of patient-recruitment or minimize inter-subject variability). The treatment effect in such a group might well be different from that

Figure 1. Mean pharmacokinetic profiles for the example bioequivalence study.

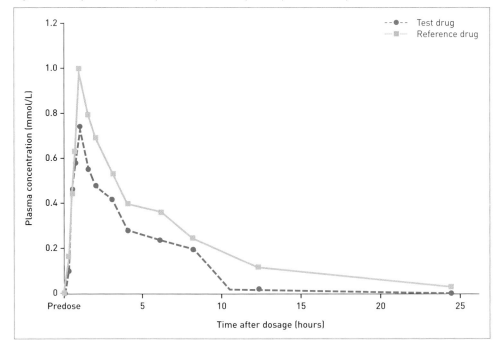

in the actual (target) population of interest. Where it is essential for the study group to closely reflect the target population, trial protocols should clearly specify and make mandatory the inclusion of a wide selection of the entire patient population.

Bias in study management

The interpretation of a randomized controlled trial relies on the assumption that any differences in outcome are the result of either chance (whose effects can be quantified) or of inherent differences between treatments. This assumption is invalid if the treatment groups are not handled equally with regard to all of the study procedures.

For instance, consider a trial conducted to compare the absorption of two dosage forms of a drug: a fast-dissolving tablet absorbed from the tongue and a regular tablet absorbed from the intestine. If, due to poorly defined study procedures or noncompliance, the subjects receiving the regular tablet are allowed to lie down following drug administration, the transit and intestinal absorption will be slowed and this might distort the overall study conclusions.

Figure 2. Mean pharmacokinetic profiles for the repeated example bioequivalence study.

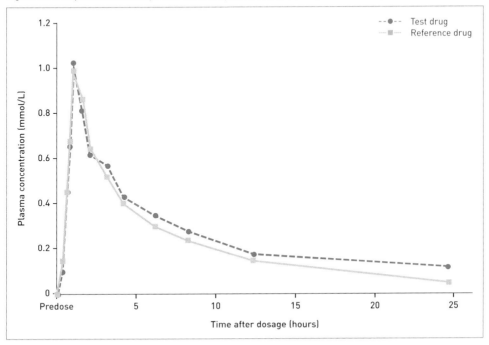

The same might happen if blood samples for pharmacokinetic analysis are not handled properly. For example, consider an anonymized study where two formulations of a drug are compared to see if they are bioequivalent. Both formulations are chemically unstable and break down very rapidly, hence certain chemicals need to be added to the blood samples as stabilizers. The pharmacokinetic analysis showed that the test formulation was significantly less bioavailable than the reference drug (see **Figure 1**). However, the study debrief showed that the test-drug blood samples had a lower concentration of stabilizer; this caused the test drug to break down more quickly than the reference drug and show falsely lower concentrations when assayed. When the study was repeated using the same drugs with adequately stabilized blood samples, the mean concentrations of the two drugs were very similar (**Figure 2**).

In order to avoid this type of bias, trials should be conducted according to standardized written protocols with clearly defined study procedures. Study personnel must be well trained and certified for particular tasks to ensure that the various measurements and assessments are performed identically on every subject and on each occasion. Study participants should be closely supervised wherever possible to ensure their compliance and to check that study restrictions are observed.

Observer (ascertainment) bias

When knowledge of the treatment assignment (by participants already recruited into a trial, investigators, or persons who analyze and report trial results) leads to systematic distortion of the trial conclusions, this is referred to as *observer* or *ascertainment* bias.

The patients' knowledge that they are receiving a 'new' treatment may substantially affect the way they feel and their subjective assessment. If the investigator is aware of which treatment the patient is receiving, this can affect the way he/she collects the information during the trial (eg, he/she asks certain questions). By the same token, the knowledge of which treatment the patient received can influence the way the assessor analyzes the study results (eg, when evaluating efficacy by selecting particular time points that favor one of the treatments over the other). In the case of laboratory-related outcomes, the knowledge of treatment assignment can have an impact on how the test is run or interpreted. Although the impact of this is most severe with subjectively graded results, such as pathology slides and photographs, it can also be a problem with more objective tests (eg, laboratory assays might be run subtly differently by the technician).

Blinding

The best way of avoiding observer bias is to conduct trials in a *blind* fashion. This means that some or all of those involved in the study (study participants, investigators, assessors, etc.) are unaware of the treatment assignment. It is important to recognise the difference between allocation concealment and blinding. Allocation concealment helps to minimize selection bias by shielding the randomization code *before and until the treatments are administered to subjects or patients*, whereas blinding helps avoid observer bias by protecting the randomization code *after the treatments have been administered* (see **Chapter 8**).

Blinding or *masking*, as it is often called, is immensely important for maintaining the integrity and validity of research results. Nonblinded studies typically favor new treatments over established ones. One meta-analysis has shown that nonblinded studies overestimate treatment effects by 17% [5].

Blinding can be performed by making study participants unaware of which treatment they are receiving (*single blind*) or by making both study participants and the investigator unaware of the treatment assignment (*double blind*). There is another level of study blinding called *triple blind* or *total blind*, which essentially means that all those involved in a study, including those responsible for data analysis, reporting, and study monitoring, have no knowledge of which treatment is being given to whom. It appears that total blinding is not as common in clinical trials as it should be. The benefit of blinding those evaluating and interpreting trial data (alongside the participants and investigators) is obvious. Similarly, usually there are no practical considerations as to why we should not blind such personnel, and we can do this by treatment coding.

To achieve blinding in a drug trial it should be impossible to distinguish between the trial medications, and, to achieve this, placebos are used. Placebos are inert substances that are identical in physical appearance to the active treatment and, if taken by mouth (eg, as tablets), they should have the smell and taste of the active treatment. In the case of an intravenous infusion, the placebo is normally the vehicle used for the active medication (the medium in which the active drug would be dissolved). One use of placebos in trials is as a direct comparison with a new medication (placebo-controlled trials), typically when there is no established active treatment that is effective and can be used as a comparator.

Achieving blinding

Effective blinding is not always easy to achieve. Patients and investigators may be clued into whether patients are taking active medication or placebo by different means. This can happen through accidental or deliberate unmasking. It can also occur as a result of practical problems in treatment administration, eg, if a patient bites the tablet and finds that it tastes different. Another source of unmasking is the fact that side-effects of the active treatment, quite understandably, are often different from those of the placebo.

Although most of these problems can be minimized by making trial procedures more stringent and improving trial participant and personnel compliance, the challenge of distinguishable side-effect profiles appear to be the most difficult to solve. It has been suggested that use of a 'three-arm design' (involving a new drug, a reference drug, and a placebo) can help to overcome this problem, whereby the third 'treatment' may make it more difficult for the patients and study personnel to ascertain the treatment allocation [6]. For instance, even if the patients guess that they are receiving an active treatment, they may not be able to tell whether they are on the 'old' or new drug. Also, noninert placebos have been used to achieve the same goal (in particular in antidepressant trials) [7]. Adding a third treatment or adding the potential for toxicity to placebo (that is, using a noninert placebo) to avoid unblinding raises some ethical issues. These need to be examined carefully before such methods are applied to a particular trial. A risk–benefit assessment should be carried out, taking into account the potential benefits of properly evaluating the new treatment on the one hand and protecting patients from any unnecessary harm on the other.

Bias introduced by exclusions after randomization

It is intended that all trial participants comply with the trial protocol and complete the trial accordingly. However, in practice (and in particular during later phases of drug development), missing data can result from some of the participants dropping-out before they complete the trial. Also, data might be missing because some of the scheduled measurements were done incorrectly or, worse, not done at all. Irrespective of their origin, inappropriate handling of the missing data can lead to bias. For example, if in a treatment comparison trial the incidence of withdrawals due to adverse events is much higher with one of the treatments, excluding withdrawn subjects from the analysis would lead to an underrating of the side-effects of that drug. Analyses that exclude all subjects who were noncompliant, have missing data, or were unable to complete their assigned treatment are called *per-protocol* analyses.

There are two bias control methods that can be used to minimize the negative impact that withdrawals and exclusions can have on the interpretation of study results (eg, as seen in per-protocol analyses).

The first is known as *intention-to-treat* analysis. In this analysis, all the study participants we intended to treat are included in the analysis, regardless of whether they completed the trial according to the protocol or not. The second method is called *worst case scenario* analysis. This involves allocating the worst possible outcomes to the missing subjects or missing time points in the group that shows the most desired results, and *vice versa*. Following this, this data set is analyzed to see whether the new analysis is in agreement with the results of the initial analysis (which did not account for the missing data). As opposed to the intention-to-treat approach, which is a way of addressing the issue of noncompliant subjects (who may or may not have missing data), the worst case scenario analysis is more specifically used to deal with missing data in a trial. There are other often-suggested methods for dealing with missing data [8,9], such as '*last observation carried forward*' and '*multiple imputation*' (see **Chapter 30**).

Publication bias

It is becoming increasingly apparent that published clinical research data do not always represent the whole truth. People involved in research, including investigators, editors, and sponsors, typically prefer positive trial outcomes, which is to some degree understandable. What is not understandable is that trials generating negative or equivocal results are less likely to be published in peer-reviewed journals, and this can seriously undermine the integrity of clinical research data [10]. This tendency to favor trials with positive results is called 'publication bias'.

Although there appears to be increasing evidence that failure to publish is not a random event [11], the lack of interest in publishing 'nonpositive trials' might, at least partly, be a result of underpowered studies. In such a trial, negative or equivocal results effectively become indeterminate, which in turn makes them of little interest to journal editors or the scientific community.

One way of tackling publication bias is by introducing the compulsory registration of trials at initiation and ensuring that the results of all trials are published. Although it remains a long-term goal, at present such a proposal is very controversial and is the subject of intense debate. Meanwhile, the reader should bear in mind that published data alone might not always provide sufficient evidence on which to make a definitive judgment about a particular treatment.

Conclusion

The types of bias described above are the most common and, arguably, the most important in clinical research. There are, however, many other biases that can be introduced in the course of, or after, a trial, and they are comprehensively described in other publications [3,12].

Randomized controlled trials are too often assumed to produce impartial evidence by eliminating bias. The truth is that randomization, treatment concealment, blinding, standardized study procedures, and other methods mentioned in this chapter help to reduce bias, but do not eliminate it completely. We may only move closer to that goal by raising awareness among scientists, investigators, peer-reviewers, and readers about the importance of bias control in clinical research, and by applying bias-control measures wherever possible.

In this chapter, we have only addressed the issue of bias. The two other sources that could still distort the true estimates of treatment effects, random error and confounding, are discussed in **Chapters 18** and **26** of this book, respectively.

References

1. Hornby AS, et al, editors. *Oxford Advanced Learner's Dictionary of Current English,* 4th edition. Oxford: Oxford University Press, 1989.
2. Altman DG, Schulz KF, Moher D, et al. The revised CONSORT statement for reporting randomized trials: explanation and elaboration. *Ann Intern Med* 2001;**134**:663–94.
3. Jadad AR. *Randomised Controlled Trials. A User's Guide.* London: BMJ Publishing Group, 1998.
4. Chalmers TC, Celano P, Sacks HS, et al. Bias in treatment assignment in controlled clinical trials. *N Engl J Med* 1983;**309**:1358–61.

5. Schulz KF, Chalmers TC, Hayes RJ, et al. Empirical evidence of bias. Dimensions of methodological quality associated with estimates of treatment effects in controlled trials. *JAMA* 1995;**273**:408–12.

6. Leber PD. Hazards of inference: the active control investigation. *Epilepsia* 1989;**30**(Suppl. 1):S57–63. Discussion: S64–8.

7. Even CE, Siobud-Dorocant E, Dardennes RM. Critical approach to antidepressant trials. Blindness protection is necessary, feasible and measurable. *Br J Psychiatry* 2000;**177**:47–51.

8. Hollis S, Campbell F. What is meant by intention to treat analysis? Survey of published randomised controlled trials. *BMJ* 1999;**319**:670–4.

9. Little R, Yau L. Intent-to-treat analysis for longitudinal studies with drop-outs. *Biometrics* 1996;**52**:1324–33.

10. Last J. Negative studies. About this "amnesty". *NCEHR Communiqué* 1998;**8**(2):1–3. Available from: URL: http://ncehr-cnerh.org/English/communique 2/Negative.html. Accessed on 21 March 2005.

11. Stern JM, Simes RJ. Publication bias: Evidence of delayed publication in a cohort study of clinical research projects. *BMJ* 1997;**315**:640–5.

12. Owen R. Reader bias. *JAMA* 1982;**247**:2533–4.

Chapter 7

Randomization

Duolao Wang and Ameet Bakhai

Randomization is the unpredictable allocation of a patient to a particular treatment strategy in a clinical trial. When a large number of patients is involved, simple randomization will balance the groups in a trial for patient characteristics and other factors that might bias outcomes (systematic error or confounding). The remaining differences in efficacy or safety outcomes between the groups can then be assumed to be due to the effects of the different treatment strategies or random error. Randomization is therefore the cornerstone of a well-conducted clinical trial. In this chapter, we describe and explain some commonly used randomization methods and their implementation.

Why should patients in a clinical trial be randomized?

The randomized controlled trial (RCT) is considered the gold standard for testing the efficacy of medical treatments [1,2]. A fundamental assumption that forms the basis of the RCT is that patients in different groups are similar for characteristics such as age, gender, social class, time of year of presentation, country of presentation, and type of hospital. In a large trial involving more than 1,000 patients, these characteristics should be balanced across each group so that any difference seen between the groups at the end of the trial is then due to the different treatment strategies (ie, if patients do better in one group we can assume that this is due to the treatment effect if not due to random error). This assumption is the basis of all comparative statistical tests performed in the trial.

To achieve this balance we randomly assign the patients (hence the term randomized in an RCT) to each treatment strategy so that, for example, men have an equal chance of being given treatment A or B, people aged over 60 years have an equal chance of being given treatment A or B, and so on. Simple randomization is one way of performing this balancing function, but other methods are needed when the number of patients is small.

Minimizing bias

A further requirement of randomization is that it must not be predictable by the person assigning patients to the treatment strategies, otherwise there is a chance that the groups will contain bias. To prevent this, certain methods of 'blinding' or 'masking' are used so that patients and staff (with the usual exception of the data and safety monitoring board) are not aware whether treatment A or B is the new treatment, or even which group patients are in (active or placebo/standard treatment), until the end of the trial. Physicians and study coordinators providing the treatments to the patients use a randomization code to find out which treatment pack has been assigned to each patient (A or B), but the code provides no information about which treatment is which (active or placebo/standard treatment). Randomization must be protected by blinding (see **Chapter 8**) so that it remains unpredictable.

How should the randomization code be determined?

A randomization code is a list of which treatment a subject should receive. It is usually determined by a statistician using computer-generated random numbers or a random-number table. Some trials use methods for assigning subjects according to date of birth (odd or even years), hospital record number, or date of screening for the study (odd or even days), but these randomization methods have a level of predictability, so strictly are not acceptable methods of randomization.

Which are the common randomization methods?

The generation of a randomization code can be achieved using one of a variety of procedures. Once a code and method of allocation are decided on, their rules must be adhered to throughout the study. Common types of randomization methods are [1,2]:

- simple randomization
- block randomization
- stratified randomization
- minimization or adaptive randomization

A combination of these methods can also be used, and other special methods do exist. Let us now discuss the more common randomization methods listed.

Simple randomization

The most common form of randomization, referred to as simple or complete randomization, is a procedure that makes each new treatment allocation without regard to those already made. The principle of this method for a trial with two treatments can be demonstrated by deciding treatment assignment by tossing an unbiased coin, eg, heads for treatment A and tails for treatment B. When the next subject is to be assigned, previous allocations are not considered.

This method is easy to implement and unpredictable. However, as it is somewhat inconsiderate to previous allocations, it can often produce small inequalities between treatment groups, eg, 200 women were assigned to treatment A and 205 women to treatment B. In a large trial this makes only a small difference, but in smaller trials at an early clinical stage that involve only a few dozen subjects, these inequalities could have a substantial impact.

Example

Consider an example trial with 12 patients. While there is an equal chance of being allocated treatment A or treatment B, the number of subjects randomly assigned to each treatment ends up being 5 and 7, respectively (**Table 1**). This imbalance in the initial allocation will result in significant difficulties in the statistics and possibly a lower power for detecting differences between the

Table 1. Example of simple randomization.

Subject	Treatment
1	A
2	B
3	A
4	A
5	B
6	B
7	B
8	B
9	A
10	A
11	B
12	B

treatments. Therefore, in cases where there are few patients, there is a need for other methods of randomization.

Block randomization

The block randomization method, also known as *permuted-block* randomization, is a popular method in clinical trials. A block randomization method can be used to periodically enforce a balance in the number of patients assigned to each treatment. The size of each block of allocations must be an integer multiple of the number of treatment groups, so with two treatment strategies the block size can be either 2, 4, 6, and so on. A block randomization can be implemented in three steps:

Step 1: Choose the block size and the number of blocks needed to cover the number of patients in the study.

Step 2: List all possible permutations of treatments in a block.

Step 3: Generate a randomization code for the order in which to select each block.

Example

Consider a clinical trial comparing treatments A and B in 24 patients. Here, we should choose a block size of 4 because the sequence would become predictable with blocks of 2, and block sizes of 6 or above are too large for this small sample size. Using this block size we must ensure that, after every fourth randomized

Table 2. Example of block randomization using a block size of 4.

Block	Permutation	Subject	Treatment
1	6	1	B
		2	B
		3	A
		4	A
2	4	5	B
		6	A
		7	A
		8	B
3	3	9	A
		10	B
		11	B
		12	A
4	1	13	A
		14	A
		15	B
		16	B
5	2	17	A
		18	B
		19	A
		20	B
6	5	21	B
		22	A
		23	B
		24	A

subject, the number of subjects in each arm is equal. Therefore, each block must contain two patients on treatment A and two on treatment B.

Step 1: Given a sample size of 24 and using a block size of 4, we need six blocks.

Step 2: There are six possible permutations that allow two As and two Bs in each box: AABB, ABAB, ABBA, BAAB, BABA and BBAA.

Step 3: The randomization code for blocks can be generated by producing a random-number list for permutations 1–6.

Table 2 provides a listing of random permutations of A and B for each subject using this method. Note that after every four patients there is a balance of subjects between treatments A and B. If we need more than six blocks (or have over 24 patients), we can continue sampling more of the six possible block permutations shown above. The procedure is repeated until all patients are randomized.

The balance forced by blocking is especially important in long-term trials if:

- recruitment is slow
- the type of patients recruited in the trial changes during the enrollment period
- the trial may be stopped early for safety or efficacy reasons
- routine practice changes for patients in both groups during the trial

The only disadvantage of blocking is that every fourth patient, and occasionally every third patient (when the sequence is AABB or BBAA), becomes predictable if the treatments are not masked and the previous allocations of that block are known.

Stratified randomization

Stratified randomization takes the balance correction suggested by blocking one step further. Not only are the numbers with treatments A and B balanced periodically, but a balance is also constantly maintained for a set of predetermined important factors that may impact on the prognosis of the patient, such as age, gender, diabetes, severity of illness, or geography. If prognostic factors are not evenly distributed between treatment groups it can give the investigator cause for concern, although statistical methods, such as the Cox regression model, are available that allow for such a lack of comparability.

Example

Stratified randomization is implemented in three steps. We can illustrate the procedures using the CF-WISE (Withdrawal of Inhaled Steroids Evaluation Study in Patients with Cystic Fibrosis) trial conducted at the Clinical Trials and Evaluation Unit of the Royal Brompton Hospital, London, UK. CF-WISE was a randomized placebo-controlled trial designed to test the feasibility and safety of periodically withdrawing inhaled corticosteroids (ICS) in 240 children and adults with cystic fibrosis who were already taking ICS. The two treatment strategies involved a return to either ICS treatment after withdrawal (A) or to placebo (B). The primary endpoint was the time to first respiratory exacerbation.

Step 1: Choose the prognostic factors that could impact on the primary endpoint.

Experience of earlier trials and literature show that atopy, forced expiratory volume within 1 second (FEV_1), and age are the most important determinants of time to first respiratory exacerbation.

Table 3. Strata definitions for the CF-WISE (Withdrawal of Inhaled Steroids Evaluation Study in Patients with Cystic Fibrosis) study show three factors for stratification.

Stratum	Atopy	FEV$_1$ (%)	Age (years)	Randomization
1	Positive	40–60	<17	ABAB, BABA, AABB...
2	Positive	40–60	≥17	
3	Positive	61–80	<17	
4	Positive	61–80	≥17	
5	Positive	81–100	<17	
6	Positive	81–100	≥17	
7	Negative	40–60	<17	
8	Negative	40–60	≥17	
9	Negative	61–80	<17	
10	Negative	61–80	≥17	
11	Negative	81–100	<17	
12	Negative	81–100	≥17	

Step 2: Determine the number of strata for each factor.

When several prognostic factors are chosen, a stratum for randomization is formed by selecting one subgroup for each factor (continuous variables such as age are split into meaningful categorical ranges). The total number of strata is therefore the product of the number of subgroups in each factor. **Table 3** describes the strata for stratified randomization in the CF-WISE study. In this example, the total number of strata is 2 (atopy) × 3 (FEV$_1$) × 2 (age) = 12.

Step 3: Generate randomization codes.

This is done by generating a randomization list for each stratum and then combining all the lists. Within each stratum, the randomization process itself could be simple randomization, but in practice most clinical trials use a blocked randomization method. In our example, three blocks of size 4 are shown for stratum 1. The key with this method is to choose the most important prognostic factors and keep the number of strata to a minimum so that randomization using blocks remains unpredictable.

Table 4. Treatment assignments based on three prognostic factors for 100 patients.

Factor	Level	Treatment A	Treatment B	Subtotal	Total
Atopy	Positive	22	21	43	
	Negative	28	29	57	100
FEV_1 (%)	40–60	19	18	37	
	61–80	20	21	41	
	81–100	11	11	22	100
Age (years)	<17	25	26	51	
	≥17	25	24	49	100

FEV_1 = forced expiratory volume within 1 second.

Minimization

Minimization – also called an adaptive randomization procedure – takes the approach of assigning subjects to treatments in order to minimize the differences between the treatment groups on selected prognostic factors. This method starts with a simple randomization method (the first of our examples) for the first several subjects, and then adjusts the chance of allocating a new patient to a particular treatment based on existing imbalances in those prognostic factors [2].

Using minimization with the CF-WISE study as an example, if treatment A has more atopy-positive than atopy-negative patients then the allocation scheme is such that the next few atopy-positive patients are more likely to be randomized to treatment B. This method is employed in situations involving many prognostic factors, and patient allocation is then based on the aim of balancing the subtotals for each level of each factor.

Example

Table 4 shows a hypothetical distribution of 100 patients according to treatment and three prognostic factors in the CF-WISE study. Consider that the next patient is atopy positive, has an FEV_1 <60% and is aged 15 years old. To find the number of similar patients already assigned to each treatment arm, the patients in the corresponding three rows of **Table 4** are added:

Sum for A = 22 + 19 + 25 = 66

Sum for B = 21 + 18 + 26 = 65

Minimization requires that the patient be given the treatment with the smallest marginal total, which in this case is treatment B. If the sums for A and B are equal, then simple randomization would be used to assign the treatment.

Although this method is mathematically uncomplicated, it has not been widely used because of the practical difficulties associated with implementing it (some patient characteristics must be collected and processed before randomization can be performed, hence slowing down the entire process). However, with increasing use of computers and, more recently, interactive voice-response systems, this method is gaining popularity, particularly in large trials, thereby removing the need for prespecified randomization lists; and to minimize influence due to imbalances in patients and baseline characteristics of patients.

Conclusion

Several commonly used methods of randomization have been described here, but there are others. Whichever method is used, the purpose of randomization remains the same: to validate the assumption that the differences seen in the outcomes are likely due to differences in the treatments and not the baseline characteristics of the patients.

References

1. Pocock SJ. *Clinical Trials: A Practical Approach*. New York: John Wiley & Sons, 1983.
2. Chow SC, Liu JP. *Design and Analysis of Clinical Trials: Concepts and Methodologies*. New York: John Wiley & Sons, 1998.

Chapter 8

Blinding

Ameet Bakhai, Sonia Patel, and Duolao Wang

Randomization can minimize the influence of bias in clinical trials by balancing groups for various characteristics. Bias can still occur, however, if study personnel and patients know the identity of the treatment, due to preconceptions and subjective judgment in reporting, evaluation, data processing, and statistical analysis. To minimize these biases, studies should be blinded, or masked, so that all participants are unaware of whether the subjects are assigned to the new or standard therapy during a trial. In this chapter, we discuss different study protocols that can be used to blind either the patients only, both patients and investigators, or a combination of investigators, patients, sponsors, trial committees, and other personnel.

Blinding or masking?

In clinical trials, the term 'blinding' has been defined as an experimental methodology in which groups of individuals involved in a trial are made unaware of which treatment the participants are assigned to. The term blinding has been challenged because it should be reserved to describe visual impairment. The term 'masking' is therefore used by some research organizations such as the US National Institutes of Health. Terms such as single blind and double blind are still ingrained in trial terminology, making it hard to replace them completely. Here, we will use the term blinding, so as to be able to appreciate the older definitions, although we would encourage the use of masking otherwise.

Why do we need blinding in studies?

Most human beings have opinions and preconceptions. When these opinions are unsubstantiated by evidence, individuals can be said to be biased. In a trial, knowledge of which treatment a patient is assigned to can lead to subjective and judgmental bias by the patients and investigators. This bias can influence the reporting, evaluation, and management of data and can distort statistical analysis of the treatment effect [1,2]. In practical terms, it is extremely difficult to quantitatively assess such bias and its impact on the evaluation of treatment effect.

Bias can occur in clinical trials because, generally, patients wish to be given the latest new treatments and doctors hope to be involved in a study that will succeed. Both patients and doctors want the effects of a new treatment to be more favorable, which can result in the underreporting of side-effects. It is therefore critical to neutralize such bias by masking the identity of treatments so that trial participants are blinded to the nature of the treatment.

At each stage of a trial, there are a variety of individuals who can introduce bias. These individuals include patients, principal investigators, physicians, surgeons, sponsors, and other healthcare professionals, local study coordinators (who may also be principal investigators themselves), core labs reporting on scans or blood samples, trial statisticians, and committees such as the adjudication or data monitoring and safety committee (DMSC). Therefore, each of these groups can be blinded.

What forms of blinding are used in a randomized study?

With respect to blinding, there are four general types of blinded studies in clinical trials [2–4]:

- open/unblinded
- single blinded
- double blinded
- triple blinded

Open/unblinded studies

On some occasions it might not be possible to use blinding. For example, if the new intervention is a surgical treatment and is being compared with tablets then the difference between the two is difficult to hide. Such studies might need to be unblinded as far as the patients and caregivers are concerned, and are known as open or unblinded studies. The advantages of unblinded studies are that they are simple, fairly inexpensive, and a true reflection of clinical practice.

The disadvantages of knowing which treatment is being given are numerous. Patients may underreport adverse effects of the new treatment. Another disadvantage is the possibility that local investigators might supply different amounts of concomitant treatments (eg, only giving analgesics to the surgical group). Therefore, some biases are unbalanced, and this must be appreciated when examining the results.

One compensation that could be made for this study design would be to blind the adjudication committee, statistics teams, and, where possible, core labs. An example of such a study would be to compare medical treatments for coronary artery disease with surgical treatments.

Single-blinded studies

In single-blinded studies, the patient should be unaware of which treatment they are taking, while the investigators are aware of whether the treatment is new, standard, or placebo [2]. The advantage here is that the design is relatively simple and allows investigators to exercise their clinical judgment when treating participants. The disadvantage is that patients might under- or overreport treatment effects and side-effects, based on some influence or response from the investigators. Investigators may give advice or prescribe additional therapy to the control group if they feel that these patients are disadvantaged in comparison to the active group, and so a number of subtle biases could be introduced either in favor of or against the new treatment depending on the investigators' opinions.

This approach might benefit treatments that have fewer side-effects. However, side-effects may be less because the treatment is less clinically effective. Safety studies often have a single-blind design that allows investigators to detect side-effects more readily.

Double-blinded studies

In double-blinded studies, neither the patient nor the investigator knows the identity of the assigned intervention [2–4]. A number of biases are thus reduced, such as investigators' preconceptions of the treatments used in the study. This reduces the ability of the investigators to monitor the safety of treatments, so a DMSC must regularly review the rate of adverse events in each arm of the trial. Operating these committees is difficult, as they must meet regularly enough to be able to detect differences promptly, avoiding needless further harm to patients, while avoiding early termination of a trial due to a chance difference.

What specific problems do double-blinded studies have?

Double-blinded studies are complex and their validity depends on the investigators and participants remaining blinded. A study of a drug is easily unblinded if the medications are not identical in appearance. Although most patients only receive one drug – unless they are involved in a crossover study, where each participant takes both the new and standard treatments – they often meet and could compare pills and tablets. Medical staff also have the opportunity to compare the medications of both groups, and can unblind the study. It is therefore important to use carefully matched medications, especially in crossover studies.

To prevent imperfect matching, a panel unconnected with the study should carry out a pre-test by comparing samples of the drugs. Perfect matches are rare, and imperfect matches are tolerated so long as they do not reveal the identity of the agent. Dyes such as vanilla can mask a distinctive odor, and quassin will give preparations a bitter taste that masks flavor and discourages the patient from biting the tablets in half, but it is usually best to avoid such extreme measures. The ideal method of blinding is to use agents that appear identical by formulating them appropriately or by enclosing them in identical capsules.

Triple-blinded studies

In triple-blinded studies, as well as the investigators and participants, all members of the sponsor's project team (eg, the project clinician, statistician, and data manager), and even the DMSC, are blinded [2]. This lessens the chance that the DMSC will stop the trial early in favor of either treatment, and makes evaluations of the results more objective. However, this hampers the DMSC's ability to monitor safety and efficacy endpoints, and some investigators might feel uncomfortable when participating because there is no one to oversee the results as they accrue. Triple blinding is appropriate for studies in which the risk of adverse events due to the new or standard treatment is low, and should not be used for treatments where safety is a critical issue. Due to the reduced ability of the DMSC to see trends early, recruitment might need to continue until statistical significance is reached for either clinical effects or adverse events.

Coding of drugs

Drug treatments involved in a study are usually known by a code (eg, study drug, identification batch 62, number 29), which is recorded with a unique patient number. This code prevents knowledge of whether the drug is the new/standard treatment or a placebo. Many drugs can still be recognized by specific side-effects, such as flushing of the face or a metallic taste in the mouth. If several participants with a similar drug code experience the same side-effects then this could unblind the study. Therefore, unique codes might be needed for each patient, but in large studies the use of unique codes might not be practical. In emergency situations, for instance when patients or investigators do not have access to their own treatment, investigators might have to 'borrow' medication from another identically coded patient until further stocks arrive.

Unblinding studies

Accidental unblinding might occur, for example, when the distribution center fails to remove all of the drug identification packing slips from the cartons, or if a blood or imaging laboratory mistakenly sends the investigators results for the participants sorted by treatment. In emergency situations it might be important for the attending investigator to know which treatment the patient is taking, but in most emergencies the medication can be withdrawn without breaking the blinding, or the specific investigator can be informed of the code without the participant or principal investigator being informed.

Methods for fast and efficient unblinding should be in place with clear guidelines as to when it is appropriate. For example, each medicine bottle used in the study could have a tear-off strip that can be kept in the pharmacy and opened in an emergency in order to reveal the identity of the drug. Care should be taken to ensure that the label cannot be read through the seal.

Assessing trial blindness

The degree to which the blinding was maintained in a study can be estimated by asking the patients to guess which group they were assigned to. If the mean result of the guesses is close to being 50% correct, the study was well blinded. A similar enquiry could be made of the patients' study investigators also.

Conclusion

The blinding of studies requires careful planning and constant monitoring to ensure that blinding is maintained, whilst also ensuring that patient safety and the validity of trial results are not compromised. Furthermore, it is vital that all study protocols clearly document who was blinded in the study and how they were blinded, as this can have a significant impact on the value of the study results.

References

1.   Pocock SJ. *Clinical Trials: A Practical Approach.* New York: John Wiley & Sons, 1983.
2.   Chow SC, Liu JP. *Design and Analysis of Clinical Trials: Concepts and Methodologies.* New York: John Wiley & Sons, 1998.
3.   Friedman LM, Furberg CD, DeMets DL. Blindness. In: *Fundamentals of Clinical Trials.* New York: Springer-Verlag, 1998:82–92.
4.   Matthews JNS. Assessment, blinding and placebos. In: *An Introduction to Randomised Controlled Trials.* London: Arnold, 2000:53–9.

Chapter 9

Sample Size and Power

Duolao Wang and Ameet Bakhai

The aim of a well-designed clinical trial is to ask an important question about the effectiveness or safety of a treatment and to provide a reliable answer by performing statistical analysis and assessing whether an observed treatment difference is due to chance. The reliability of the answer is determined by the sample size of the trial: the larger a trial, the less likely we are to miss a real difference between treatments by chance. In this chapter, we review the issues that determine an appropriate sample size for a randomized controlled trial.

What is 'sample size' for a randomized study?

The sample size of a randomized controlled trial (RCT) is the number of subjects that are to be enrolled in the study. Choosing the right sample size is critical for a study, and is based on key assumptions: the size of the benefit we anticipate with the new treatment compared to standard (or placebo) treatment (the 'expected treatment effect'); and the amount of certainty we wish to have with which to capture the treatment benefit (the 'power' of the study).

The larger the sample size, the better the power with which to detect a treatment effect, which means that smaller treatment effects can be detected as statistically significant. In the same way, the smaller the sample size, the less power we have with which to detect a treatment effect, meaning that the effect must be greater in order to be detected as significant. The calculation used to find the required sample size for a trial is also influenced by the trial's design, so the method by which the primary outcome is to be determined must also be clarified in advance of determining the sample size.

Why do we have to choose a sample size?

When resources are limited we must decide how best to invest them in order to maximize the benefits received. For example, should we use treatment X or treatment Y? To answer this question, we need to decide how hard we will look for the answer. Until we do, people will continue to be given or refused a treatment without evidence. We might decide that it is only worth looking at the question if we are fairly likely to detect a 10% improvement with the new treatment. To improve the chance that such a difference is detected (if it exists) we have to choose the sample size wisely, based on realistic initial assumptions. More importantly, it is unethical to carry out a study that is unlikely to capture a real difference since we will have spent precious resources on performing a study for no gain. From this, we can appreciate that choosing an appropriate sample size for a study is dependent on good judgment, which is critical to a trial's success.

What factors determine the sample size?

Several factors are considered when determining the appropriate sample size to use for an RCT [1,2]:

- the expected summary measure of the primary endpoint (such as event rate) in the control or standard treatment arm of the trial

- the smallest treatment effect or benefit that we are trying to detect
- the significance level at which we will reject the null hypothesis that there is no difference in the treatment effects
- the power with which we want to detect an effect
- the design of the study (parallel or crossover, etc.)
- the expected dropout rate of subjects during the study

Example

An RCT is planned to evaluate the effect of a new drug on reducing the death rate, at 12 months' follow-up, of subjects with severe coronary heart disease.

Determine the expected event rate in the control arm

To estimate the expected rate of death at 12 months (the mortality rate) in the control group, we must review previous studies and registries of subjects with severe coronary disease. In this example, the mortality rate at 12 months is 12%, denoted by π_1.

Evaluate the smallest treatment effect that is clinically worth detecting

When determining the size of a clinically relevant treatment effect, it helps to systematically review the literature on previous studies and to discuss trial design with experts. In this example, the mortality rate seen in the treatment group might be 10% (denoted by π_2). Therefore, the absolute treatment effect that we are trying to detect is 2% (12%–10%), denoted by δ. At this point in the trial it is not known whether the new drug will be beneficial or not, but we need enough subjects enrolled in the trial to have a good chance of being able to detect such a difference. By 'detect', we mean that if a treatment benefit is seen, it should be of such a magnitude to be statistically significant (ie, it should have a calculated P-value <0.05).

Determine the significance level for rejecting the null hypothesis (Type I error)

Consider a study that is performed on all individuals in the world who have severe coronary disease. The study finds that the mortality rate for the new treatment is the same as that for the standard treatment, so in this case we would say there is no real difference due to the new treatment. Imagine that we then do an RCT on a sample of the whole suitable population (those with severe coronary heart disease) and that we see a statistically significant difference between the mortality rates for the two treatments. The RCT result would therefore be a false-positive result, which is also known as a Type I error. By setting a significance threshold of 0.05, the chance of seeing this false-positive is 5%, ie, there is a Type I error threshold of 5%. More subjects will be needed in the study if we want a lower rate for these 'false alarms'. Conventionally, a level of 5% is chosen and is denoted by the term α.

Choosing the power of a trial (Type II error)

Consider the reverse situation to the above, that is, in the study on the whole population the new treatment produces a 2% absolute reduction in the mortality rate and in our RCT we did not find a statistically significant difference. We would call this a false-negative result, or a Type II error. Conventionally, the Type II error rate is set at 20%, and this is represented by the constant β. The power of a study (the ability to find a significant difference if it exists) is $100\% - \beta$, which in this case is $100\% - 20\% = 80\%$.

The higher we choose to set the power, the more subjects we will need in the study. Using a power of 80% (in this case to capture a 2% minimum benefit as significant), there is a one in five chance of failing to detect the difference. This might appear high, but the chance of missing larger effects is smaller. It should be noted that the error rate for a Type I error is set lower than that for a Type II error since in medicine we conventionally have a higher threshold for switching to a new treatment than for keeping the traditional treatment.

Study design

The calculation of the sample size is dependent on the design of the study. A standard parallel arm RCT, with the standard treatment group acting as the control, will require more subjects than a 'before and after treatment' type of study in which the subjects act as their own controls. Even with a standard RCT, as in our example, we might choose to have two subjects on the new treatment for every subject on the standard treatment in order to give us more safety information and experience with the new treatment. If the ratio is higher than 1:1, more subjects will be required. A further component of trial design is whether the outcome is a categorical event such as death, a continuous variable such as cholesterol level, or the time to the first event, as in a survival analysis. The features of these outcomes will dramatically influence the sample size. In our example, the event of interest is survival (or mortality) at 12 months, a relatively simple, clear, and meaningful endpoint.

To calculate the sample size we can apply the equation shown in **Figure 1**. In our RCT we can see that a sample size of 3,842 subjects is required. For any combination of the four basic elements (α, β, π_1 and δ) there is a corresponding number of patients per group. **Figure 2** shows how the number of patients per treatment group varies with respect to π_1 and δ while α and β remain at 5% and 20%, respectively.

The most important observation made from this figure is that the number of patients required per treatment group decreases as the smallest treatment effect to be detected increases. For example, for $\pi_1 = 50\%$, as δ changes from 10% through 20%, 30%, and 40%, the sample size decreases from roughly 500 through 100, 50, and 25.

Figure 1. Calculating the sample size. The following formula can be used to calculate the sample size that is required in each arm of the example randomized controlled trial.

$$n = \frac{\left[z\,(\alpha/2)\,\sqrt{2\pi\,(1-\pi)} + z\,(\beta)\,\sqrt{\pi_1\,(1-\pi_1) + \pi_2\,(1-\pi_2)}\,\right]^2}{\delta^2}$$

α = the Type I error rate
β = the Type II error rate
π_1 = the expected event rate in the control group
π_2 = the expected event rate in the treatment group
$\pi = (\pi_1 + \pi_2)/2$
$\delta = \pi_1 - \pi_2$
$z\,(\alpha/2)$ = constant from the standard normal distribution depending on the value of α
$z\,(\beta)$ = constant from the normal distribution depending on the value of β

For this example:
α = 5% = 0.05
β = 20% = 0.20
π_1 = 12% = 0.12
π_2 = 10% = 0.10
$\pi = (\pi_1 + \pi_2)/2 = (12\% + 10\%)/2 = 11\% = 0.11$
$\delta = \pi_1 - \pi_2 = 12\% - 10\% = 2\% = 0.02$
$z\,(\alpha/2) = 1.96$
$z\,(\beta) = 0.842$

$$n = \frac{\left[1.96\,\sqrt{2 \times 0.11\,(1-0.11)} + 0.842\,\sqrt{0.12\,(1-0.12) + 0.10\,(1-0.10)}\,\right]^2}{0.02^2} = 3,842$$

Therefore for our RCT, a sample size of 3,842 subjects is required for each group.

Taking subject dropout into account

During any clinical study, subjects might leave the study due to a variety of reasons, such as loss to follow-up, noncompliance with treatment, or moving away geographically. The sample size should therefore be increased to allow for this. If our RCT has a likely dropout rate of 20% (a ratio of 0.20) within the first year of the trial, the sample size per group should be adjusted accordingly, ie, $3,842/(1-0.20) = 4,803$. Our RCT therefore requires a total of 9,606 subjects, or 4,803 subjects in each treatment group.

Are negative trials due to small sample sizes?

A negative clinical trial is a trial in which the observed differences between the new and standard treatments are not large enough to satisfy a specified significance level (Type I error threshold), so the results are declared to be not statistically significant [2]. With the benefit of hindsight, analyses of negative clinical trials have shown that the assumptions chosen by investigators often lead

Figure 2. The relationship between the number of patients required per treatment group and the smallest anticipated treatment effect, with a 5% significance level and 80% power.

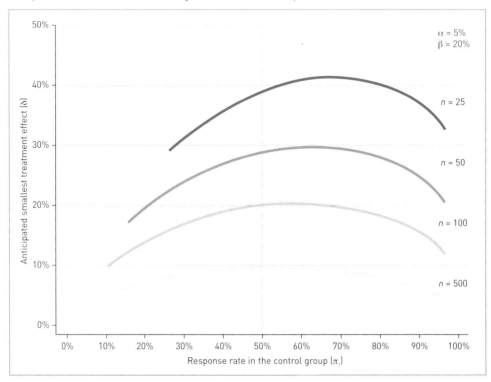

them to choose a sample size that is too small to offer a reasonable chance of avoiding a false-negative error (a Type II error).

Not all negative trials are due to insufficient power. In some cases it might be that the event rate in the control group was lower than expected or that there were confounding factors, such as changes to routine treatment methods during the duration of the study. A branch of medical statistics known as meta-analysis combines the results from many such small studies to try to estimate a true mean effect more closely. If this analysis shows that the new treatment has a favorable benefit, then this should be verified by performing a larger, definitive RCT. However, one must always take into consideration the outlay of resources required to realize the potential benefit, and even then, large RCTs might produce unexpected results.

So is that it – just apply the formula?

Statisticians have developed various methodologies for determining sample sizes, depending on the number of treatments compared, the type of primary endpoint measured, the statistical analysis method used to analyze outcomes, and the design of the study. Detailed formulas for various endpoints can be found in reference [3].

When determining the sample size it is wise to finalize the main objective of the protocol and then to look at a range of assumptions by working with a medical statistician. This approach will suggest a range of sample sizes and a balance can then be struck between the ideal statistical power, the available resources, and the length of time before the sample size can be finalized. Even then, interim analyses of overall event rates during an RCT (at this point in the trial we are still unaware of event rates in each treatment group) will provide a guide as to whether the sample size needs to be altered as the RCT proceeds. If event rates are measured by treatment arm during the course of a study, the data and safety monitoring board might recommend the early termination of the study if a large benefit or element of harm is seen with the new treatment.

Conclusion

The sample size is the most important determinant of the statistical power of a study, and a study with inadequate power is unethical unless being conducted as a safety and feasibility study. However, the calculation of sample size is not an exact science. It is therefore important to make realistic and well-researched assumptions before choosing an appropriate sample size. This sample size should account for dropouts, and there should be a consideration for interim analyses to be performed during the study, which can be used to amend the final sample size.

References

1. Pocock SJ. *Clinical Trials: A Practical Approach*. New York: John Wiley & Sons, 1983.

2. Moher D, Dulberg CS, Wells GA. Statistical power, sample size, and their reporting in randomized controlled trials. *JAMA* 1994;**272**:122–4.

3. Chow SC, Shao J, Wang H. *Sample Size Calculation in Clinical Research*. New York: Marcel Dekker, 2003.

Part II

Alternative Trial Designs

Chapter 10

Crossover Trials

Duolao Wang, Ulrike Lorch, and Ameet Bakhai

Crossover trials are designed so that each recruited patient receives both active and control treatments in either order for a specified duration, with a 'washout' period between treatments when no treatment is administered. In such trials, patients act as their own controls, therefore fewer patients are required to evaluate the effects of different therapies than in a trial with a parallel design. There are also limitations to the crossover design, however, and here, in this chapter, we discuss the advantages and disadvantages of crossover trials.

What is a crossover trial?

There are two commonly used types of study design in clinical research: *parallel* and *crossover*. In a parallel study design, each subject is randomized to one and only one treatment. Most large clinical studies adopt this approach. On the other hand, in a crossover trial, each subject receives more than one treatment in a specified sequence. In other words, a crossover trial is a study that compares two or more treatments or interventions in which subjects, on completion of a course of one treatment, are switched to another. This effectively means that each subject acts as his/her own control. The fundamental assumption of crossover trials is that patients usually have a chronically stable condition that will not vary between when they are taking the first and second treatments. Therefore, crossover trials are, by necessity, short-term trials.

Typically, each treatment is administered for a selected period of time and, often, there is a 'washout' or 'restabilization' period between the last administration of one treatment and the first administration of the next treatment, allowing the effect of the preceding treatment to wear off. Where possible, allocation of the treatment sequences in crossover trials is a randomized, blinded process.

Example study 1: Bioequivalence evaluation of two brands of cefuroxime 500 mg tablets (Julphar's Cefuzime® and GlaxoSmithKline's Zinnat®) in healthy human volunteers [1]

Cefuroxime axetil is a semisynthetic, broad-spectrum cephalosporin antibiotic for oral administration. A single-dose, two-treatment crossover design was carried out to evaluate the bioequivalence between two varying oral formulations of 500 mg cefuroxime axetil in 24 healthy volunteers. The two formulations used were Cefuzime as the test product and Zinnat as the reference product.

Each treatment was administered to subjects after an overnight fast on two treatment days separated by a 1-week washout period. After treatment administration, serial blood samples were collected for a period of 8 hours. Various pharmacokinetic parameters including AUC_{0-t}, $AUC_{0-\infty}$, C_{max}, T_{max}, $T_{1/2}$ and λ were determined from plasma concentrations of both formulations. The results demonstrated that Cefuzime was bioequivalent to Zinnat since the 90% confidence intervals for the test/reference ratios of the relevant pharmacokinetic parameters were within the bioequivalence acceptance range of 80–125% (see **Chapter 13** for more about bioequivalence studies).

Table 1. A summary of the key features of two example crossover studies.

	Study 1	Study 2
Design	2×2 crossover	2×2 crossover
Objective	Bioequivalence evaluation	Efficacy assessment
Endpoint	Pharmacokinetic parameters $(AUC_{0-t}, AUC_{0-\infty}, C_{max}, T_{max}, T_{1/2},$ and $\lambda)$	Plasma concentration of activated protein C
Treatment A	500 mg Cefuzime tablets	150 mg levonorgestrel and 30 mg ethinylestradiol
Treatment B	500 mg Zinnat tablets	150 mg desogestrel and 30 mg ethinylestradiol
Sequence 1	AB	AB
Sequence 2	BA	BA
Period 1	1 day	2 consecutive menstrual cycles
Period 2	1 day	2 consecutive menstrual cycles
Washout period	1 week	2 consecutive menstrual cycles
Sample size	24 subjects	33 subjects
Conclusion	Bioequivalence between A and B	Lower efficacy of B than A

Example study 2: Low-dose oral contraceptives and acquired resistance to activated protein C: a randomized crossover study [2]

A randomized crossover trial was carried out to assess how the use of second-generation oral contraceptives (treatment A: 150 mg levonorgestrel and 30 mg ethinylestradiol) and third-generation oral contraceptives (treatment B: 150 mg desogestrel and 30 mg ethinylestradiol) varies with respect to their resistance to the anticoagulant action of activated protein C (APC). Thirty-three healthy female volunteers between the ages of 18 and 40 years and without menstrual irregularities were assigned the two oral contraceptive preparations in random order (AB or BA).

The first oral contraceptive (A or B) was used for two consecutive menstrual cycles (Period 1) and, after a washout of a further two menstrual cycles (much longer than the half-life of each preparation), the volunteers were switched to the second preparation (B or A) for two cycles (Period 2). Blood samples were obtained between days 18 and 21 of all six menstrual cycles – one at baseline before starting either treatment, two during administration of the first preparation, one during the last cycle of the washout period, and two during administration of the second preparation. The study concluded that, compared with levonorgestrel (A), the desogestrel-containing oral contraceptive treatment (B) conferred significant additional resistance to APC. A summary of the key features of the two crossover studies is given in **Table 1**.

Figure 1. A standard two-sequence, two-period crossover design.

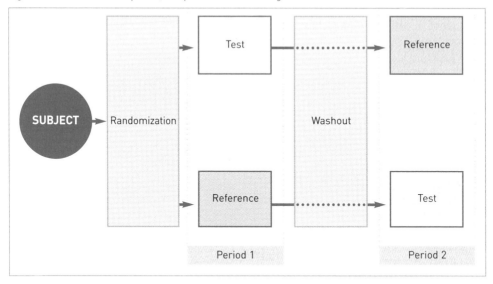

Classification of crossover trials

Crossover trials are classified according to the number of treatments given to a subject and according to whether a given subject receives all (*complete crossover*) or just some (*incomplete crossover*) of the study treatments.

The simplest crossover design is a two-treatment, two-period crossover trial in which each subject receives either the test (A) or reference (B) treatment in the first study period and the alternative treatment in the succeeding period. These trials are often referred to as *2 × 2* or AB/BA trials. The order in which the treatments A and B are administered to each subject is random; typically, half the subjects receive the treatment in the sequence AB and the other half in the sequence BA. An example of a standard *2 × 2* crossover design is given in **Figure 1**.

Where appropriate, the crossover design can be extended to include more than two treatments per subject in consecutive periods or more than two sequences. If a trial has *p* sequences of treatments administered over *q* different dosing periods, the trial is referred to as having a *p × q* crossover design.

Table 2 lists some commonly used higher-order crossover designs. Each design depends on the number of treatments to be compared and the duration of the study [3].

Table 2. Examples of high-order crossover trial designs.

Design type	Order	Treatment sequence
Two-sequence dual design	2 × 3	ABB, BAA
Doubled design	2 × 4	AABB, BBAA
Balaam's design	4 × 2	AA, BB, AB, BA
Four-sequence design	4 × 4	AABB, BBAA, ABBA, BAAB
Williams' design with three treatments	6 × 3	ABC, ACB, BAC, BCA, CAB, CBA
3 × 3 Latin square design	3 × 3	ABC, BCA, CAB
4 × 4 Latin square design	4 × 4	ABDC, BCAD, CDBA, DACB

Advantages of crossover trials over parallel studies

Since each subject in a crossover trial acts as his/her own control, there is an assessment of both (all) treatments in each subject. This means that treatment differences can be based on *within-subject* comparisons instead of *between-subject* comparisons. As there is usually less variability within a subject than between different subjects, there is an increase in the precision of observations. Therefore, fewer subjects are required to detect a treatment difference. If $N_{parallel}$ is the total number of subjects required for a two-way parallel trial to detect a treatment effect (δ) with 5% significance and 80% power, then the total number of subjects $N_{crossover}$ required for a 2 × 2 crossover trial to detect the same effect (δ) is approximately:

$$N_{crossover} = (1 - r) N_{parallel} / 2$$

where r is a correlation coefficient among the repeated measurements of the primary endpoint in a crossover trial. The above equation indicates that as the correlation increases towards 1, fewer subjects are needed for a crossover trial. **Figure 2** illustrates sample sizes for a crossover trial for some selected values of r and the sample size ($N_{parallel}$ = 100) required by a parallel design trial for detecting the same clinical effect. The graph shows that:

- A crossover trial only needs half the sample size of that used in a parallel trial if there is no correlation among repeated measurements of the primary endpoint.
- If the correlation coefficient is 50%, a crossover trial only needs a quarter of the sample size of a parallel design.
- Sample size can be drastically reduced in a crossover trial if the correlation increases towards 1.

Figure 2. Sample sizes required for a crossover design to detect the same treatment effect as that seen with a parallel design with a sample size of 100, given different correlation values (r) among the repeated measurements of the primary endpoint in a crossover trial.

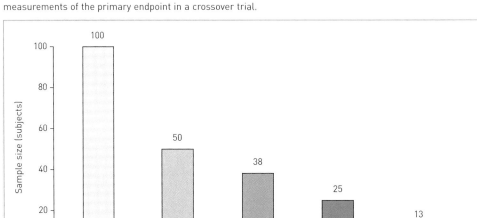

In addition, a crossover design provides the least-biased estimates for the difference between treatments assuming that the response of subjects to treatment is consistent. Take as an example the previously mentioned Study 2: if a parallel design were used for the study, observed differences in APC between two contraceptives could be subject to unknown bias or uncontrolled effects of the menstrual cycle. By conducting this cycle-controlled randomized crossover trial, this study has effectively reduced this potential source of bias.

Main limitations of crossover trials

The main limitation of crossover trials is that they pose greater inconvenience to the subjects because multiple treatments are given and the subjects will therefore be exposed to various transitions between treatment phases. This longer period of study involvement increases the chance of subject withdrawal from the study. Censored observations due to subject withdrawal have a higher impact in a crossover design study, particularly if unequal numbers of subjects have completed different phases of the trial, meaning that even partially complete data could produce biased results.

For crossover studies, it is essential that subjects are in a comparable condition at the start of each treatment period, otherwise the validity of treatment comparisons is compromised. Crossover design is therefore more appropriate for chronic diseases that have a stable set of symptoms (such as rheumatoid arthritis), while acute conditions (such as heart attacks) are less appropriate. Similarly, the crossover design is not suitable either for primary outcomes that are permanent or for terminal events (such as pregnancy or death).

Although crossover trials require fewer patients, this might not always be appropriate, such as for Phase III studies where a large body of evidence of patient exposure is needed to satisfy regulatory requirements regarding drug safety, tolerability, and the likelihood of unpredictable side-effects with the new treatment.

The most significant problem of crossover trials is the 'carryover' effect. The carryover effect is defined as the persistence (whether physically or in terms of effect) of treatment applied in one treatment phase of the study to subsequent treatment phases [4]. In a bioequivalence study this would arise if, for example, the pre-dose blood sample in the second period contained any measurable amount of the study drug administered in the previous period. If this is the case, it is right to conclude that the half-life of the study drug has been underestimated and, consequently, that the washout period between the two periods was not sufficiently long for there to be near-complete elimination of the drug from the subject (pharmacokinetic study) or for the subject to return to baseline values of outcome parameters (pharmacodynamic study). Psychological carryover is also possible, where some memory of the therapeutic experience under the previous treatment affects the patient's present judgment, ie, his / her perception of the next treatment. This memory may be either positive or negative [5].

Where it occurs, the consequence of carryover is that the investigators will be measuring the combined effects of two or more treatments, which in turn (if undetected) will lead to a biased evaluation. There are statistical methods that can help compensate for the lack of return to baseline for individual treatment effects in the event of a carryover [3,4,6]. However, these make further assumptions, thereby weakening the study results. The ideal scenario is to ensure that an adequate washout period is predetermined for each drug or that there is continued monitoring throughout the washout period until all subjects have returned to baseline.

Another potential problem with crossover trials is the period effect (treatment by period interaction). Even after an adequate washout interval, the effect of either treatment can be influenced simply by whether it is administered first or second. For example, in a crossover trial testing two antihypertensive drugs, both drugs might be more effective in the second period than in the first (beyond even differences due to different patients) due to the effect of being in the trial itself. If this period effect is large, it can be minimized by allocating equal numbers of subjects to different sequences and some form of statistical adjustment might then be required [4–6].

Where are crossover trials useful?

Crossover trials are most commonly used in early drug development, especially in Phase I pharmacokinetic, bioequivalence, dose-proportionality, and dose-escalation studies (for investigating the maximum–tolerated dose), and in Phase II pharmacodynamic studies. In later phases of drug development, as well as in other clinical studies, a crossover design is suitable for trials that involve relatively stable conditions such as asthma, rheumatism, migraine, mild-to-moderate hypertension, and angina.

Treatments with a quickly reversible effect (eg, bronchodilators) are more suited for investigation under crossover design than those with a more persistent effect (eg, steroids). Furthermore, this design is more applicable to single-dose studies than to long-term repeat-administration studies.

Conclusion

The crossover design for trials is a valuable tool in clinical research when applied in the correct setting. Its main advantage is that it evaluates within-subject treatment comparisons rather than between-subject comparisons, as in studies with a parallel design. Consequently, the data variability in crossover trials is lower, which is reflected in there being more robust data with narrower confidence intervals, and which reduces the number of study subjects needed to test hypotheses in clinical settings. The main limitation of the crossover design is the possibility that a carryover effect could occur, but this can be avoided by ensuring that there is a sufficient washout interval between the different treatment periods.

Crossover trials are widely used in the earlier phases of clinical drug development (pharmacokinetic, bioequivalence, and pharmacodynamic Phase I studies) and are clinically useful in studies involving stable chronic conditions and/or drugs with short-lived effects.

References

1. Al-Said MS, Al-Khamis KI, Niazy EM, et al. Bioequivalence evaluation of two brands of cefuroxime 500 mg tablets (Cefuzime® and Zinnat® in healthy volunteers). *Biopharm Drug Dispos* 2000;**21**:205–10.

2. Rosing J, Middeldorp S, Curvers J, et al. Low-dose oral contraceptives and acquired resistance to activated protein C: a randomised crossover study. *Lancet* 1999;**354**:2036–40.

3. Chow SC, Liu JP. *Design and Analysis of Clinical Trials: Concepts and Methodologies*. New York: John Wiley & Sons, 1998.

4. Senn S. *Crossover Trials in Clinical Research*, 2nd edition. Chichester: John Wiley & Sons, 2002.

5. Senn S. Crossover design. In: Chow SC, editor. *Encyclopedia of Biopharmaceutical Statistics*. New York: Marcel Dekker, 2000:142–9.

6. Jones B, Kenward MG. *Design and Analysis of Cross–over Trials*, 2nd edition. London: Chapman and Hall/CRC, 2003.

Chapter 11

Factorial Design

Zoe Fox, Dorothea Nitsch, Duolao Wang,
and Ameet Bakhai

In a clinical trial, a situation may arise where the nature of the
study calls for the evaluation of more than one treatment for
safety and/or efficacy compared to a control. Possible solutions
include conducting a multiple-arm parallel trial or several
separate trials to evaluate the effect of each treatment
individually. A more economic way to approach this problem
is to conduct a factorial trial. By using a factorial design, it is
possible to evaluate individual treatment effects for more than
one treatment within the same trial. Although factorial studies
appear extremely useful on the surface, there are a number
of issues that we need to consider during their study design
and analysis. In this chapter, we discuss and illustrate
advantages and problems of factorial design trials.

What is a factorial study?

The simplest factorial design takes a *2 × 2* format, and throughout this chapter we will refer to *2 × 2* factorial studies unless otherwise specified. In a factorial design clinical trial with a *2 × 2* format, individuals are randomly assigned to two separate interventions (eg, interventions A and B) and these interventions are each compared with their corresponding control(s).

In a balanced *2 × 2* factorial design, this would mean that from a total of N individuals, $N/2$ are randomly allocated to receive intervention A and $N/2$ are randomly allocated not to receive intervention A. Correspondingly, $N/2$ individuals are allocated to receive intervention B or to not receive intervention B. Overall:

- $N/4$ individuals are allocated to no treatment (control group).
- $N/4$ individuals are allocated to intervention A only.
- $N/4$ individuals are allocated to intervention B only.
- $N/4$ individuals are allocated to the combination of A + B simultaneously.

The benefit in terms of sample size or power of the factorial trial becomes apparent in the analysis. The usual method is to compare individuals who are randomized to intervention A (ie, those who receive A and those who receive A + B) with those who are not randomized to A (ie, those receiving either intervention B or no treatment at all). Similarly, individuals who are randomized to intervention B are compared with those who are not randomized to B. In a factorial design, it is usual to assume A and B to have independent effects from each other, ie, that there is no interaction between treatment A and B.

Example

In a *2 × 2* factorial trial set up to investigate the effects of multivitamins excluding vitamin A (factor 1) and including vitamin A (factor 2) on birth outcomes of HIV-1 infected women, each woman was allocated once to each treatment [1]. Therefore, every mother was randomized twice overall, resulting in the following four treatment groups:

- Women who received vitamin A only.
- Women who received multivitamins but no vitamin A.
- Women who received both multivitamins and vitamin A.
- Women who received neither.

By using a factorial trial, it is possible to perform two comparisons simultaneously at the cost of one experiment. In this example, it is possible to compare birth outcomes for mothers who received vitamin A with those who did not by

Table 1. Treatment groups after randomization in a *2 × 2* factorial study comparing the effects of vitamin supplements on pregnancy outcomes in 1,075 Tanzanian women infected with HIV-1 [1].

Multivitamins	Vitamin A		Overall
	Yes	No	
Yes	Vitamin A + multivitamins (n = 270)	Multivitamins (n = 269)	Treated with multivitamins (n = 539)
No	Vitamin A (n = 269)	Placebo (n = 267)	No multivitamins (n = 536)
Overall	Treated with vitamin A (n = 539)	No vitamin A (n = 536)	Total women (n = 1075)

comparing column margins. Similarly, by comparing row totals, it is possible to evaluate the effect of using multivitamins during pregnancy (see **Table 1**).

It is also possible to analyze this as a four-way study by investigating each cell of the contingency table separately; however, the number of individuals included in each comparison is reduced, and consequently the study loses power. All *2 × 2* factorial studies can be laid out in the same format as **Table 1**.

Why should we consider a factorial design?

A factorial design allows two treatments to be evaluated with a trial budget for a single comparison, providing both treatments have similar expected benefits. This is important because trials are becoming increasingly expensive as higher standards are expected and larger trials are needed. A trial involving 1,000 patients currently costs approximately US$4 million, assuming the trial investigates a new agent, involves evaluations every 6 months, and is partly conducted in Western countries.

Such an expense is unlikely to be spared to answer questions concerning relatively cheap treatments that could never hope to recoup the investment from profits. For example, no commercial company would finance a trial for aspirin because there is no profit to be made from aspirin and such expenditure could not be regained. Therefore, questions about the benefits of cheap, traditional agents are often appended onto trials of more commercially viable agents.

A factorial design presents the opportunity for an investigator to answer a question from both commercial and noncommercial angles. For example, in the ISIS-4 (Fourth International Study of Infarct Survival) trial, investigators assessed the benefits of captopril (a new blood-pressure–lowering agent), oral mononitrate (an old anti-angina drug), and intravenous magnesium (an old agent) in 58,043 patients with suspected acute myocardial infarction. While captopril showed a small but significant reduction in mortality at 5 weeks, neither of the older agents showed significant benefit. This trial was a *2 × 2 × 2* factorial design. [2].

A further example was the HOPE (Heart Outcomes Prevention Evaluation) study, which compared ramipril and vitamin E supplementation, both against control; the latter agent proved ineffective as opposed to the considerable benefit seen with ramipril, in patients with coronary disease [3].

How do we randomize for a factorial design?

For a factorial design, randomization can be performed using the same methods as in a two-arm parallel study; however, individuals have to be randomized multiple times, depending on the number of interventions used. In a *2 × 2* factorial study, participants are first randomized to either intervention A or its control, and then to either intervention B or its control in a second randomization. Alternatively, individuals can be randomized to one of the following four arms to avoid the need to randomize twice: A, B, A + B, or placebo.

How do we calculate sample size for a factorial study?

The most common technique used to calculate the sample size for a *2 × 2* factorial study is to first think of the study as consisting of two individual two-arm trials. Sample size calculations are carried out for the target effect size of each intervention separately, assuming the same power and level of statistical significance. The final number of individuals that need to be recruited is taken from the comparison that provides the larger sample size – this will ensure enough power to assess the effect of the remaining comparison. Sample sizes are calculated in the usual way for parallel-arm randomized controlled trials, so the power to detect a treatment difference is dependent on the number of individuals in the groups being compared, not on the overall number of individuals in the study.

The aforementioned calculations are based on the assumption that there is no interaction between interventions A and B; however, this will not necessarily be true. An interaction between interventions means that the effect of treatment A depends on the presence or absence of treatment B (or *vice versa*). In this case, it is more appropriate to consider the study as a multiple-arm study and ensure enough power to detect the smallest treatment difference among all possible pair-wise comparisons. As a result, the trial can be viewed as a four parallel-arm study instead of a factorial trial, depending on the comparison of interest. With the presence of an interaction effect, sample size calculations will depend on the aim of the study. The possibilities are as follows:

- To compare three active treatments with control and to show that any of the treatment combinations is effective compared with the control.
- To compare two active treatments with control and to show that either intervention is effective on its own compared with the control.
- To make six pair-wise comparisons between all four groups.

The final sample size for the four-arm study is determined using the same method as above by using the largest sample size as the final trial size.

How do we analyze a factorial study?

It is sometimes assumed that a *2 × 2* factorial study can be analyzed by handling the four different treatment groups separately. However, such an analysis lacks power since it excludes a number of individuals and does not take into account the benefits of the factorial design. On the other hand, if the study subsequently finds an unexpected interaction effect then this might be a viable approach.

In general, however, the analysis should reflect the initial aim and design of the trial when assumptions seem tenable. To incorporate the full potential of a simple *2 × 2* factorial study, all individuals should be included in the analyses.

Example
The aim of the Canadian Trial in Threatened Stroke was to investigate the use of aspirin and sulfinpyrazone for preventing strokes and deaths [4]. The number of strokes or deaths in relation to the number of individuals is outlined in **Table 2**. These data were initially analyzed by comparing the odds of stroke or death for individuals on aspirin and individuals not on aspirin (odds ratio 0.63; $P = 0.03$). The odds ratio of stroke or death for patients who received sulfinpyrazone compared with those who did not was not significant. Thus, it was concluded that aspirin, but not sulfinpyrazone, had a protective effect against stroke and death.

Treatment interaction
The underlying assumption of no treatment interaction in the analysis of conventional factorial studies needs to be validated; it is possible to test for the presence of an interaction by including an interaction term between treatments in a regression model, and comparing the same model without the interaction term (see **Chapter 27**). If the interaction term is a significant part of the model,

Table 2. Number of strokes or deaths / number of individuals in the Canadian Trial in Threatened Stroke [4].

Sulfinpyrazone	Aspirin	
	Yes	No
Yes	20 / 146	38 / 156
No	26 / 144	30 / 139

The odds of stroke or death for individuals on aspirin was (20 + 26) / ([144 + 146] – [20 + 26]) = 46 / 244.

The odds of stroke or death for individuals not on aspirin was (38 + 30) / ([139 + 156] – [38 + 30]) = 68 / 227.

an interaction between treatments exists and the study results must be presented separately for each treatment combination.

For example, in the GISSI (Gruppo Italiano per lo Studio della Streptochinasi nell'Infarto Miocardico) trial, the data were initially analyzed using a two-way method and then by a four-way method, looking at the outcome in individual cells compared with the control [5]. The interaction effect was found to be nonsignificant and the results from the main effects model were therefore presented as the main study result. Difficulties arise if the interaction test results in a low, but nonsignificant, P-value (eg, between 0.05 and 0.10) – this can indicate that the study is underpowered to detect an interaction, rather than establishing the absence of an interaction effect.

Different types of factorial designs

The notation of a factorial study is rather mathematical; the number of interventions in a factorial study is represented by a product term, which also contains the number of levels of that intervention. Each number refers to the different levels of each intervention; for example, treatment 'yes' / 'no' represents two levels, whereas treatment 'none' / 'dose 1' / 'dose 2' corresponds to three levels. In an investigation of two treatments an $I \times J$ factorial study is required, where the first treatment has I levels and the second has J levels.

An $I \times J \times K$ factorial study refers to an evaluation of three treatments, with the third treatment having K levels. A $2 \times 2 \times 2$ notation would be suitable for an evaluation of three drugs given at a single dose for each drug; that is, the levels would correspond to the dose and the control. If two dosages of two drugs are to be simultaneously evaluated and compared with their baseline value, a 3×3 notation would be used where each drug is given at three different levels (control, dose 1, and dose 2). The number of treatment arms can be deduced by solving the product of the notation: eg, a 2×2 factorial study results in four treatment groups, a 2×3 design in six groups, a $2 \times 2 \times 2$ notation in eight groups, and so on.

Example

A *2 × 3* factorial design was used in the evaluation of several drug regimens as initial antiretroviral therapy for HIV-1 infection [6].

- The first randomization step assigned HIV-1-infected individuals to treatment with either didanosine and stavudine (DDI + D4T) or zidovudine and lamivudine (ZDV + 3TC).
- The second randomization step evaluated the effect of efavirenz alone (EFV), nelfinavir (NFV) alone, or the combination of both (EFV + NFV).

Thus, the first randomization step contained two levels, and the second randomization assigned individuals to three groups: a *2 × 3* factorial study resulting in six different treatment groups (see **Table 3**).

In the previously mentioned ISIS-4 study, a *2 × 2 × 2* factorial design was used to evaluate 58,050 individuals with suspected acute myocardial infarction who were randomized to receive oral captopril (OC), oral mononitrate (OM), and/or intravenous magnesium sulfate (IMS) [2]. This design required three randomization steps, and over 7,000 individuals were randomized to each of the resulting eight treatment groups (see **Table 3**):

- placebo
- OC alone
- OM alone
- IMS alone
- OC + OM
- OC + IMS
- OM + IMS
- OC + OM + IMS

Increasing the interventions

Since a factorial design makes it is possible to analyze more than one intervention in a single trial, it is tempting to extend the design to a study that investigates three or more interventions by performing an expanded factorial design. As outlined above, for every additional two-level intervention evaluated, there is a resulting two-fold increase in the final number of treatment groups. Moreover, the more interventions evaluated, the more likely it is to uncover an interaction between interventions. It is therefore advisable to keep the number of interventions as low as possible, unless there is certainty that all of the interventions will work independently.

Table 3. Examples of factorial trial notations.

Factorial design	Example	Resulting intervention groups		
$2 \times k$, eg, 2×3	Comparison of sequential three-drug regimens as initial therapy for HIV-1 infection [6]		Treatment 1	
		Treatment 2	DDI + D4T	ZDV + 3TC
		NFV	NFV + DDI + D4T	NFV + ZDV + 3TC
		EFV	EFV + DDI + D4T	EFV + ZDV + 3TC
		NFV + EFV	EFV + NFV + DDI + D4T	EFV + NFV + ZDV + 3TC

		OC = Yes:			OC = No:		
$2 \times 2 \times 2$	ISIS-4: A randomized factorial trial assessing early OC, OM, and IMS in 58,050 individuals with suspected myocardial infarction [2]		OM			OM	
		IMS	Yes	No	IMS	Yes	No
		Yes	OC + OM + IMS	OC + IMS	Yes	OM + IMS	IMS
		No	OC + OM	OC	No	OM	Placebo

$2 \times 2 \times 2$ $\times 2 \times 3 \times 2$	A factorial trial of six interventions for the prevention of postoperative nausea and vomiting [10]	See below

3TC = lamivudine; D4T = stavudine; DDI = didanosine; EFV = efavirenz; IMS = intravenous magnesium sulfate; NFV = nelfinavir; OC = oral captopril; OM = oral mononitrate; ZDV = zidovudine [2,6,10]. The table below row 3 is reproduced with permission from the Massachusetts Medical Society [10].

Incomplete or partial factorial studies

Studies that evaluate every combination of factors, such as those described above, are sometimes referred to as *fully crossed* factorial designs. *Incomplete* or *partial* factorial studies exclude some treatment groups for reasons such as suitability, feasibility, or ethics. For example, specific combinations of treatments might result in excess toxicity, and it would therefore be unethical to evaluate them in a clinical trial. Alternatively, it might not be feasible or necessary to make certain treatment comparisons [7]. In such cases, it is possible to economize if cells are left blank intentionally by not allowing recruitment to those combinations, thereby reducing the total number of groups under comparison and consequently the total number of individuals.

For example, in a study that evaluated the effect of different percentage levels of dietary calcium (Ca) and phosphorus (P) on performance, structural soundness, and bone characteristics of growing pigs at different stages of their development, there were four different available diets with Ca:P ratios of 0.45:0.32, 0.52:0.40, 0.65:0.50, and 0.80:0.60. For simplicity, the authors used the weights of the animals to define their stage of development. A total of 664 pigs were initially fed one of three diets with higher Ca:P phosphate content (0.52:0.40, 0.65:0.50, 0.80:0.60) during growth (19–56 kg body weight). This was followed by one of three diets with lower Ca:P levels (0.45:0.32, 0.52:0.40, 0.65:0.50) until the pigs reached their market weight. This was analyzed as an incomplete 3×3 factorial study because comparisons for the more extreme Ca:P diets at both ends of the range were omitted [8].

Unbalanced factorial studies

Another design variation is the *unbalanced* factorial study, where different numbers of individuals are randomized to each cell. These studies commonly occur in investigations of combination antihypertensive drugs. Dose combinations that are expected to be employed as initial therapy may be given a larger sample size to ensure there is enough power to detect any additional effect of a third treatment. It is more complicated to analyze an unbalanced factorial study than a balanced design, yet various approaches to dealing with problems related to different sample sizes have been suggested [9].

Complicated factorial design

An example of a more complicated factorial design, including several interventions as well as imbalances between groups, is a study evaluating nausea and vomiting after elective surgery with general anesthetic [10]. This trial was set up to examine six interventions as a 2^6 ($2 \times 2 \times 2 \times 2 \times 2 \times 2$) format; however a third arm, containing 10% of the individuals, was added for the fifth intervention, which resulted in a $2^5 \times 3$ ($2 \times 2 \times 2 \times 2 \times 3 \times 2$) format (see **Table 3**).

As prior information was available on the risk of postoperative nausea and vomiting for one treatment group, in order to quantify this effect appropriately there were twice as many people randomized to one arm of the intervention compared with the other. The trial was powered to allow for interactions between a maximum of three interventions; however, since no interaction effect was present, the trial provided an estimate of the combined effect of interventions in addition to individual effects. It was also not feasible for one study site to randomize individuals to all six interventions; however, even with a reduced number of individuals, there were enough individuals for the planned comparisons to be viable.

What are the advantages of a factorial design?

Cost

The main advantage of a factorial design is its relative economy: it is possible to evaluate two or more interventions within the same trial at less than the cost of two separate trials, and possibly with only a marginal additional cost to a single trial of one intervention. Rather than omitting treatment comparisons in order to perform a conventional parallel-arm study, or expanding the sample size to a multiple-arm study, it is possible to evaluate multiple treatments within the same trial using fewer patients than individual comparisons.

Sample size

Take, for example, the previously mentioned trial of multivitamins and vitamin A in HIV-1-infected women [1]. If the same study had been performed as a three-arm parallel study with the same sample size, N, then a third of the individuals would have been randomized to receive multivitamins, a third would have received vitamin A, and the remaining third would have received neither. In the factorial design used, however, half of the women were randomized to each treatment irrespective of the other treatment. Therefore, a three-arm parallel trial has less power to make comparisons; moreover, to achieve the same power as in a 2×2 factorial trial, the three-arm parallel trial would need to randomize $1.5N$ women. Hence, substantially fewer individuals are needed in a factorial trial than in a multiple-arm parallel study with the same power.

Exploring interaction effects

A second, often-quoted advantage is that factorial designs are useful to crudely evaluate the combination of interventions. If the aim of the study is to accurately quantify the interaction effect, many more individuals are required. Quantifying the effect of a combination of treatments is represented by a multiple-arm trial that tests the treatment combination in a distinct arm. It follows that, in the above example, we would need to increase our original sample size by a factor of four to investigate whether women on vitamin A and multivitamins have improved birth outcomes compared with either intervention separately.

What are the limitations of a factorial design?

Interactions

The main disadvantage of factorial trials is that the possibility of interaction effects can usually only be determined at the end of the study. If such an interaction effect is present then the usual way of analysis – ignoring the other treatment assignment by summing up over the table margins – becomes invalid, since each cell by itself is meaningful.

Since factorial trials are often designed with the assumption of the absence of a treatment interaction, they are not powered to detect interactions, unless they are substantially over-powered or the initial assumptions were very conservative. It follows that, in order to test the validity of assumptions of the analysis, interactions need to be tested for, but often they cannot be completely excluded. A more detailed description of power associated with a test for interaction in factorial design can be found elsewhere [11,12].

Compliance

Another notable disadvantage is that individuals randomized to only one or two interventions will find it easier to comply with treatment than individuals randomized to several different interventions. In the analysis of a factorial design, individuals are combined across treatment groups and then compared to calculate the effect of each intervention at a time. Therefore, if adherence is reduced in an imbalanced way, it could strongly influence the overall findings. A possible practical solution is to manufacture study medication that contains all the different drug combinations/placebo within a single pill; however, this might not be economical or profitable if certain biochemical interactions occur by combining the different drug formulations in the manufacturing process.

Conclusion

Most trials consider a single treatment factor where an intervention is compared with one or more alternatives or placebo. Factorial studies are an efficient and economical way of comparing multiple interventions because they combine two or more trials into a single study for little more than the cost of the first study. Participants are randomly allocated to one or more overlapping intervention combinations. It is then possible to test the independent effect of each intervention on the expected outcome, in addition to the combined effect of both interventions. Such trials allow investigators a golden opportunity to test commercially profitable and nonprofitable therapies together.

In the analysis and reporting of a factorial design trial, it should be stated that the potential interaction effect between treatments has been tested for and excluded. The economical advantage and simplicity of these studies usually outweigh the complications that arise due to unexpected treatment interactions, and these studies should be used more frequently in clinical practice where appropriate.

References

1. Fawzi W, Msamanga G, Spiegelman D, et al. Randomised trial of effects of vitamin supplements on pregnancy outcomes and T cell counts in HIV-1-infected women in Tanzania. *Lancet* 1998;**351**:1477–82.
2. ISIS-4 (Fourth International Study of Infarct Survival) Collaborative Group. ISIS-4: A randomised factorial trial assessing early oral captopril, oral mononitrate, and intravenous magnesium sulphate in 58,050 patients with suspected acute myocardial infarction. *Lancet* 1995;**345**:669–85.
3. Yusuf S, Dagenais G, Pogue J, et al. Vitamin E supplementation and cardiovascular events in high-risk patients. The Heart Outcomes Prevention Evaluation Study Investigators. *N Engl J Med* 2000;**342**:154–60.
4. The Canadian Cooperative Study Group. A randomized trial of aspirin and sulfinpyrazone in threatened stroke. *N Engl J Med* 1978;**299**:53–9.
5. Gruppo Italiano per lo Studio della Streptochinasi nell'Infarto Miocardico. Dietary supplementation with n-3 polyunsaturated fatty acids and vitamin E after myocardial infarction: results of the GISSI-Prevenzione trial. *Lancet* 1999;**354**:447–55.
6. Robbins G, De Gruttola V, Shafer RW, et al. Comparison of sequential three-drug regimens as initial therapy for HIV-1 infection. *N Engl J Med* 2003;**349**:2293–303.
7. Pocock SJ. *Clinical Trials: A Practical Approach*. New York: John Wiley & Sons, 1983.
8. Cera KR, Mahan DC. Effect of dietary calcium and phosphorus level sequences on performance, structural soundness and bone characteristics of growing-finishing swine. *J Anim Sci* 1988;**66**:1598–605.
9. Hung HM. Evaluation of a combination drug with multiple doses in unbalanced factorial design clinical trials. *Stat Med* 2000;**19**:2079–87.
10. Apfel CC, Korttila K, Abdalla M, et al. A factorial trial of six interventions for the prevention of postoperative nausea and vomiting. *N Engl J Med* 2004;**350**:2441–51.
11. Montgomery AA, Peters TJ, Little P. Design, analysis and presentation of factorial randomised controlled trials. *BMC Med Res Methodol* 2003;**3**:26.
12. Green S, Liu PY, O'Sullivan J. Factorial design considerations. *J Clin Oncol* 2002;**20**:3424–30.

Chapter 12

Equivalence Trials

Ameet Bakhai, Rajini Sudhir, and Duolao Wang

Clinical trials are usually conducted to detect the superiority of one treatment over another. However, compounds often undergo alterations to either their release mechanism, formulation, or manufacturing process, and some are modified chemically, resulting in related compounds. It can then become necessary to conduct a trial to compare the altered versus the original compound or drug to demonstrate that there has been no loss of effectiveness or increase in side-effects. Such trials are known as equivalence trials, and their place in the clinical trial armamentarium is explained here.

Glossary	
Superiority	Demonstration of improved efficacy of a new treatment over placebo/standard treatment meeting statistical significance
Equivalence	Demonstration that the absolute reduction of events achieved by one treatment is similar to that achieved by another treatment, with the difference being within a predefined range
Noninferiority	Demonstration that the average efficacy of a new treatment, while being less than that of the standard treatment, is still within a predefined range and is not clinically significantly lower
Clinical equivalence	Therapeutic equivalence based on clinical outcomes such as reduced deaths or strokes
Bioequivalence	Therapeutic equivalence based on pharmacokinetic parameters such as blood concentrations or receptor occupancy rates

Introduction

Clinical trials, particularly Phase II (small patient groups) and Phase III (large patient groups) studies, usually aim to demonstrate improved efficacy of a new treatment over placebo/standard treatment. This type of trial is known as a *superiority trial*. In other cases, such as when it is unethical to use a placebo control, it can be necessary to show that a new drug is comparable to an existing one. Such studies are known as *equivalence trials*. An example of this is the CANDLE (Candesartan versus Losartan Efficacy) study, in which two angiotensin II receptor blockers for reducing hypertension were tested [1].

Reasons for equivalence trials

Improved methods of drug delivery or manufacturing are also sometimes developed, producing new forms of existing drugs. An equivalence trial can be used here to check that this change in formulation (eg, sustained release versus rapid release given more often) does not change the efficacy of the compound. Equivalence trials are also used when the efficacy of a drug needs to be demonstrated across varying patient groups, as occurred in the Syst-Eur (Systolic Hypertension-Europe) substudy. Here, the effect of nitrendipine – a calcium antagonist that lowers blood pressure – was compared in diabetic versus non-diabetic patients [2].

Another application of equivalence trials is assessing whether generic and original drugs have identical therapeutic effectiveness. It is important that patients experience the same efficacy from both formulations and ensure that they are interchangeable without a change in side-effect profiles, given that generic drugs will be produced by companies whose manufacturing processes may not be as complex as those of the parent company.

What types of equivalence trials are there?

Clinical equivalence
Equivalence trials based on clinical outcomes such as death, stroke, heart attack, or hospitalization are termed *clinical equivalence trials*. However, some outcomes, such as death, are not always practical due to the timescale involved, and outcomes such as improvement in depression are difficult to measure objectively and reproducibly.

Bioequivalence
An alternative method is to use a pharmacokinetic (PK) approach, which compares the PK parameters derived from plasma or blood concentrations of the compound. Here, the outcomes are more objective and measurable. Trials based on PK parameters are called *bioequivalence trials*. The major advantages of a PK approach are the clear definition of the outcomes (PK parameters) and the lower variability of these outcomes.

The basic assumption underlying the PK approach to bioequivalence studies is that the same number of drug compound molecules occupying the same number of receptors will have similar clinical effects. The bioequivalence problem is then reduced to proving that equal numbers of drug compound molecules reach the receptors. From administration of the drug to the molecules reaching the receptors, factors of drug distribution, metabolism, and elimination now come into play. If the chemical nature of the compound in the two different (generic and original) formulations is identical, the distribution and elimination patterns are assumed to be the same once the drugs are absorbed. Any change in the number of drug molecules reaching the receptors is then due to differences in absorption profiles. For that reason, the US Food and Drug Administration believes that if the absorption properties of two drugs based on the same compound are similar, then the two drugs will produce similar effects [3–6]. Bioequivalence trials are discussed further in the following chapter.

Design issues for equivalence trials

How does design affect equivalence trials?
Equivalence trials can be of parallel or crossover design. The two designs differ mainly in the way they deal with intersubject variability. *Between-subject* variability is a measure of the differences between subjects, whereas *within-subject* variability is a measure of the differences within each subject. Subject validity has a large statistical influence on the equivalence result, so the design chosen is important. Both types of variability are present in each trial, but in the crossover design –

where each subject receives both treatments in a random order – the between-subject variability is minimized because the same subject is given both treatments. Assuming that the subject remains in similar health at the beginning of each arm of the study, he/she acts as his/her own reference or control group. This makes the crossover design more efficient in terms of sample size. If a parallel design were used, more volunteers would be needed to reach equivalence with the same power.

In some cases, if the within-subject variability is high (eg, nifedipine and acyclovir have highly variable effects whereby the same dose and drug given to the same subject on different occasions will have differing absorption, metabolism, and clinical effects), the advantage of using a crossover design is minimal.

Noninferiority

There are instances in which the efficacy of a drug needs to be shown to be not inferior to that of another drug, and equivalence trials designed to detect this are said to be *noninferiority trials*. TARGET (Do Tirofiban and ReoPro Give Similar Efficacy Outcomes Trial) is an example of a noninferiority trial. This study compared two glycoprotein IIb/IIIa receptor blockers with similar mechanisms of action but different chemical structures, platelet-cell adherence profiles, and durations of action [7]. Although the trial was designed to show the noninferiority of tirofiban as compared with abciximab, the trial results demonstrated that tirofiban had higher ischemic event rates than did abciximab, failing to show noninferiority.

Interpreting results

Equivalence trials

The definition of an endpoint can also vary depending on the drug/disease in question. In an equivalence trial in a disease that has a major impact on the patient, an absolute reduction of events of within 1% of the established/reference treatment might be acceptable for equivalence. So, if the established/reference treatment achieved a 10% reduction in events, the new treatment must achieve an absolute reduction of events of between 9% and 11%. However, for a disease with a relatively small impact on the patient, such as the common cold, a result within 5% of the reference treatment might be considered equivalent.

Noninferiority trials

When two treatments are compared, a single trial gives one estimate of the true difference between them. A range can be determined from that single estimate to capture the true effect (see **Chapter 18**). Consider an example trial that shows that a new treatment is 10% less effective than an established treatment, with

Table 1. Features of equivalence and noninferiority trials.

Assumptions	Let π_N and π_S be the rates of outcomes (eg, deaths or myocardial infarctions) with the new and standard treatments, respectively, and let a smaller value mean better efficacy	
	Equivalence	Noninferiority
Statistical test	Two-sided equivalence test	One-sided equivalence test
Null hypothesis	$H_0 : \pi_N - \pi_S \leq -D$ or $\pi_N - \pi_S \geq D$ Where D is the magnitude of prespecified difference between outcome rates with the new and standard treatments. The null hypothesis (H_0) implies that the new and standard treatments have differing outcome rates.	$H_0 : \pi_N - \pi_S \geq M$ Where M is the prespecified maximum allowable limit of difference in outcome rates between the new and standard treatments. The null hypothesis (H_0) implies that the new treatment is inferior to the standard one.
Alternative hypothesis	$H_a : -D < \pi_N - \pi_S < D$ The new treatment is statistically similar in outcome rates to the standard treatment, within a predefined range $(-D$ to $D)$.	$H_a : \pi_N - \pi_S < M$ The new treatment is clinically noninferior to the standard treatment within the predefined allowable range (M) of clinical significance.
Example	In an equivalence trial, the standard treatment has an event rate of 10% (π_S). Medical experts in that field agree that an absolute reduction of events within 1% (D) of the standard treatment might be acceptable to determine the new treatment as having an equivalent efficacy. So we have $(-D, D) = (-1\%, 1\%)$. The result shows that the 95% CI for $\pi_N - \pi_S = (-0.5\%, 0.5\%)$. As this interval falls within $(-D, D)$, equivalence between the new treatment and the standard one can be established. If the 95% CI for $\pi_N - \pi_S = (-2\%, 2\%)$, then equivalence between the new treatment and standard one cannot be concluded.	Consider a trial in which we would prespecify that if the effectiveness of the new treatment is 20% (M) less than that of the standard treatment, then we would consider the new treatment to be clinically inferior. The result shows that a new treatment is 10% less effective than standard treatment $(\pi_N - \pi_S = 10\%)$, with a one-sided 95% CI for $\pi_N - \pi_S$ being 5–15%. As the upper limit of the 95% CI (15%) is $< M$ (20%), the new treatment is deemed to be noninferior to the standard treatment. If the prespecified limit (M) is 12%, then the new treatment fails the noninferiority test as 15% is higher than the predefined 12% threshold.

a 95% confidence interval (CI) of 5–15% less. The prespecified definition of noninferiority (see **Chapter 14**) for this trial might state that the upper limit of the 95% CI must be <20%. Here, the new treatment cannot be called inferior to the existing treatment as its upper limit is 15%. If the prespecified definition used a 12% cutoff then the new treatment would have failed the noninferiority test and, in this scenario, the existing treatment would therefore be deemed superior to the new treatment. The features of equivalence and noninferiority trials are shown in **Table 1**.

Conclusion

Equivalence studies have important uses in clinical trials:

- They are used for comparing similar treament compounds.
- They are used for comparing the efficacy of the same treatment compound in differing formulations or in different cohorts of patients.

The key things to remember are that:

- They can have either an equivalence or a noninferiority endpoint.
- The outcomes can be clinical or pharmacokinetic.

While most published works concentrate on superiority endpoints, equivalence studies are performed in large numbers, particularly for regulatory submissions, so understanding the basic issues related to these approaches is therefore important. Other variables involved include scientific and ethical issues, and statistical assessment of superiority, equivalence, and noninferiority.

References

1. Gradman AH, Lewin A, Bowling BT, et al. Comparative effects of candesartan cilexetil and losartan in patients with systemic hypertension. *Heart Dis* 1999;**1**:52–7.
2. Tuomilehto J, Rastenyte D, Birkenhager WH, et al. Effects of calcium-channel blockade in older patients with diabetes and systolic hypertension. Systolic Hypertension in Europe Trial Investigators. *N Engl J Med* 1999;**340**:677–84.
3. Guidance for industry: Bioavailability and bioequivalence studies for orally administered drug products – general considerations. Rockville: US Department of Health and Human Services, Food and Drug Administration and Center for Drug Evaluation and Research, 2000.
4. Guidance for industry: Statistical procedures for bioequivalence studies using a standard two-treatment crossover design. Rockville: US Department of Health and Human Services, Food and Drug Administration and Center for Drug Evaluation and Research, 1992.
5. Guidance for industry: Statistical approaches to establishing bioequivalence. Rockville: US Department of Health and Human Services, Food and Drug Administration and Center for Drug Evaluation and Research, 2001.
6. Ware JH, Antmann CG. Equivalence trials. *N Engl J Med* 1997;**337**:1159–62.
7. Topol EJ, Moliterno DJ, Herrmann HC, et al. Comparison of two platelet glycoprotein IIb/IIIa inhibitors, tirofiban and abciximab, for the prevention of ischemic events with percutaneous coronary revascularization. *N Engl J Med* 2001;**344**:1888–94.

Chapter 13

Bioequivalence Trials

Duolao Wang, Radivoj Arezina,
and Ameet Bakhai

Bioequivalence studies are, by and large, conducted to compare a generic drug preparation with a currently marketed formulation – typically an innovator drug product. In a bioequivalence study, blood samples are collected just before the administration of a drug and for a period of time after administration. The drug concentrations are then plotted against time in order to derive pharmacokinetic parameters and evaluate the bioequivalence of the drugs under study. In this chapter, we describe some of the practical issues involved in the design and evaluation of bioequivalence studies and show how inappropriate design of such studies can lead to erroneous conclusions.

What is a bioequivalence trial?

A bioequivalence trial is a study of presumed therapeutic equivalence based on pharmacokinetic (PK) parameters rather than on clinical, or other, endpoints. There are several *in vivo* and *in vitro* methods that can be utilized to evaluate therapeutic equivalence between two medicinal products. In ascending order of preference, these include:

- *in vitro* studies
- comparative clinical studies
- pharmacodynamic (PD) studies
- PK studies

While some of these methods are appropriate only in certain circumstances (eg, *in vitro* dissolution tests can be used to evaluate the therapeutic equivalence of highly soluble, rapidly dissolving, orally active drugs), others (comparative clinical and PD studies) are considered less reliable and are generally only recommended if the PK approach is not possible [1–3]. Quite often, comparisons based on PD endpoints and, in particular, clinical endpoints, prove to be very difficult. Such studies are frequently hindered by factors such as a lack of clearly defined endpoints and huge variability in the measured parameters. Hence, the PK approach is commonly accepted as the method of choice for evaluating therapeutic equivalence between a generic and an innovator (reference) medicinal product. Bioequivalence studies compare PK parameters such as peak concentration (C_{max}) derived from plasma, serum concentrations, and blood concentrations, as described below.

Which PK parameters are used in a bioequivalence study?

To illustrate the PK parameters used, data from an anonymous study of the bioequivalence of generic and reference anagrelide products (used to decrease platelet count) will be used. An anagrelide 'plasma concentration over time' profile of a volunteer is shown in **Figure 1**. The raw PK data are also given in the first three columns of **Table 1**. In a PK study, the following parameters are usually derived from the PK profile in order to describe the drugs studied:

- *AUC*: the area under the 'plasma concentration over time' curve, which describes the total number of drug molecules present in the plasma, thereby providing information on the extent of absorption.

Figure 1. An example of a subject's anagrelide concentration profile.

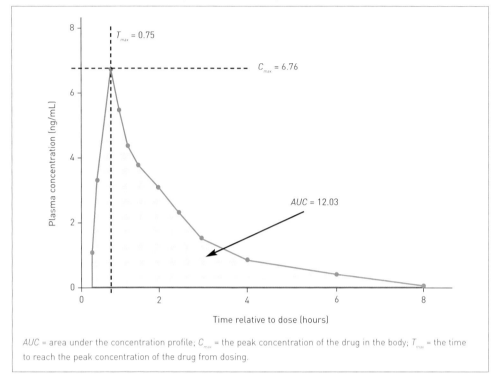

$T_{max} = 0.75$

$C_{max} = 6.76$

$AUC = 12.03$

Plasma concentration (ng/mL)

Time relative to dose (hours)

AUC = area under the concentration profile; C_{max} = the peak concentration of the drug in the body; T_{max} = the time to reach the peak concentration of the drug from dosing.

- C_{max}: the peak concentration of the drug in the body.
- T_{max}: the time, from dosing, to reach C_{max} (C_{max} and T_{max} together are indirect indicators of the rate of absorption).
- λ: the elimination constant, which describes the loss of drug activity from the body per time unit (eg, per hour).
- $T_{1/2}$: the elimination half-life. This is the time required for the amount (or concentration) of the drug in the body to decrease by half.

These parameters fully describe the shape of the 'plasma concentration over time' profile of a study drug. The absorption and elimination phases of a drug are distinguished by the parameters C_{max} and T_{max}. When the amount of the drug absorbed equals the amount eliminated, C_{max} is reached. Before C_{max} is reached, absorption is higher than elimination, and after C_{max} is reached, the situation is reversed.

Table 1. Anagrelide concentration and calculation of *AUC*.

Samples	T_i (h)	C_i (ng/mL)	$(C_i + C_{i-1}) / 2$	$T_i + T_{i-1}$	AUC_i (ng.h/mL)
1	0.00	<LLQ	NA	NA	NA
2	0.25	0.96	NA	0.25	NA
3	0.50	3.19	2.08	0.25	0.52
4	0.75	6.76	4.97	0.25	1.24
5	1.00	5.24	6.00	0.25	1.50
6	1.25	4.20	4.72	0.25	1.18
7	1.50	3.61	3.91	0.25	0.98
8	2.00	2.96	3.29	0.50	1.64
9	2.50	2.24	2.60	0.50	1.30
10	3.00	1.60	1.87	0.50	0.94
11	4.00	0.95	1.28	1.00	1.23
12	6.00	0.29	0.62	2.00	1.18
13	8.00	0.09	0.16	2.00	0.32
14	10.00	<LLQ	NA	2.00	NA
15	12.00	<LLQ	NA	2.00	NA
Total					12.03

AUC = area under the curve; *C* = concentration; LLQ = lower limit of quantitation (0.05 ng/mL); NA = not applicable; *T* = time.

Calculation of PK parameters

C_{max} and T_{max}

The parameters C_{max} and T_{max} can be directly observed from the PK profile for a subject. For the anagrelide data in **Table 1** or **Figure 1**, it is easy to see that C_{max} = 6.76 ng/mL and T_{max} = 0.75 hours.

AUC_{0-t}

AUC_{0-t} stands for the area under the PK concentration profile from time zero to time *t*, where *t* is the last time point at which there is a quantifiable plasma concentration. AUC_{0-t} is usually calculated by the so-called linear trapezoidal rule using the following formula:

$$AUC_{0-t} = \sum_{1}^{t} \left(\frac{C_i + C_{i-1}}{2} \right) (T_i - T_{i-1})$$

Columns four to six in **Table 1** show the calculation procedure for the anagrelide data, yielding a value of AUC_{0-t} = 12.03 ng.h/mL

λ and T$_{1/2}$

For calculating the remaining PK parameters, a statistical model must be established. In general, there is no special parametric PK model that fits the 'plasma concentration over time' profile for the whole time interval. Nevertheless, it is empirically accepted that a single exponential model can be fitted to describe the 'plasma concentration over time' profile during the so-called terminal or elimination phase, and that this declining exponential curve will continue even beyond the observation interval. In other words, it is assumed that the disappearance of the drug molecules follows the most simple linear one-compartmental model (treating the body as a single compartment) during the elimination phase, but not for the entire interval. Based on the above assumption, the other PK parameters can be derived.

In most cases, elimination of the drug is a first-order process (ie, the rate of drug elimination is directly proportional to the concentration of the drug), and a log transformation makes it possible to draw a straight line through data from the elimination phase. The slope of this regression line in the elimination phase is equivalent to the elimination rate constant [1,2].

A log transformation of the concentration values in **Table 1** is plotted in **Figure 2**, from which the elimination phase and rate constant can be determined. It is crucially important to select the correct starting point for the elimination phase – ie, where elimination is no longer influenced by absorption and after which the transformed concentration values tend to be linear. This time point is the first point of the elimination phase, while the last data point measured is the last point of the elimination phase. From the anagrelide data in **Figure 2**, it is obvious that the elimination phase is from 2 to 8 hours and that the log concentration data are very close to the fitted regression line:

$$\text{Log}(C_i) = 2.25 - 0.58 \times T_i \text{ with } R^2 = 0.9998$$

This gives $\lambda = 0.58$ (the loss of drug activity per hour). R^2 is a measurement of the goodness-of-fit of the regression line (a value close to 1 means that the regression line is a very good fit to the data), 2.25 is the intercept, and –0.58 is the slope of the fitted regression line.

As elimination is a first-order process, by simply dividing 0.693 (ln 2) by the estimated λ value, the half-life ($T_{1/2}$) can be calculated [1,2]:

$$T_{1/2} = \ln 2 / \lambda = 0.693 / 0.58 = 1.19$$

Figure 2. Determination of the elimination phase and elimination rate constant.

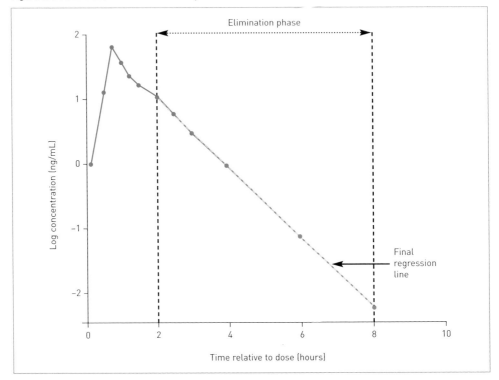

AUC$_{0-\infty}$

The next step in the PK parameter calculation is to obtain the AUC$_{0-\infty}$ – the total amount of drug present in the blood – by extending the 'plasma concentration over time' profile to infinity.

Assuming that the exponential elimination process will continue beyond the last observed concentration at time t, the extended area after t is C_t / λ [1–4]. This gives:

$$AUC_{0-\infty} = AUC_{0-t} + AUC_{t-\infty} = AUC_{0-t} + C_t / \lambda$$

For the anagrelide data, we get:

$$AUC_{0-\infty} = 12.03 + 0.09 / 0.58 = 12.18$$

How to collect PK samples correctly

The success of a bioequivalence trial depends on many factors, such as:

- the standardization of study procedures
- demographic and dietary factors
- analytical work

Among these factors there are two basic study-design issues related to blood sampling that deserve special attention, since they determine whether the samples can be used to fully describe the absorption, distribution, and elimination phases of the drug.

Sampling times

The sampling times at which the blood samples are collected have a decisive impact on the calculation of the PK parameters for the study drug. Ideally, the samples should be collected as frequently as possible during the study period so as to give an accurate PK profile. However, in practice, a relatively small number of blood samples are usually collected at selected time points due to ethical and financial considerations.

The US Food and Drug Administration (FDA) requires that sample collection should be spaced in such a way that the maximum concentration of the drug in the blood (C_{max}) and the terminal elimination rate constant (λ) can be accurately estimated [1–3]. It is important that there are enough sampling times clustered around C_{max}. For example, in **Figure 1**, the blood samples were collected every 0.25 hours from 0 to 1.5 hours around the T_{max} value (0.75 hours), meaning that the anagrelide PK profile is correct. However, occasionally, not enough blood samples are collected around C_{max} and, consequently, false C_{max}, T_{max} and AUC values are obtained. **Figure 3** shows an incorrect sampling scheme missing the time point at 0.75 hours. As a consequence of missing just this one time point, the PK parameters derived from this scheme, such as C_{max}, T_{max}, and AUC_{0-t}, are severely biased, and therefore erroneous conclusions about bioequivalence could be drawn from them.

The sampling period

The FDA requires that, to obtain an accurate estimate of λ from linear regression, sampling should continue for at least three terminal half-lives of the drug, and that at least three to four samples should be obtained during the terminal log-linear phase [1,2]. In the case of anagrelide, for example, empirical studies had shown that the half-life for this drug ranges from 1 to 2 hours, so a sampling period of 12 hours was planned for the anagrelide trial. The profiles for anagrelide from this trial show that this sampling period was long enough to obtain an accurate estimate of λ because, after 8 hours, the anagrelide plasma concentrations were no

Figure 3. A concentration profile from an incorrect sampling design.

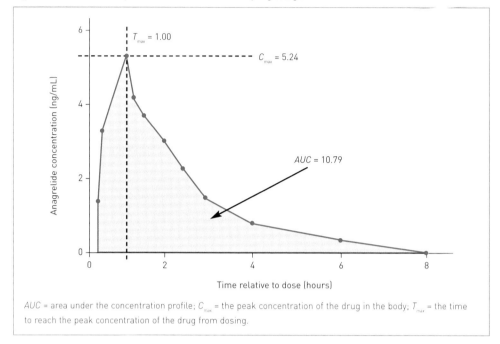

AUC = area under the concentration profile; C_{max} = the peak concentration of the drug in the body; T_{max} = the time to reach the peak concentration of the drug from dosing.

longer quantifiable for most subjects. This is displayed for one subject in **Figure 1**. Also, the terminal phase has 6 samples, as shown in **Figure 2**, which is much greater than the required minimum of four, yielding a reliable estimate of λ for this PK profile.

What basic designs are used for bioequivalence trials?

Due to large between-subject variability in PK parameters, it is advantageous to plan bioequivalence studies with a randomized crossover design. When two drug formulations are compared, the standard two-way crossover design is often appropriate. If more than two formulations are involved in a bioequivalence study, Latin square design, which balances the period and sequence effects, becomes attractive.

A $K \times K$ Latin square design is a way of putting K replicates of each of K treatments in a $K \times K$ array such that in each row and column, all the treatments are different. A 3×3 Latin square design is shown in **Table 2** and this pattern can be extended to any size. In some crossover trials, eg, those involving nifedipine (a calcium channel blocker) and acyclovir (an antiviral drug), the PK within-

Table 2. A *3 × 3* Latin square design.

	Period 1	Period 2	Period 3
Sequence 1	A	B	C
Sequence 2	B	C	A
Sequence 3	C	A	B

subject variability (the variability of a drug's effect within a single subject) is very high. In these cases, a crossover design is no longer advantageous and a parallel design could be an alternative choice.

How do we evaluate the bioequivalence between two drugs?

Standard statistical methodology based on a null hypothesis is not an appropriate method to assess bioequivalence [4,5]. The FDA has therefore employed a testing procedure – termed the 'two one-sided tests procedure' [1–4,6] – to determine whether average values for PK parameters measured after administration of the test and reference products are equivalent. This procedure involves the calculation of a 90% confidence interval (CI) $[\theta_1, \theta_u]$ for the ratio (θ) between the test (T)- and reference (R)-product PK-variable averages [4,7]. The FDA guidance requires that to reach an average bioequivalence, $[\theta_1, \theta_u]$ must fall entirely within a range of 0.80–1.25. This is known as the bioequivalence criterion [1–3].

How do we calculate the 90% confidence interval, $[\theta_1, \theta_u]$?

The FDA recommends that parametric (normal-theory) methods should be used to derive a 90% CI for the quantity $\mu(T) - \mu(R)$, the mean difference in log-transformed PK parameters between the T and R products [1–3]. The anti-logs of the confidence limits obtained constitute the 90% CI $[\theta_1, \theta_u]$ for the ratio of the geometric means between the T and R products. The 90% CI for the difference in the means of the log-transformed data should be calculated using statistical models that are appropriate to the trial design.

For example, for replicated crossover designs, the FDA recommends that the linear mixed-effects model (available in PROC MIXED in SAS or equivalent software [3]) should be used to obtain a point estimate and a 90% CI for the adjusted differences between the treatment means. Typically, the mixed model includes factors accounting for the following sources of variation: sequence, subjects nested in sequences, period, and treatment. The mixed model also treats the subject as a random effect so that the between-subject and within-subject variability can be measured.

Table 3. Point estimates and 90% confidence intervals for the bioavailability ratio $\mu(T) / \mu(R)$.

Parameter	Point estimate, θ	Lower 90% CI, θ_l	Upper 90% CI, θ_u
$AUC_{0-\infty}$	0.9796	0.9151	1.0485
C_{max}	1.1237	0.9959	1.2681
AUC_{0-t}	0.9804	0.9155	1.0498
$T_{1/2}$	0.9734	0.9165	1.0338
λ	1.0273	0.9673	1.0911
T_{max}	0.9450	0.6609	1.3511

AUC_{0-t} = area under the concentration profile, ie, the amount of drug present in the blood, from 0 to t hours; $AUC_{0-\infty}$ = area under the curve from 0 to ∞ hours, ie, the total amount of drug present in the blood; C_{max} = the peak concentration of the drug in the body; $T_{1/2}$ = the elimination half-life; T_{max} = the time to reach the peak concentration of the drug from dosing; λ = the elimination rate constant; $\mu(R)$ = mean pharmacokinetic parameter for the reference product; $\mu(T)$ = mean pharmacokinetic parameter for the test product; θ = ratio of the geometric means between the test and reference products.

Figure 4. Ratios of pharmacokinetic parameters and their 90% confidence intervals.

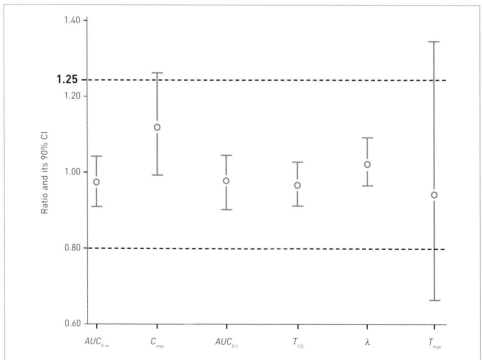

O = point estimate; ⊤ = upper limit of 90% CI; ⊥ = lower limit of 90% CI; AUC_{0-t} = area under the concentration profile from 0 to t hours; $AUC_{0-\infty}$ = area under the curve from 0 to ∞ hours; C_{max} = the peak concentration of the drug in the body; $T_{1/2}$ = the elimination half-life; T_{max} = the time to reach the peak concentration of the drug from dosing; λ = the elimination rate constant.

In **Table 3**, the ratios and 90% CIs for six PK parameters are presented as a hypothetical study of bioequivalence between test (T) and reference (R) products. These values are also displayed in **Figure 4**. For example, for $AUC_{0-\infty}$ the ratio between treatments T and R has a parametric point estimate of 0.98 and a 90% CI of 0.95–1.05. As this interval falls well within 0.80–1.25, the bioequivalence between treatments T and R can be established with respect to $AUC_{0-\infty}$. Similarly, bioequivalence holds true for AUC_{0-t}, $T_{1/2}$, and λ. However, as the 90% CIs for C_{max} and T_{max} are not completely covered by the bioequivalence acceptance range of 0.80–1.25, a conclusion of bioequivalence cannot be reached regarding the rate of absorption of the study products. Two drugs can only be considered to be bioequivalent when the rate and extent of absorption are equivalent. With respect to generic drugs it would be useful to know which statistical ranges the manufacturers adhere to.

Conclusion

We have highlighted the importance of a correctly designed bioequivalence study with respect to sampling times and sampling period. We have also demonstrated how easily biased PK parameters can be generated as a result of an inappropriate sampling scheme, leading to erroneous conclusions regarding the bioequivalence.

The typical approach to bioequivalence described in this chapter focuses on the comparison of population averages for a PK parameter. Developments in bioequivalence have included the concepts of individual and population bioequivalence that compare not only population averages, but also variance of PK parameters. Detailed discussions of these issues can be found in reference [3].

References

1. Guidance for Industry: Bioavailability and bioequivalence studies for orally administered drug products – general considerations. Rockville, MD: US Department of Health and Human Services, Food and Drug Administration and Center for Drug Evaluation and Research, 2000.
2. Guidance for Industry: Statistical procedures for bioequivalence studies using a standard two-treatment crossover design. Rockville, MD: US Department of Health and Human Services, Food and Drug Administration and Center for Drug Evaluation and Research, 1992.
3. Guidance for Industry: Statistical approaches to establishing bioequivalence. Rockville, MD: US Department of Health and Human Services, Food and Drug Administration and Center for Drug Evaluation and Research, 2001.
4. Chow SC, Liu JP. *Design and Analysis of Bioavailability and Bioequivalence Studies*, 2nd edition. New York: Marcel Dekker, 2000.

5. Hauck WW, Anderson S. A new statistical procedure for testing equivalence in two-group comparative bioavailability trials. *J Pharmacokinet Biopharm* 1984;**12**:83–91.

6. Schuirmann DJ. A comparison of the two one-sided tests procedure and the power approach for assessing the equivalence of average bioavailability. *J Pharmacokinet Biopharm* 1987;**15**:657–80.

7. Westlake WJ. Statistical aspects of comparative bioavailability trials. *Biometrics* 1979;**35**:273–80.

Chapter 14

Noninferiority Trials

Sam Miller, Colin Neate, and Duolao Wang

A noninferiority trial aims to demonstrate that the effect of a new treatment is as good as, or better than, that of an active comparator. This is assessed by demonstrating that the new treatment is not worse than the comparator by more than a specified margin (the noninferiority margin [δ]). In this chapter, we discuss in detail, using a recent trial, situations where noninferiority trials are appropriate, factors to be considered when choosing an appropriate δ, methods for sample size determination, and the issues involved in the analysis and evaluation of noninferiority.

What is a noninferiority trial?

Noninferiority trials aim to show that an experimental treatment is not worse than an active control by more than a predefined noninferiority margin, which is often denoted by the symbol δ. This margin is the largest reduction in efficacy that can be judged as clinically acceptable [1]. It is not the case that the lack of a statistically significant difference in a superiority trial demonstrates noninferiority. From the outset, the trial must be designed to conclusively show that the new treatment's effect is worse by no more than an agreed, prespecified amount.

A noninferiority trial is a specific type of trial known as an equivalence trial (see **Chapter 12**). For an equivalence trial, interest lies in whether the effect of the two treatments differs by more than the equivalence margin in either direction, and not solely in whether the new treatment is not worse. Care needs to be taken with interpreting the terminology used – the term 'equivalence' is often used (incorrectly) when the trial's aim is specifically *noninferiority*. It is usual for the term noninferiority to be used in therapeutic studies and for *equivalence* to be used in pharmacokinetic (such as 'bioequivalence') studies or in safety studies.

The following study will illustrate issues relating to the design and analysis of noninferiority clinical trials.

Example
A randomized, double-blind, multicenter, parallel-group study was undertaken to assess the efficacy and safety of oral Augmentin SR 2000/125 mg (pharmacokinetically enhanced amoxicillin/clavulanate) twice daily versus oral Augmentin 875/125 mg (amoxicillin/clavulanate) twice daily for 7 days in the treatment of adults with bacterial community-acquired pneumonia (CAP) [2].

The objective of this study was to demonstrate that, in adults, oral Augmentin SR 2000/125 mg is at least as effective clinically as oral Augmentin 875/125 mg in the treatment of CAP in terms of clinical response (success/failure) at test of cure at 4 weeks posttreatment (primary endpoint). Further details of this study are summarized in **Table 1**.

Noninferiority trials are also used in other therapeutic areas. For example, an asthma trial might be conducted with bronchodilator drugs in order to demonstrate the noninferior efficacy of a novel delivery method in comparison with a conventional inhaler. A typical primary endpoint might be improvement in peak expiratory flow, with a δ of –12 L/min.

Table 1. A summary of the key features of the bacterial community-acquired pneumonia (CAP) trial example [2].

Design	Randomized, double-blind, multicenter, parallel group
Objective	To demonstrate that oral Augmentin SR 2000/125 mg twice daily for 7 days is at least as effective clinically as oral Augmentin 875/125 mg twice daily for 7 days in the treatment of CAP in adults
Primary endpoint	Clinical response (success/failure) at test of cure at 4 weeks posttreatment
Treatment	
New treatment	Oral Augmentin SR 2000/125 mg twice daily
Standard treatment	Oral Augmentin 875/125 mg twice daily
Noninferiority margin	$\delta = -10\%$
	The prespecified maximum allowable limit of difference in success rates between the new and standard treatments
Null hypothesis	$H_0 : \pi_N - \pi_S \le \delta$
	Where π_N and π_S represent the rates of success at test of cure with the new and standard treatments, respectively
	The null hypothesis (H_0) implies that the new treatment is inferior to the standard one
Alternative hypothesis	$H_a : \pi_N - \pi_S > \delta$
	The new treatment is clinically noninferior to the standard treatment within the predefined allowable range (δ) of clinical significance
Sample size	Approximately 592 patients with CAP were required so as to provide 444 evaluable patients (222 per treatment arm), with which the study will have 90% power to assess that Augmentin SR 2000/125 mg is noninferior to Augmentin 875/125 mg
Analysis method	Two-sided 95% confidence interval for the difference in the proportion of successes between the treatment groups, calculated using the normal approximation to the binomial distribution
Results	Estimated difference in the proportion of successes between the treatment groups and 95% confidence interval
	Per-protocol: 2.7% (–3.0%, 8.3%)
	Intention-to-treat: 7.0% (0.9%, 13.0%)
Conclusion	Augmentin SR 2000/125 mg, twice daily for 7 days, is at least as effective clinically as Augmentin 875/125 mg, twice daily for 7 days, in the treatment of CAP in adults

When are noninferiority trials used?

A number of important factors contribute to choosing a noninferiority design. Primarily, noninferiority trials are employed in situations where efficacious treatments already exist. Where this is the case, it will often be unethical to carry out a randomized, placebo-controlled clinical trial. The new treatment might be tested to establish that it matches the efficacy of the standard, and at the same time has secondary advantages (eg, in terms of safety, convenience to the patient, or cost-effectiveness). Alternatively, it might have potential as a second-line therapy to the standard (in cases where the standard fails or is not tolerated).

Noninferiority trials do not conform to the definition of 'gold standard' trials (ie, randomized, double-blind, placebo-controlled trials) [1]. However, it is sometimes possible to incorporate a third, placebo, arm into the trial in order to demonstrate internal validity within the trial. Noninferiority trials also suffer from the criticism that no naturally conservative analysis exists (in the sense that a true treatment effect can be diluted by poor investigator conduct and patient compliance). This is discussed further later in this chapter.

Example (continued)

A number of antibiotics exist for bacterial infections (such as CAP), offering ≥85% clinical efficacy at 4 weeks posttreatment. Demonstrating superior efficacy on the primary endpoint (ie, clinical response at test of cure) in the general population would be difficult given such an excellent success rate. However, since drug resistance is an increasing problem, new antibiotics are required, and so it is considered appropriate to show noninferiority to an active comparator and to demonstrate activity against resistant pathogens.

How is the noninferiority margin chosen?

The choice of δ is a critically important aspect of the study design. The value is typically chosen using clinical judgment, with reference to relevant regulatory guidance [1,3] and, if appropriate, to guidance for the particular indication. A margin should be chosen such that a difference in treatments of such a magnitude would be considered clinically irrelevant, and anything greater would be unacceptably large. The value of δ is likely to be smaller than the difference looked for in a placebo-controlled superiority trial, since this would be a value of undisputed clinical importance.

An alternative way to arrive at a δ is to think of the study as attempting to show that the new compound is superior to a historical control. A δ of half the difference previously demonstrated in a superiority trial might, therefore, seem appropriate. Other factors that might influence the choice of δ are the degree of risk associated with treatment failure for the indication, relative toxicity, ease of use of the new treatment compared with the control, and, possibly, feasibility of the study in terms of enrolling the required number of subjects.

Example (continued)

Success rates of 80–90% are typical for currently approved antibiotics in the treatment of CAP [4]. As such, a δ of –10% is considered clinically irrelevant, so this is the margin recommended in regulatory guidelines [5].

Biocreep

There is some concern about noninferiority studies regarding the occurrence of a phenomenon known as 'biocreep'. This is where a slightly inferior new drug becomes the comparator for the next generation of compounds and so on, sequentially, until the new drugs of the future only have efficacy close to that of placebo. Biocreep can occur if a new drug with a lower efficacy rate than the comparator is approved with a wide δ. The concern can be alleviated when the chosen active comparator is the current gold standard treatment, and δ is chosen appropriately for the indication in question and further reduced if a placebo arm is incorporated into the study design.

How is the sample size calculated?

Conventionally, the sample size of a clinical trial is powered based on the primary endpoint, with the aim of obtaining a confidence interval (CI) for the treatment difference that shows the new treatment's efficacy to be worse by, at most, δ [1]. As in conventional trials, the following statistics are required to determine the sample size (see **Chapter 9**):

- anticipated efficacy of the comparator (ie, proportion for a binary endpoint, and mean and standard deviation for a continuous endpoint)
- significance level or threshold (α, Type I error)
- power ($1 - \beta$, $1 -$ Type II error)

In addition, the clinically relevant δ needs to be specified.

As further illustrated by later examples, the resultant sample size is particularly sensitive to the anticipated efficacy of the comparator, the anticipated effect of the experimental treatment relative to this, and the choice of δ.

Since δ is often assumed to be a fraction of the treatment difference on which a placebo-controlled superiority trial would be powered, noninferiority trials often require much larger sample sizes. Conversely, they may require smaller sample sizes than if an active-controlled superiority trial was to be designed, since the superiority margin for such a trial may be smaller than δ [6].

For noninferiority, the conventional null hypothesis of a superiority trial (ie, that the true treatment difference is zero) and the alternative (that it is positive) is essentially replaced by a null hypothesis that it is inferior by an amount of more than the defined δ and an alternative that it is not. Guidance recommends

Table 2. Examples of noninferiority sample sizes.

	Assumptions				
Example	π_N	π_S	δ	N_E	N_T
A	88%	88%	–10%	222	592
B	88%	88%	–12%	155	414
C	85%	85%	–10%	268	716
D	90%	88%	–10%	143	382

π_N = rate of success with the new treatment; π_S = rate of success with the standard treatment; δ = noninferiority margin; N_E = number of evaluable subjects per arm; N_T = total number of subjects enrolled accounting for dropouts. Assumptions for sample size calculation: H_a one-sided alternative hypothesis; α = 2.5%; power = 90%; dropout rate = 25% (to allow for subjects not eligible for efficacy analyses); confidence interval calculation method = normal approximation.

that, conventionally, a one-sided CI is used to assess noninferiority [1]. In the anti-infectives therapeutic area, a 2.5% significance level has regularly been used to assess the null hypothesis. This corresponds to assessing noninferiority based on a one-sided 97.5% CI. However, estimation is often best based on a two-sided 95% CI and sample sizes for this are very similar. **Table 2** gives some examples of sample size calculations [7].

Example (continued)
The total number of patients required for the study is 592 (see **Table 2**, row A). This is based on the following assumptions: one-sided H_a, α = 2.5%, power = 90%, dropout rate = 25%, π_N = 88%, π_S = 88%, δ = –10%, CI calculation method = normal approximation, $N_S = 2 \times (N_E / [1 - 0.25])$.

The choice of δ has a large impact on the number of subjects required for the trial, as seen when using a value of –12% rather than –10% (see **Table 2**, row B). Therefore, this clinical information is of high importance.

The anticipated efficacy rates also strongly influence the required sample size, as can be seen by the increase in sample size when efficacy is assumed to be 85% instead of 88% (see **Table 2**, row C). On the probability scale, variance (and hence width of the CI) is a function of the efficacy rate. Therefore, larger sample sizes are required for efficacy rates towards the center of the 0–100% probability scale, where variance is greatest.

If the clinician truly believes that a small advantage in efficacy will be observed for the experimental treatment, but the primary goal remains to demonstrate noninferiority, the calculation should be performed under an assumption of unequal efficacy. By assuming the efficacy for the experimental treatment is superior (90% vs 88%), a smaller sample size is required to obtain a CI with a lower limit at or above –10% (see **Table 2**, row D).

A noninferiority trial (by design) includes the possibility of superiority under the alternative hypothesis. Therefore, when calculating the sample size, it might be reasonable to assume that the experimental treatment has a small advantage. It is then possible to test for both noninferiority and superiority. However, unequal efficacy should not be assumed simply to reduce sample size, as, if the assumption is found not to hold, then the study will not be powered to meet the primary objective of enabling a clinically conclusive assessment of noninferiority.

A further consideration is the methodology that will be used to calculate the CI for assessing noninferiority. Specifically, there is a need to avoid using an analysis method that has the property of being more conservative (ie, leads to a wider CI) than that used in calculating the sample size. For the analysis of probability differences, approximation methods (such as the normal approximation to the binomial distribution) can be unreliable for extreme probabilities (where the expected frequency of events for analysis is small and event probabilities are approaching asymptotic limits). This can lead to substantial differences in the sample size estimates obtained when the calculations are made using another method (eg, the score method [8]).

How are noninferiority trials analyzed?

Noninferiority and superiority trials differ in terms of the standard method of analysis. Superiority is usually demonstrated by reference to a *P*-value (the probability of seeing the observed treatment difference, or a more extreme difference, calculated under the null hypothesis of no difference between treatments), with a CI also used in order to estimate the range of plausible values for the treatment difference. The smaller, or more significant, the *P*-value, the more confidence in the conclusion of superiority. However, the reverse does not apply – a large *P*-value does not necessarily correspond to a clinically insignificant treatment difference.

In noninferiority trials, a CI is calculated to estimate the range of values in which the treatment difference is likely to lie. This CI is used to provide the basis for drawing the study's conclusions. If the CI does not include any values for the treatment difference that are more extreme than the noninferiority limit, then noninferiority is demonstrated. The confidence level of the CI is usually set at 95%, corresponding to a 2.5% one-sided significance level. The specific method for calculating the CI will depend on the study design and the endpoints, but the

Figure 1. Examples of noninferiority study results.

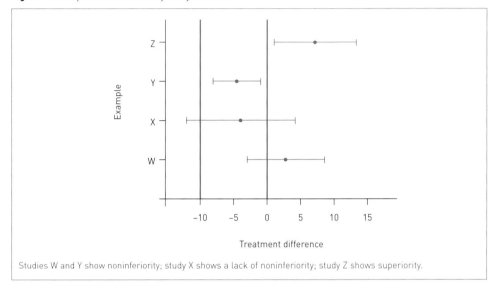

Studies W and Y show noninferiority; study X shows a lack of noninferiority; study Z shows superiority.

principles underlying the drawing of conclusions will be the same. Some typical noninferiority study CIs are shown in **Figure 1**.

Example (continued)

The 95% CI for the difference in success rate (Augmentin SR 2000/125 mg – Augmentin 875/125 mg), calculated using the normal approximation to the binomial distribution, is (–3.0%, 8.3%) (per-protocol [PP] population) (see **Figure 1**, study W). This lies entirely above the specified noninferiority limit of –10%, so the study demonstrates that Augmentin SR 2000/125 mg is noninferior to Augmentin 875/125 mg.

Had the lower limit of the CI been below the noninferiority limit, then the study would not have demonstrated noninferiority (see **Figure 1**, study X). Note that lack of noninferiority does not necessarily imply inferiority, since the CI does include some positive values for the treatment difference. The reverse is also true (see **Figure 1**, study Y). These results would lead to a conclusion of noninferiority (since the CI lies above –10%), though they also show a statistically significant (clinically insignificant) difference in favor of the standard therapy.

Patient population

Another key issue in analysis is the choice of patient population. The intention-to-treat (ITT) principle is widely recognized as the most valid analytical approach for superiority trials that involve long-term follow-up, because it adheres to the randomization procedure and is generally conservative [1]. Although some might argue that ITT analysis is overly conservative, most would agree that a positive outcome of an ITT analysis in a superiority trial is convincing.

Unfortunately, no such conservative analysis exists for noninferiority trials. Including data after study drug discontinuation in the analysis, as ITT does, tends to give a conservative estimate of the treatment difference, which could make a truly inferior treatment appear noninferior. Alternatively, excluding data from patients with major protocol violations – PP analysis – can bias the results in either direction (eg, in a situation where dropout is related to efficacy outcome). Therefore, noninferiority trials are generally analyzed using both ITT and PP approaches, and conclusions can be considered more robust when both approaches support the noninferiority of the treatment.

The CI for the ITT population is (0.9%, 13.0%) (see **Figure 1**, study Z). This supports the conclusion of noninferiority from the PP population, since the CI lies entirely above –10%.

Example (continued)
In the CAP example, although the study was set up to show noninferiority, it may have been possible to 'switch' to a conclusion of superiority (had the PP analysis (W) also supported this conclusion). In situations where the CI only includes positive values of the treatment difference, a statistically significant benefit of the new treatment over the comparator is demonstrated. The clinical significance of a treatment difference of this size would need discussion.

Conclusion

Noninferiority trials provide an alternative study design for indications where superiority trials would not be appropriate (due to ethical or practical constraints). They are often used where efficacious treatments already exist, and the demonstration of noninferiority, as well as secondary benefits, is sufficient for regulatory approval. However, noninferiority trials suffer from the criticism that trial results do not show internal validity (since they provide no direct comparison with placebo), and also that the analysis approach is not naturally conservative [9].

These criticisms can be overcome by [10]:

- incorporating a placebo arm into the trial
- ensuring that the comparator used is the current standard of care
  and previously demonstrated as superior to placebo

- ensuring that the trial is well monitored
- ensuring that the results of the two analysis populations (PP and ITT) do not conflict

The choice of δ is critically important, and needs to be prespecified and justified when designing the trial. Although the choice of δ is dependant on the indication and available regulatory guidance, sound clinical judgment is always required.

References

1. International Conference on Harmonisation of Technical Requirements for Registration of Pharmaceuticals for Human Use. ICH Harmonised Tripartite Guideline: Statistical Principles For Clinical Trials E9. Recommended for Adoption at Step 4 of the ICH Process on 5 February 1998 by the ICH Steering Committee. Available from: www.ich.org/MediaServer.jser?@_ID=485&&@_MODE=GLB. Accessed May 6, 2005.
2. File TM Jr, Lode H, Kurz H, et al. Double-blind, randomized study of the efficacy and safety of oral pharmacokinetically enhanced amoxicillin-clavulanate (2000/125 milligrams) versus those of amoxicillin-clavulanate (875/125 milligrams), both given twice daily for 7 days, in treatment of bacterial community-acquired pneumonia in adults. *Antimicrob Agents Chemother* 2004;**48**:3323–31.
3. Committee for Proprietary Medicinal Products. Points to Consider on the Choice of Non-Inferiority Margin. Efficacy Working Party, EMEA. Draft released for consultation, February 2004. Available from: www.emea.eu.int/pdfs/human/ewp/215899en.pdf. Accessed June 10, 2004.
4. Garau J. Treatment of drug-resistant pneumococcal pneumonia. *Lancet Infect Dis* 2002;**2**:404–15.
5. Committee for Proprietary Medicinal Products. Note for guidance on evaluation of medicinal products indicated for treatment of bacterial infections. Efficacy Working Party, Note for Guidance, European Commission. Draft 1996. Available at www.emea.eu.int/pdfs/human/ewp/055895en.pdf. Accessed June 14, 2004.
6. Snapinn SM. Noninferiority trials. *Curr Control Trials Cardiovasc Med* 2000;**1**:19–21.
7. Makuch R, Simon R. Sample size requirements for evaluating a conservative therapy. *Cancer Treatment Reports* 1978;**62**:1037–40.
8. Farrington CP, Manning G. Test statistics and sample size formulae for comparative binomial trials with null hypothesis of non-zero risk difference or non-unity relative risk. *Stat Med* 1990;**9**:1447–54.
9. Hauck WW, Anderson S. Some issues in the design and analysis of equivalence trials. *Drug Inf J* 1999;**33**:109–18.
10. Jones B, Jarvis P, Lewis JA, et al. Trials to assess equivalence: the importance of rigorous methods. *BMJ* 1996;**313**:36–9.

Chapter 15

Cluster Randomized Trials

Umair Mallick, Ameet Bakhai, Duolao Wang, and Marcus Flather

While conventional trials randomize individual subjects to different treatments, cluster randomized trials use a group of individuals, a hospital, or a community as the unit of randomization. Cluster randomized trials are increasingly used in primary care, health promotion, and public health, where the methodological superiority of these trials has been proven when compared with conventional randomized trials. Cluster randomized trials potentially require a much larger number of individuals in the trial if there is a high likelihood for similar outcomes between individuals, since otherwise the power of such trials to detect a significant difference is much lower than conventional randomized trials. In this chapter, we provide an overview of cluster randomized trials along with their design, analysis, and ethical implications.

Introduction

In conventional randomized trials, the unit of randomization is usually the individual subject. In interventions that address organizational changes, however, it is not always feasible to randomize at the individual level. Trials that randomize groups of subjects are called *cluster randomized trials* (CRTs). When individual randomization proves inappropriate, CRTs can be used to reduce the potential for contamination within treatment groups (see **Table 1**). Examples of clusters are shown in **Table 2**.

In recent years, CRTs have become an important tool in clinical research, particularly since the interventions being evaluated tend to be relatively complex and diversified. CRTs are particularly used in the evaluation of health care, screening, and educational interventions, where patients are nested within larger group settings such as practices, hospitals, or communities.

Design of cluster randomized trials

The methodological quality of these trials is diverse. Due to the dual nature of CRTs – focusing on both the cluster and the individual – the design, size, and analysis of these trials can be complex [1–3]. Therefore, there should be a clear justification and rationale for using the CRT design.

Cluster effect

Individuals randomized in a clinical trial are assumed to have an independent chance of being given a placebo or active treatment, and an independent progression through the trial. However, if the intervention cannot be blinded (eg, a counseling service for a disease) then patients and clinicians are likely to influence the outcome of this intervention.

For example, a physician might show frustration at having to give additional reassurance to a patient who is not being counseled, or make earlier therapy decisions for patients who are being counseled. Patients being counseled might report fewer side-effects of other therapies or be more compliant, or be receiving support from other patients who are also in counseling. This exchange of information will bias the effect of the intervention, and so it is easier to offer all of the patients of one hospital counseling, while those in a similar, nearby hospital receive no counseling. This enables us to see the impact of this intervention without the trial being contaminated by the *cluster effect*.

Table 1. Why use cluster randomization?

• To evaluate health care interventions in practices, hospitals, regions, or communities
• Patients in one cluster are more likely to have similar outcomes
• To eliminate contamination of the intervention effects between patients within a cluster

Table 2. Potential units of randomization in cluster randomized trials.

• Groups of individuals chosen by a specific link (eg, geographic location)
• Primary care practices
• Hospitals
• Communities

Note: Intervention is usually applied at the cluster level.

It is important to ensure that enough similar hospitals exist to enable balance when randomized as a cluster; the size of each cluster must also be similar (eg, 20 patients recruited at each hospital). Randomizing by cluster must now be accounted for in the design, analysis, and reporting of a trial, since the lack of independence between patients in a CRT has important statistical implications [4].

Selection bias

In conventional trials, selection bias can be minimized by the randomized allocation of individual subjects [5]. However, trials in cluster settings are prone to contamination effects due to correlations among individuals within clusters in the trial – eg, patients attending an affluent hospital are more likely to be compliant and to report side-effects.

This bias can be partially offset by using each cluster as a unit of randomization (rather than the individual subject), providing enough similar clusters can be identified. However, CRTs are less efficient than conventional trials since the number of clusters randomized is smaller than when randomizing at the individual patient level. This can generate a trade-off between an individual randomized trial and a CRT [6]. For example, in studies at the primary care level that randomize physicians of a practice as the unit of clustering – rather than as individual physicians – the sample size, interpretation, and analysis can all be affected [7–9].

Confounding

As in a simple randomized trial, the effect of a treatment in CRTs can be influenced by the presence of possible confounding factors due to imbalances in the baseline characteristics of patients (or *covariates*) between treatment groups (see **Chapter 25**).

It has been argued that the results of CRTs are more subjective to imbalance at baseline than simple randomized trials, as it can be impossible to know the clusters well enough to be able to assure an adequate balance of clusters to each treatment arm. For example, one cluster might have a heavy bias toward ethnic minority individuals or older patients. Therefore, proper randomization schemes should be implemented in order to minimize the possible confounding effect on the outcome variables.

Example

The PROMIS (Prospective Registry of Outcomes and Management in Acute Ischaemic Syndromes)-UK study illustrates the use of CRT design in an ongoing study [10]. In this trial, the strategy under investigation is a guideline adherence educational program on enhancing the use of evidence-based treatments (aspirin, heparin, beta-blockers, clopidogrel, and statins) to improve the outcomes of patients admitted with acute coronary syndromes. Individual centers are either randomized to the education program or not.

The primary outcome is defined as a composite score of all five treatments being prescribed during the in-hospital phase (1 point for each treatment on a patient, with a range from 0 to 5). In this CRT, the primary objective is to compare the composite score for the five evidence-based treatments between the education group and the control group.

Since it is likely that many of the same health professionals will look after different patients within a hospital entering the study, the patients cannot be treated as having independent outcomes on an individual basis – hence, the choice of a CRT design is justified. To control for possible confounding, the investigators have employed a stratified randomization scheme. This aims to achieve a balanced distribution of hospitals between two treatment groups with regard to geographic distribution, teaching hospital status, and whether a hospital has the facilities to perform invasive therapies for an acute coronary syndrome, since such hospitals are more likely to also use more drug interventions.

Impact of clustering on sample size

In CRTs, statistical power is greatly reduced in comparison with a similarly sized individually randomized trial due to randomizing by cluster – therefore, the sample size calculations need to be inflated, using a cluster inflation factor to accommodate for the clustering.

Another factor to consider is that although the unit of randomization is the cluster (eg, hospital), the unit of outcome measure is the patient. Therefore, we need to adjust for the cluster size and number, as well as how closely related the patients' outcomes are within a cluster. This correlation can be measured by a statistic called the *intra-cluster correlation coefficient* (ICC), which can be calculated using different formulas for different types of outcome variables [1–4].

The impact of using a CRT design on sample size can be substantial; it depends on the size of the clustering effect, as measured by the ICC, and the number of clusters available, as seen in the following formula:

$$N_{cluster} = (1 + [m - 1] \times ICC) \times N_{simple}$$

where:

- N_{simple} and $N_{cluster}$ are the sample sizes for simple randomization and cluster randomization, respectively
- m is the number of subjects in each cluster
- $(1 + [m - 1] \times ICC)$ is the design effect
- ICC measures the correlation of the patient's outcome within a cluster

The *design effect* indicates the amount by which the sample needs to be multiplied. Thus, a CRT with a large design effect will require many more subjects than a trial of the same intervention that randomizes individuals.

Example

Consider the PROMIS-UK study, a trial of an educational intervention to implement a clinical guideline. An individual randomized trial would require 348 patients (N_{simple}) to detect a change of 0.30 in the composite score for patients who are managed with all five therapies (with 80% power and 5% significance). However, this design would be inappropriate because of the potential for contamination.

For this study, it was estimated that the ICC was about 0.15 and 20 patients were available per cluster (ie, $m = 20$). Based on these assumptions, the sample size adjusting for clustering is 67 clusters or 1,340 patients ($N_{cluster}$), ie, almost four times that of the individual randomized trial. We can also see from the formula that the larger the ICC, the more patients are needed.

Analysis of cluster randomized trials

In analyzing CRTs, the experimental unit is often used as the unit of analysis, although summary statistics can be made for each cluster. In PROMIS-UK, although randomization was at the level of the hospital, it was planned that guideline adherence would be measured at both the patient and hospital levels, but analysis of subsequent outcome variables be done at the patient level.

Cluster effect

In the analysis of CRTs, failure to control for the cluster effect (correlation between individuals within the same cluster) can lead to a biased estimate of treatment effect, such as a *P*-value and confidence intervals that overstate the significance of the result, and hence have an inflated Type I error rate (rejection of a true null hypothesis) [11,12]. This, in turn, increases the chances of spurious significant findings and misleading conclusions.

Donner showed, using data from Murray et al., that the *P*-value for this specific study changed from 0.03 if the effect of clustering is ignored to >0.10 after adjusting for the effect of clustering [8,13]. This example is typical, and shows that the evidence for a statistically significant treatment effect can be exaggerated if the cluster effect is not taken into account in a CRT design.

Statistical methods and models

The classic statistical methods and models, such as the *t*-test (see **Chapter 19**), are not appropriate for the analysis of CRTs because they are based on a strong assumption that all individuals in a sample are independent from each other (ie, there is no cluster effect in the sample). Fortunately, many advanced statistical methodologies have been developed to address the cluster effect in CRTs. These approaches include the robust variance estimate method and the random effect (multilevel), general estimating equation, and Bayesian hierarchical models [11,12]. The common thread of these techniques is to take into account the cluster effect by relaxing the independence assumption in their methodological developments.

Of these models, the *random effect* model has been widely used because it not only controls for a cluster effect, but also provides an estimate of the cluster effect. By applying a random effect model, we can assess to what extent the treatment effect could be contaminated by the cluster effect. Another advantage of this model is its ability to take into account heterogeneity due to other unobservable factors. In addition, appropriate exploratory covariate adjustments can be made, adjusting for any major imbalances in the groups – including the type of hospital, the case mix of physicians treating patients (specialists versus nonspecialists), and patient characteristics.

Table 3. How to improve precision of the treatment effect in cluster randomized trials.

- Have clear justification for the use of the cluster randomized trial design
- Carefully select the outcome measures
- Adjust the sample size according to the size and number of clusters
- Take into account the clustering aspect of the design in the analysis
- Carry out sensitivity analyses to assess the robustness of results, using various statistical methods specified in the protocol

Sensitivity analysis

Sensitivity analyses assess how estimated treatment effects vary with different statistical methods, in particular methods that do and do not take the cluster effect into consideration. If the estimates of treatment effect are sensitive to a cluster effect in a CRT, it would suggest that the CRT design is important.

A sensitivity study that compared analytical methods in CRTs showed that results from different approaches that address the cluster effect are less sensitive when outcomes are continuous than if outcomes are binary [12,14].

Bias in published cluster randomized trials

Although there is increasing recognition of the methodological issues associated with CRTs, many investigators are still not clear about the impact of this design on sample size requirements and the results of analysis.

A retrospective review of CRTs from January 1997 to October 2002 examined the prevalence of a risk of bias associated with the design and conduct of CRTs [15]. The study showed that, out of 36 trials at the cluster level, 15 trials (42%) provided evidence for appropriate allocation and 25 (69%) used stratified allocation. Few trials showed evidence of imbalance at the cluster level. However, some evidence of susceptibility to risk of bias at the individual level existed in 14 studies (39%). The authors concluded that some published CRTs might not have taken adequate precautions against threats to the internal validity of their design [15].

Similarly, another review explored the appropriate use of methodological and analytical techniques used in reports of CRTs of primary prevention trials [16]. Out of 24 articles identified, only four (19%) included sample size calculations or discussions of power that allowed for clustering, while only 12 (57%) took clustering into account in the statistical analysis. The authors concluded that design and analysis issues associated with CRTs generally remain unrecognized (see **Table 3**) [16].

Table 4. Reporting cluster randomized trials.

- Explain the baseline distribution of important characteristics of the population
- Include sample size calculations and assumptions of correlation with a cluster
- Provide values of the cluster effect, as calculated for the primary outcome variables
- Explain how the reported statistical analyses account for the cluster effect

The CONSORT (Consolidated Standards of Reporting Trials) statement on trial conduct and reporting has now been extended to take into account the special features of CRTs, such as rationale for the cluster design, and implications of the cluster effect in design and analysis. These changes hope to increase the reporting quality of these trials [17].

Reports of CRTs should include sample size calculations and statistical analyses that take clustering into account. Information regarding other details (eg, estimates of design effects, baseline distribution of important characteristics in the intervention group, number of clusters, and average cluster size for each group) can guide researchers to design better trials and avoid key errors when conducting and reporting CRTs (see **Table 4**) [18]. Indeed, the ideal scenario would be to publish and submit the design of a CRT for open peer review before the trial gets under way; this would allow assumptions to be adequately challenged by experts in the field.

Ethical issues in cluster randomized trials

Several reports, guidelines, and codes provide an extensive overview of the importance of ethical issues in individual patient randomized trials. However, the ethical issues raised by CRTs have also drawn the attention of experts.

Individuals consenting in conventional randomized trials are likely to consent with a higher degree of freedom and independence compared to those who participate in CRTs. In these trials, participants are likely to impinge on each other's choices when informed consent for trial entry (that is, for randomization) is obtained. The decision to participate in the trial or intervention may depend not just on the individual, but also on the guardian (eg, the hospital chief executive or managing partner of the primary care trust) in the CRT. For example, a hospital manager may agree to have a counseling service for all patients with a stroke, and, since this intervention will be accessible to all patients admitted to that hospital, it might become protocol rather than a specific consent-requiring therapy – although the trial design will, of course, have been approved by an ethics committee [19].

Table 5. Main advantages and disadvantages of cluster randomized trials.

Advantages	Disadvantages
• Optimal design for evaluating quality improvement strategies in health care intervention and education program studies	• Larger sample size is required than for a simple randomized trial
• Account for contamination between patients within a cluster	• The patients and clinicians may recognize whether they are in the active or placebo arm
• Easier to administrate the randomization and centers	• Clinicians might transfer information between clusters

Issues related to the nature and practice of informed consent in CRTs raise new questions that need to be properly addressed. Other ethical implications of these trials, such as principles relating to the quality of the scientific design and analysis, balance of risk and benefit, liberty to leave a trial, early stopping of a trial, and the power to exclude people from potential benefits, also need careful consideration [20].

Advantages and limitations of using cluster randomized trials in clinical research

CRTs represent an important type of design that can be considered complementary to conventional randomized trials. CRTs have certain advantages over conventional randomized trials. For instance, CRTs help to account for the potential for contamination between treatments when trial patients are managed within the same setting. Moreover, the outcomes of patients in a cluster are likely to be influenced by a number of similar factors. Thus, these patients cannot be treated as having independent outcomes on an individual basis. CRTs are especially useful for evaluating quality improvement strategies in health care interventions and education programs.

On the other hand, when choosing a design between individual randomized trials and CRTs, one should be ready for some trade-off due to the limited efficiency of CRTs. There is potentially a considerable loss of power between a conventional randomized controlled trial and a CRT for the same number of patients. Therefore, in the statistical analysis and estimation of trial power, the clustering aspect of the design should not be ignored. Some main points about CRTs discussed in this chapter are summarized in **Table 5**.

Conclusion

In clinical research, CRTs have already become an important tool for the effective evaluation of health care interventions, in particular at the level of primary and secondary health care institutes across a certain geographical area. In this chapter, we have illustrated various aspects of design and analysis using appropriate statistical methods particular to CRTs, and discussed the ethical implications of this experimental design.

We have highlighted that a cluster effect can influence or bias trial outcomes, particularly when the intervention cannot be blinded (such as organizational interventions offering additional services), and can lead to an over-inflation of a treatment effect if this bias is not accounted for. It is also important to recognize that publication of CRT results need to follow CONSORT guidelines, and include (in particular) power calculations and statistical methods dealing with the cluster effect. Further advanced issues regarding CRTs can be found in references [12,21,22].

References

1. Campbell M, Grimshaw J, Steen N. Sample size calculations for cluster randomized trials. Changing Professional Practice in Europe Group (EU BIOMED II Concerted Action). *J Health Serv Res Policy* 2000;**5**:12–16.

2. Donner A, Klar N. Methods for comparing event rates in intervention studies when the unit of allocation is a cluster. *Am J Epidemiol* 1994;**140**:279–89.

3. Donner A, Birkett N, Buck C. Randomization by cluster: sample size requirements and analysis. *Am J Epidemiol* 1981;**114**:906–14.

4. Campbell MK, Grimshaw JM. Cluster randomized trials: time for improvement. The implications of adopting a cluster design are still largely being ignored. *BMJ* 1998;**317**:1171–2.

5. Fayers PM, Jordhoy MS, Kaasa S. Cluster-randomized trials. *Palliat Med* 2002;**16**:69–70.

6. Chuang JH, Hripcsak G, Heitjan DF. Design and analysis of controlled trials in naturally clustered environments: implications for medical informatics. *J Am Inform Assoc* 2002;**9**:230–8.

7. Cornfield J. Randomization by group: a formal analysis. *Am J Epidemiol* 1978;**108**:100–2.

8. Donner A. An empirical study of cluster randomization. *Int J Epidemiol* 1982;**11**:283–6.

9. Kerry SM, Bland JM. The intra-cluster correlation coefficient in cluster randomization. *BMJ* 1998;**316**:1455.

10. Clinical Trials and Evaluation Unit. Study Protocol: PROMIS-UK 'Prospective Registry of Outcomes and Management in acute Ischaemic Syndromes-in United Kingdom.' An ongoing trial. Designed by: Clinical Trials and Evaluation Unit, Royal Brompton and Harefield NHS Trust, Sydney Street, London. Personal communication, May 5, 2005.

11. Mollison JA, Simpson JA, Campbell MK, et al. Comparison of analytical methods for cluster randomized trials: an example from a primary care setting. *J Epidemiol Biostat* 2000;**5**:339–48.

12. Donner A, Klar N. *Design and Analysis of Cluster Randomization Trials in Health Research*. London: Arnold, 2000.

13. Murray DM, Perry CL, Griffin G, et al. Results from a statewide approach to adolescent tobacco use prevention. *Prev Med* 1992;**21**:449–72.

14. Donner A, Klar N. Issues in the meta analysis for cluster randomized trials. *Stat Med* 2002;**21**:2971–80.

15. Puffer S, Torgerson D, Watson J. Evidence for risk of bias in cluster randomized trials: review of recent trials published in three general medical journals. *BMJ* 2003;**327**:785–9.

16. Simpson JM, Klar N, Donnor A. Accounting for cluster randomization: a review of primary prevention trials, 1990 through 1993. *Am J Public Health* 1995;**85**:1378–83.

17. Campbell MK, Elbourne DR, Altman DG; CONSORT group. CONSORT statement: extension to cluster randomised trials. *BMJ* 2004;**328**:702–8.

18. Donner A, Brown KS, Brasher P. A methodological review of non-therapeutic intervention trials employing cluster randomization, 1979–1989. *Int J Epidemiol* 1990;**19**:795–800.

19. Edwards SJL, Braunholtz DA, Lilford RJ, et al. Ethical issues in the design and conduct of cluster randomized controlled trials. *BMJ* 1999;**318**:1407–9.

20. Hutton JL. Are distinctive ethical principles required for cluster randomized controlled trials? *Stat Med* 2001;**20**:473–88.

21. Murray DM. *The Design and Analysis of Group-Randomized Trials*. Oxford: Oxford University Press, 1998.

22. Bland JM. Cluster randomised trials in the medical literature: two bibliometric surveys. *BMC Med Res Methodol* 2004;**4**:21.

Chapter 16

Multicenter Trials

Ann Truesdale, Ameet Bakhai, and Duolao Wang

A multicenter study has several advantages over a single-center study, namely: it allows a large number of patients to be recruited in a shorter time; the results are more generalizable and contemporary to a broader population at large; and such studies are critical in trials involving patients with rare presentations or diseases. In this chapter, we discuss how multicenter trials are conducted (reviewing the reasons for using the multicenter design), and how such trials are organized, and explain the practical issues involved in planning, conducting, and analyzing such studies.

What is a multicenter trial?

A multicenter trial is a trial that is performed simultaneously at many centers following the same protocol. The activity at these centers is synchronized from a single command center – the coordinating center. A multicenter trial is not equivalent to a number of separate single-site trials, since the data collected from the different centers are analyzed as a whole.

The earliest documented randomized trial was a multicenter study conducted in 1948 by the UK Medical Research Council, evaluating streptomycin for the treatment of pulmonary tuberculosis. This was discussed in a theme issue of the *BMJ* published to mark the 50th anniversary of this trial [1]. Since then, there have been hundreds more multicenter trials, mainly in the form of large randomized controlled trials [2].

The majority of these trials have commercial funding and are driven by pharmaceutical sponsors, but in **Table 1** we have listed some multicenter trials undertaken by independent clinical investigators. Most of these studies are unique as they are pragmatic trials with little commercial interest, designed with primary outcomes such as death. Such trials are usually published on behalf of all the investigators, acknowledging the team effort involved.

Why are multicenter trials conducted?

Multicenter rather than single center trials are carried out for several reasons:

- When studying rare diseases, there will be a larger pool of patients to recruit from when using a multicenter trial. Therefore, the patient recruitment target will be reached more quickly than in a single-center study [3,4].
- For diseases with low event rates, treatments are likely to have a small absolute benefit and so large numbers (thousands) of patients might be needed in order to see a significant benefit.
- Multicenter trials provide a better basis for the subsequent generalization of the study findings [3,4] since the treatment benefits are not dependent on one specific center and, therefore, should be reproducible at other centers.
- Any bias that might be related to the practice methods of a single unit – where methods may be tailored to address local issues – will be reduced.
- Using many investigators to simultaneously evaluate a treatment gives more sources of feedback, allows more doctors and healthcare professionals to gain experience and confidence with the experimental intervention, and highlights any problems earlier. For example, the

Table 1. Examples of multicenter trials undertaken by independent clinical investigators.

Trial	Number of centers (countries involved)	Number of patients recruited/sample size for ongoing trial	Outcome	Reference
CESAR	98 online and recruitment of centers ongoing (UK)	180	Death or severe disability at 6 months post-randomization	www.cesar-trial.org
CRASH	239 online and recruitment of centers (UK and overseas)	10,008	Death from any cause within 2 weeks of injury Death or neurological deficit at 6 months	[5,6]
MAGPIE	193 (33 countries)	10,141	Eclampsia Death of baby	[7]
ORACLE	161 (15 countries)	4,826	Neonatal death/ chronic lung disease or major cerebral abnormality on ultrasonography before discharge	[8]
OSIRIS	229 (21 countries)	6,774	Death or oxygen dependence at 28 days Death or oxygen dependence at expected date of delivery	[9]
RITA 3	56 (UK)	1,810	Death, myocardial infarction, or refractory angina at 4 months Death or myocardial infarction at 1 year	[10]
TMC	8 (UK and Republic of Ireland)	606	Death, retransplantation, or treatment failure for immunologic reasons	[11]
UK collaborative trial of neonatal extracorporeal membrane oxygenation	55 (UK)	185	Death or severe disability at 12 months	[12]

CESAR = Conventional Ventilation or Extra Corporeal Membrane Oxygenation for Severe Adult Respiratory Failure; CRASH = Corticosteroid Randomisation After Significant Head Injury; MAGPIE = Magnesium Sulphate or Placebo for Women with Pre-Eclampsia; ORACLE = Broad Spectrum Antibiotics for Preterm, Prelabour Rupture of Fetal Membranes; OSIRIS = Open Study of Infants at High Risk of or with Respiratory Insufficiency – the Role of Surfactant; RITA 3 = Noninvasive Versus Invasive (Angiography) in Patients with Unstable Angina or Non-Q Wave Infarct; TMC = Tacrolimus Versus Microemulsified Cyclosporin in Liver Transplantation.

CRASH (Corticosteroid Randomisation After Significant Head Injury) trial was a large randomized controlled trial that examined whether an infusion of corticosteroids can reduce the immediate risk of subsequent death and neurologic disability when given to adults with head injury and impaired consciousness [5]. This large, multicenter trial aimed to gain feedback from many investigating clinicians, which is particularly useful since this intervention is conducted in a relatively high-risk situation [6].

- In certain cases, a difference in therapeutic approaches is being tested and multiple centers that have different facilities or access to treatments are needed. For example, the PCI-CURE (Percutaneous Coronary Intervention and Clopidogrel in Unstable Angina to Prevent Recurrent Ischemic Events) substudy compared patients given the antiplatelet agent clopidogrel or placebo and a routine coronary angiography and revascularization strategy as needed with patients in the main study comparing clopidogrel and placebo in a setting of angiography driven by clinical need only. Therefore, this trial needed centers both with and without access to angiography facilities [13].

How is a multicenter trial organized?

Once a specific question to test using a clinical trial structure has been identified, there is a well-defined procedure for planning and executing the trial [14]. A critical issue in multicenter trials is the coordination of the many investigators involved, all of whom are adhering to a single protocol. In **Figure 1** we outline the main steps and stages involved in a multicenter trial and give a typical timeline for such studies. **Figure 2** shows a typical organizational structure for a multicenter trial. Such large trials tend to have 5-year timelines, and therefore require an experienced coordinating team. The skills of such teams are being increasingly acknowledged and deserve some further explanation [15].

Role of the coordinating team in multicenter trials

The coordinating team for an investigator-led multicenter trial is often attached to a clinical or academic center. Many essential functions are the same regardless of whether the trial is single-center or multicenter. However, there are certain aspects that are unique to multicenter trials:

- site selection
- site recruitment
- obtaining national or regional ethics approvals
- constructing a multicenter randomization process for patient allocation to treatments

Figure 1. Typical timeline for a multicenter trial with the primary outcome assessed at 6 weeks. The activities will vary with each individual trial.

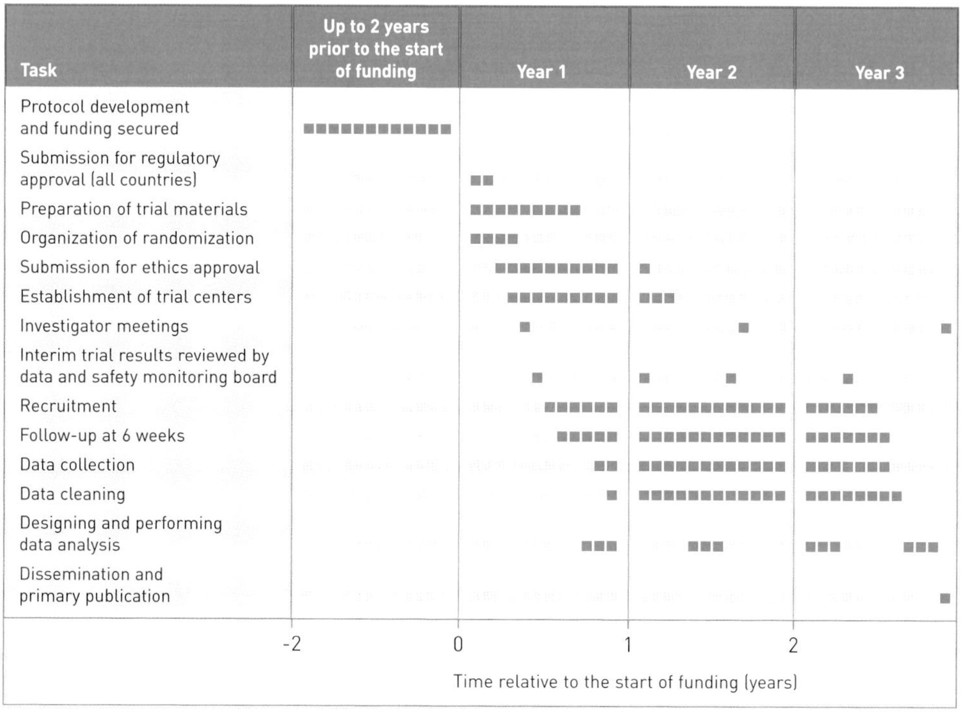

Task	Up to 2 years prior to the start of funding	Year 1	Year 2	Year 3
Protocol development and funding secured	▪▪▪▪▪▪▪▪▪▪▪▪▪			
Submission for regulatory approval (all countries)		▪▪		
Preparation of trial materials		▪▪▪▪▪▪▪▪▪		
Organization of randomization		▪▪▪▪		
Submission for ethics approval		▪▪▪▪▪▪▪▪▪▪	▪	
Establishment of trial centers		▪▪▪▪▪▪▪▪▪	▪▪▪	
Investigator meetings		▪	▪	▪
Interim trial results reviewed by data and safety monitoring board		▪	▪ ▪	▪
Recruitment		▪▪▪▪▪▪	▪▪▪▪▪▪▪▪▪▪▪▪	▪▪▪▪▪▪
Follow-up at 6 weeks		▪▪▪▪▪	▪▪▪▪▪▪▪▪▪▪▪▪	▪▪▪▪▪▪▪
Data collection		▪▪	▪▪▪▪▪▪▪▪▪▪▪▪	▪▪▪▪▪▪▪
Data cleaning		▪	▪▪▪▪▪▪▪▪▪▪▪▪	▪▪▪▪▪▪▪▪
Designing and performing data analysis		▪▪▪	▪▪▪	▪▪▪ ▪▪▪
Dissemination and primary publication				▪

-2	0	1	2

Time relative to the start of funding (years)

- site monitoring visits
- organizing local and international meetings for investigators and trial committees such as the steering, events adjudication, and data and safety monitoring board committees

Coordinating teams will also need to tag each item of data so that the center generating that item can be identified, and edit-queries regarding missing or incorrect data will need to be directed to the appropriate center. Throughout the trial, the coordinating team will maintain communications with all relevant parties (eg, from sites to academic institutions, from ethics and safety committees to sponsors), all of whom are likely to be independent of each other.

Finally, the coordinating team may assist with the dissemination of the results through further meetings or publications and presentations. Established and experienced coordinating teams are particularly successful because they are familiar with the many national ethics bodies and their requirements, and will be able to recruit centers that have already demonstrated an ability to meet recruitment targets and send data with minimal editing queries.

Figure 2. The typical life cycle of a multicenter clinical trial.

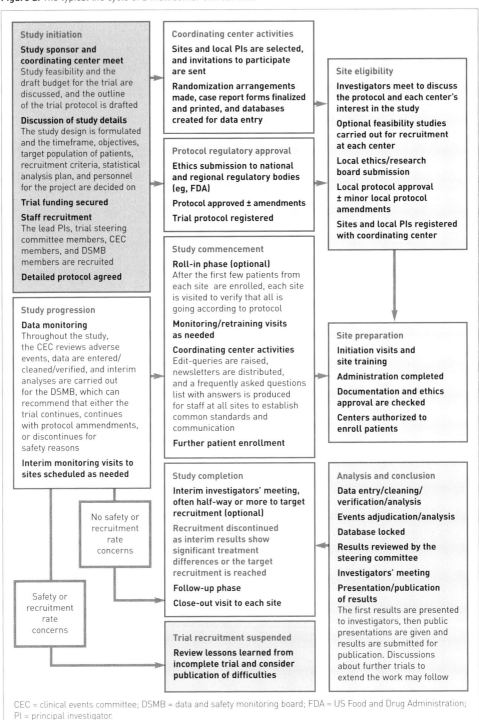

CEC = clinical events committee; DSMB = data and safety monitoring board; FDA = US Food and Drug Administration; PI = principal investigator.

Facilitating collaboration

Multicenter trials clearly involve more personnel than single-center studies, including a range of investigators and their research teams. The coordinating center must maintain records for all of these individuals, including their resumés and signatures. Such information is needed in order to conduct an audit at each stage of a trial to ensure that every piece of data can be linked to a specific researcher.

If there are any queries, the coordinating center will communicate with the local lead investigator who has responsibility for the actions of a center and its personnel. These local lead investigators will be identified in reports and acknowledged in publications of the primary results from the study. Coordinating centers should also confirm that 'black-listed' researchers do not participate in their studies. The US Food and Drug Administration (FDA) and other national agencies make available lists of clinicians who are suspended from performing certain types of research.

Meeting recruitment targets and maintaining morale in multicenter trials

In large trials, motivating centers to meet or maintain recruitment targets is essential because, once a few centers slow down, others might follow suit in a 'domino effect'. This task is made considerably harder by the large number of individuals involved in the trial. In a clinical setting, performing a randomized trial requires time and enthusiasm from already over-committed clinicians and nurses. Therefore, it is essential to market a trial in an imaginative (but ethical) way. Studies performed in key disease areas where there is a lot to gain by improving patients' quality of life tend to be successful. Such studies have greater impact and encourage the participation of centers and investigators.

The coordinating team can also boost morale with newsletters and meetings. Once the study is underway, an eye-catching trial newsletter can become an excellent source of study-specific information and can provide a source of answers to frequently asked questions. Anything that will raise the trial's profile should be considered, such as posters, pens, and promotional stands at appropriate conferences. If recruitment targets are being met, then it is important to keep the recruiting centers informed and to thank them. If targets are not being met, league tables of how many patients each center has recruited can be presented to act as a stimulus to slower recruiting centers. A trial-specific web site is also helpful, allowing investigators from different sites to communicate and raise protocol queries more effectively.

The logistics of organizing a multicenter trial

Ethics approval

Before a patient can be invited to take part in a trial, approval must be granted by the participating institution's ethics board. If such a board does not exist, independent ethics boards can be approached. Often, approval is also needed from the research and finance departments of each institution. Even before institutional approval is arranged, a national or regional ethics board might need to be approached for multicenter trials in some countries. Each country has its own particular system, and it is the role of the coordinating team to discover and get to know the requirements and help local collaborators to work their way through the approval process.

In the UK, for any trial conducted at five or more sites, an application must first be submitted for approval to a regional multicenter research ethics committee, and then to the relevant local research ethics committees covering each collaborating site. The documentation includes an approval application, the protocol, the drug/device specifications, and any prior research information and documentation intended for potential trial participants.

In the US, clinical trial protocols are submitted simultaneously to institutional review boards (IRBs) and the FDA, even before the centers are approached. The FDA submission is critical if data from the trial are to be later submitted to the FDA for regulatory approval of a new therapy or device. The FDA has a 30-day waiting period in which it can request further details of the protocol or ask for amendments before the trial can begin at centers. The FDA may advise on any aspect of the protocol, but particularly on whether sufficient data will be captured for later regulatory submission, such as toxicology and adverse event data, and the results of biochemical assays.

Two broad types of IRB exist: those that are based within academic institutions and those that are commercially operated. The former are responsible for ethics approvals for the hospitals within an academic network, while commercial IRBs make their ethics assessments irrespective of which sites will be recruiting. The approval that commercial IRBs provide can subsequently be used by any number of site management organizations (SMOs) without each SMO having to reapply to their own IRB.

IRBs and ethics boards are particularly interested in the safety and ethical aspects of trials (eg, consent procedures and incentives used to recruit subjects). They may request changes to consent documents, or changes in the trial design or protocol. This process can take several months, requiring further submissions and numerous negotiations. The consent form and case report forms might then have to be translated for use in multinational studies and minority ethnic communities. Protocols might also need to be translated for use by international researchers.

Selection of centers

The sites that are invited to participate can impact a trial in several ways. The sites invited should be both competent at undertaking the research and able to meet recruitment targets for the trial. The competency of centers can be determined both by external regulatory bodies – such as the FDA in the USA – or by internal audit committees. The purpose of such audits is to protect the rights, safety, and well-being of trial subjects, particularly as they might be vulnerable due to illness. Most sites now adhere to international codes of conduct for research, such as the International Conference on Harmonisation guidelines for Good Clinical Practice [14].

The number of centers needed for a multicenter trial will depend on the estimated number of eligible patients at each center. While some coordinating units keep records of recruitment rates from each site, other coordinating units perform a survey prior to authorizing sites to recruit patients, saving considerable time, frustration, and embarrassment later if recruitment rate projections are over-ambitious. Such surveys help to keep trials within their budgets.

Randomization of patients and interim analyses

The presence of additional sources of variability not present in single-center trials (due to variations in protocol adherence or the level of skill of the investigators at centers) is a specific drawback of multicenter trials. To minimize this variability, multicenter trials are designed to use a randomization method that equally distributes patients from each center to each treatment strategy (see **Chapter 7**). In this way, missing data from a single center are also distributed equally across the treatment groups.

Telephone randomization is currently the gold standard (with Internet and interactive voice-randomization services becoming increasingly popular), and imbalances in randomization can be dealt with by minimization criteria set out in the protocol. At an early stage in recruitment, the independent data and safety monitoring board will view the data by center if the sample size is large. Centers with large deviations in results will be scrutinized in more detail to ensure that there are no particular biases or problems. Towards the end of the study, statistical tests called *interaction tests* are performed to confirm that treatment outcomes are similar across all of the centers and that they are not unique to a few centers.

Financial considerations

Multicenter trials require more resources than single-center trials. Budgets for multicenter trials are more complex and usually require that several years of funding are secured from the start of the trial. Rarely can a multicenter trial be performed in under 1 year (although for the same protocol design, a multicenter trial will still be faster than a single-center trial). Also, start-up costs are often considerable, with compilation of a protocol, securing a center and personnel to manage the trial, designing and printing case report forms, invitation of researchers, and multiple ethics submissions required. Events such as investigator meetings, site authorization, and start-up visits will also need to be budgeted for. Often, large trials now have a 'roll-in' phase for the first few patients from each center before the trial gets into full swing. At the end of the roll-in phase, each site is visited to verify that all is going according to the protocol. At this stage, protocol deviations will trigger protocol amendments. In a multicenter trial, amendments are extremely troublesome as each ethics review board or IRB has to be notified of the amendment and all sites have to be sent revised paperwork.

The amount of data that a multicenter trial is to collect has an important bearing on funding. Large amounts of data are only necessary if they are to be used for regulatory submissions. Collecting, entering, and cleaning data is expensive, so it is important only to collect data that will be used in the final analysis.

For every trial that completes successfully, a number fail due to recruitment problems. If a trial is falling behind recruitment targets then it is essential to see this early on so that remedial measures can be taken such as adding centers.

Publication policy

In a multicenter trial there is usually a manuscript writing committee or group. This group helps to facilitate a standardized approach to all the statistical analyses, ensures that conclusions from the results are appropriate, recommends which investigators should be lead authors on publications, and deals with other authorship issues. The key publications from multicenter studies will usually acknowledge all participating investigators and may be authored simply as 'the "X" trial investigators'.

Conclusion

In recent years an increasing number of multicenter trials have been performed in medical research. Such trials bring with them a host of practical problems in terms of their design, conduct, and analysis because of their size, organizational complexity, and the large number of investigators involved. In this chapter we have examined some key issues, such as the need for, design of, and practicalities of coordinating multicenter trials. Careful consideration of these issues during the various stages of trial protocol development and coordination is important to the success of multicenter trials.

References

1. Chalmers I. Unbiased, relevant, and reliable assessments in health care: important progress during the past century but plenty of scope for doing better. *BMJ* 1998;**317**:1167–8.
2. Yusuf S, Collins R, Peto R. Why do we need some large, simple randomized trials? *Stat Med* 1984;**3**:409–20.
3. Friedman LM, Furberg CD, DeMets DL. *Fundamentals of Clinical Trials*. New York: Springer-Verlag, 1998.
4. Pocock SJ. *Clinical Trials: A Practical Approach*. New York: John Wiley & Sons, 1983.
5. MRC CRASH Trial Collaborative Group. Effect of intravenous corticosteroids on death within 14 days in 10,008 adults with clinically significant head injury (MRC CRASH trial): randomised placebo-controlled trial. *Lancet* 2004;**364**:1321–8.
6. Wasserberg J. Assessing corticosteroid treatment for severe head injury. *Clinical Researcher* 2001;**1**(3):21–5.
7. The Magpie Trial Collaborative Group. Do women with pre-eclampsia, and their babies, benefit from magnesium sulphate? The Magpie Trial: a randomised placebo controlled trial. *Lancet* 2002;**359**:1877–90.
8. Kenyon SL, Taylor DJ, Tarnow-Mordi W (for the ORACLE Collaborative Group). Broad spectrum antibiotics for preterm, prelabour rupture of fetal membranes: The ORACLE 1 randomised trial. ORACLE Collaborative Group. *Lancet* 2001;**357**:979–88.
9. The OSIRIS Collaborative Group. Early versus delayed neonatal administration of a synthetic surfactant – the judgment of OSIRIS. The OSIRIS Collaborative Group (open study of infants at high risk of or with respiratory insufficiency – the role of surfactant). *Lancet* 1992;**340**:1363–9.
10 Fox KAA, Poole-Wilson PA, Henderson RA. Interventional versus conservative treatment for patients with unstable angina or non-ST-elevation myocardial infarction: the British Heart Foundation RITA 3 randomised trial. *Lancet* 2002;**360**:743–51.
11. O'Grady JG, Burroughs A, Hardy P, et al. (for the UK and Republic of Ireland Liver Transplant Study Group). Tacrolimus versus microemulsified ciclosporin in liver transplantation: the TMC randomised controlled trial. *Lancet* 2002;**360**:1119–25.
12. UK Collaborative ECMO Trial Group. UK collaborative randomised trial of neonatal extracorporeal membrane oxygenation. *Lancet* 1996;**348**:75–82.
13. Mehta SR, Yusuf S, Peters RJ, et al. Effects of pretreatment with clopidogrel and aspirin followed by long-term therapy in patients undergoing percutaneous coronary intervention: the PCI-CURE study. *Lancet* 2001;**358**:527–33.
14. Flather M, Aston H, Stables RH, editors. *Handbook of Clinical Trials*. London: Remedica, 2001.
15. Farrell B. Efficient management of randomised controlled trials: nature or nurture. *BMJ* 1998;**317**:1236–9.

Part III

Basics of Statistical Analysis

Chapter 17

Types of Data and Normal Distribution

Duolao Wang, Ameet Bakhai, and Ashima Gupta

In a clinical trial, substantial amounts of data are recorded on each subject at randomization, such as the patient's demographic characteristics, disease-related risk factors, medical history, biochemical markers, and medical therapies, as well as outcome or endpoint data at various time points. These data can be quantitative or qualitative. Understanding the types of data is important as they determine which method of data analysis to use and how to report the results. In this chapter, we introduce data types and demonstrate ways of summarizing and presenting data in clinical research. In addition, we describe the fundamentals of the normal distribution theory and its applications.

What are data and variables?

In a clinical trial, a large amount of information is collected on various characteristics of subjects at randomization, as well as on efficacy and safety during follow-up visits. Sometimes, information on the participating centers in a multicenter study is also collected.

'Data' is a collective term for information gathered under various headings or variables. Variables may be related to demographic characteristics, such as age, gender, height, weight, and so forth; or be disease specific, such as the presence of a torn anterior cruciate ligament, coronary disease, or severity of breathlessness; or related to treatment response, such as reduction in pain, improvement of disease, return to work or sport, prolongation of life, or improvement in quality of life.

For example, in a clinical trial evaluating the effect of cardiac medications in patients with heart failure there will be two types of variables (data) collected:

- qualitative (or categorical) data; these characterize a certain quality of a subject (eg, gender, age group, or disease severity group)
- quantitative (or continuous or numerical) data; these represent a specific measure or count (eg, heart size, blood pressure, or heart rate)

Qualitative data can be classified further into three main groups:

- binary: only two possible responses (eg, gender)
- unordered: many equal responses (eg, race)
- ordered: responses have some form of increasing value (eg, disease severity)

To demonstrate some of the above concepts, let us consider data from an anonymized randomized clinical trial, conducted to assess physical exercise intervention on reducing the risk of coronary artery disease (CAD) among people aged between 60 and 70 years. **Table 1** provides baseline data for 10 participants, and the occurrence of CAD during the 5-year study period.

In the table, there are three binary variables (gender, treatment, and CAD status at 5 years), one unordered categorical variable (race), one ordered categorical variable (chest pain symptoms), and three numerical variables (age, systolic blood pressure [SBP], and heart rate). Each row in the dataset represents the values of all the variables for one subject – called an 'observation'. Each column represents the range of values for a specific variable. If the variable is quantitative, it can be numerically summarized by means, medians, modes, and standard deviations.

Table 1. Data from a hypothetical, randomized clinical trial, conducted to assess the administration of a new agent to reduce systolic blood pressure (SBP) among people aged between 60 and 70 years.

Subject	Age (years)	Gender	SBP (mm Hg)	Heart rate (bpm)	Chest pain symptoms	Race	Treatment	CAD present?	CAD-free time (days)
1	65.9	Male	189	62	No chest pain	White	Intervention	Yes	1,657
2	65.2	Female	207	60	Nonanginal pain	White	Control	Yes	283
3	66.8	Male	152	80	Atypical chest pain	Asian	Control	Yes	188
4	63.7	Male	154	60	Typical chest pain	Asian	Intervention	No	1,657
5	69.8	Male	158	65	No chest pain	Other	Control	Yes	1,257
6	68.1	Male	177	88	Nonanginal pain	White	Intervention	No	228
7	63.5	Female	99	100	Atypical chest pain	Other	Control	No	1,657
8	63.3	Male	153	94	No chest pain	White	Control	Yes	827
9	67.2	Male	123	72	Nonanginal pain	Asian	Intervention	No	1,656
10	68.6	Female	120	72	Atypical chest pain	White	Intervention	No	1,027

bpm = beats per minute; CAD = coronary artery disease.

The next concept we shall consider is that there might be relationships between these variables.

What are dependent and independent variables?

Multivariate regression techniques (see **Chapter 24**) are tools to explore relationships among a set of variables, particularly when at least three variables are involved. In regression analysis, one variable (the dependent variable) is usually taken to be the response or outcome variable, to be predicted by the other variables. These other variables are called *predictor* or *explanatory* variables or, sometimes, *independent* variables because multivariate regression analysis aims to separate the independent contribution of each of these variables to the outcome variable. For example, if we are interested in predicting the likelihood of a patient having CAD, then the CAD variable ('yes' or 'no') is the response variable, whereas age, gender, SBP, heart rate, chest pain symptoms, race, and smoking status may all be predictors or independent variables. If the relationship between these variables and CAD is strong then one can confidently predict the likelihood of being CAD-'yes' or CAD-'no' given the other variable values.

What are survival data?

In some medical research, the response variable indicates not only whether an event occurs, but also the time it takes for an event to occur. This kind of data requires a combination of a binary (event status) and a continuous variable (time). In the above example, investigators are interested in the factors that predict CAD-free time from the start of this study. In some instances, the event of interest is death (such as cardiovascular death), but it might be the end of a period of remission from a disease, the relief of symptoms, or a further admission to hospital. These types of data are generally referred to as 'time-to-event data' or most frequently 'survival data', even when the endpoint or the event being studied is something other than death. The terms 'survival analysis' or 'time-to-event analysis' encompass the methods and models that are applied to survival data.

Presenting summaries of variables

In medical reports, data are summarized for presentation by groups (such as the age-specific group for age distribution) using frequency distributions. These present the distribution of both qualitative and quantitative data, summarizing how often each value of a variable is repeated. With quantitative data, we mostly present a grouped frequency distribution table from which we can appreciate:

- the frequency (number of cases) occurring for each category or interval (eg, number of 70- to 74-year-old patients)
- the relative frequency (percentage) of the total sample in each category or interval (eg, 70- to 74-year-old patients comprised 10% of the overall sample)
- the highest and lowest or the range of possible values from our patient groups (eg, the oldest patient was aged over 95 years and the youngest patient was aged below 25 years)

Although a frequency table provides a detailed summary of the distribution of the data, the message from the data can be made more immediate by presenting the distribution in a graph or a chart. The type of graph presented depends on the type of data. Generally, for categorical data we prefer to use a bar chart or a pie chart. For continuous data, a histogram or frequency polygon is more appropriate; this can either represent data from the entire treatment group of patients or from smaller subgroups of interest. This gives an immediate way of seeing broad similarities or differences between treatment groups. We can then use statistical tests to ascertain whether any differences between the groups are significant.

Figure 1. Pie chart and bar chart for percentage distribution by gender and New York Heart Association (NYHA) class.

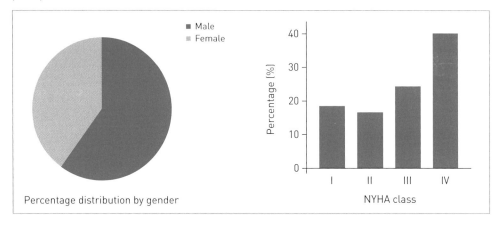

Figure 2. Histogram for systolic blood pressure (SBP) and polygon for heart rate.

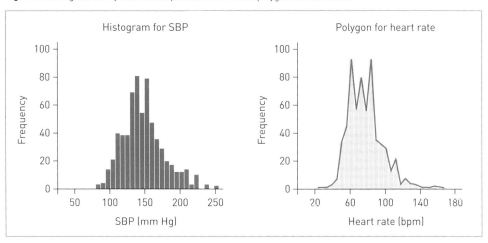

Box plots are another tool for conveying location and variation information for continuous data, particularly for detecting and illustrating location and variation changes between different groups of data.

Figure 1 shows a pie chart and a bar chart comparing the percentage distributions by gender and New York Heart Association class, respectively, of patients with heart failure. In **Figure 2**, a histogram and a frequency polygon are displayed to describe the SBP and heart rate, respectively.

Categorical variables are most conveniently summarized and presented in terms of percentages and compared by treatment groups. For quantitative variables we can do more than this, as we have other measures with which to summarize the data (summary measures). From the observed data, we can calculate the location (or central tendency) that summarizes where the center of the distribution lies and we can also summarize the spread, range, or variation of the distribution, and describe how widely the values are spread above and below the central value.

There are three measures commonly used to describe the location or 'center' of a distribution of a quantitative variable:

- mean: the mean can be calculated by summing all the values of observations and dividing by the total number of observations
- median: the median is the value that divides the distribution into equal numbers of observations. The median can be more appropriate for distributions that are skewed, such as physical fitness. When the distribution is symmetrical, the median equals the mean
- mode: the mode is the value that occurs most frequently, ie, the most typical value. There may be more than one mode if two values are equally frequent

The main differences between these measures of location are:

- the mean is sensitive to outliers, but the median and mode are not
- the mean and median are not affected by small changes in the data, while the mode may be

So which one should be presented? Generally, for skewed distributions (ie, asymmetrical distributions with extreme values) the median is a better measure of central location than the mean, though ideally it is worth presenting both. For statistical analysis and inference, the mean is more commonly used, although if the data are considerably skewed then statistical techniques based on medians should be employed.

Percentiles are also sometimes used to describe a variable distribution, giving proportions of the data that should fall above and below a given value. The pth percentile is a value such that at most $p\%$ of the measurements are less than this value and at most $(100 - p)\%$ are greater. The 50th percentile is the median. The most frequently used percentiles are the 25th, 50th, and 75th.

Table 2. Summary of systolic blood pressure (SBP) (mm Hg) by treatment and visit in a drug trial.

Statistics	Visit 1 (Baseline)		Visit 2 (2 weeks)		Visit 3 (4 weeks)		Visit 4 (6 weeks)	
	Drug	Placebo	Drug	Placebo	Drug	Placebo	Drug	Placebo
No. of patients	1,013	1,015	1,001	994	978	969	975	958
No. of unknowns	0	0	12	21	35	46	38	57
Mean	129.94	130.32	124.54	129.46	123.19	129.72	121.42	127.90
Standard deviation	18.97	18.52	20.05	18.51	20.48	19.34	20.60	18.71
25th percentile	117	118	110	116	110	118	108	114
Median	130	130	122	130	120	130	120	128
75th percentile	140	140	140	140	138	141	134	140

There are three measures commonly used to summarize the spread of a variable:

- standard deviation: this gives an indication of the average distance of all observations from the mean. The standard deviation has an important role in statistical analysis
- range: the difference between the highest and lowest values is known as the full range of values
- range between percentiles: percentiles are the value below which a given percentage of the data observations occur. A common range used is the interquartile range, which is the range between the 25th and 75th percentile. Using this overcomes the problem of extreme data values away from the mean or median

Each measure has its own advantages, but the standard deviation is more commonly used and is more often applied in statistical inference. For survival data, the median and range are often used to describe the central location and spread.

Example

In the clinical report of a pharmaceutical trial, descriptive statistics are often provided, such as number of observations, mean, standard deviation, median, and 25th and 75th percentiles by treatment. **Table 2** is such a table extracted from a clinical report, summarizing the SBP change at different visits in a randomized placebo-controlled clinical study assessing the effect of a study drug on reducing SBP. The table was designed to provide a quick reference to summary measures across the treatment groups at each visit. Three types of summary measures are tabulated.

Figure 3. Box plots of systolic blood pressure (SBP) data from Table 2.

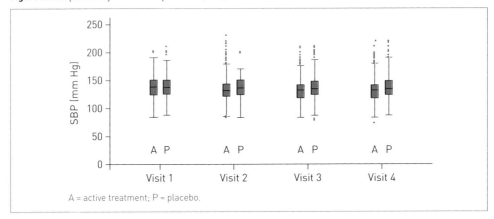

The first is the number of observations together with the number of missing observations. This sample size information is important in determining the strength of observed evidence and illustrating the dynamics of patient follow-up.

The second group of summary measures includes the mean and standard deviation. The former is the average level of SBP for the respective group, which shows that, after the baseline, patients on the study drug have a consistently lower SBP than the placebo group. The standard deviation provides a measure of the spread of SBP for the respective groups.

The third category of summary measures are three percentiles. The 25th percentile of SBP for the active treatment group at visit 2 is 110 mm Hg: 25% of patients had an SBP below 110 mm Hg (in the placebo group, 25% of patients had an SBP below 116 mm Hg). **Table 2** shows that the active treatment group has a consistently lower SBP than the placebo group after randomization in terms of the 25th, 50th, and 75th percentiles.

The SBP data in **Table 2** can also be summarized visually in a box plot (**Figure 3**), in which the vertical axis represents the SBP and the horizontal axis represents the factors of interest (treatment and visit). The box plot shows the main body (covering 50% of data values around median with the top of the box marking the 75th percentile and the bottom the 25th percentile) as well as individual values outlying the main body. This box plot, comparing SBP by treatment and visit, shows that the study drug has some effect on SBP after randomization with respect to both location and variation.

Figure 4. Histogram and fitted normal distribution curve for systolic blood pressures (SBPs) from 4,000 subjects.

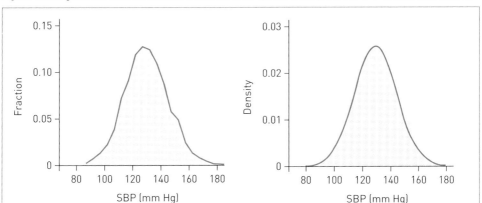

The normal distribution

In medical research, most quantitative variables have a range of values that occur with the highest frequency at a mean value and less frequently further away from this mean value, yielding a symmetric, bell-shaped frequency distribution. This is known as a *normal distribution*. The assumption of a normal distribution for outcome variables is a key prerequisite for various statistical analysis methods and models.

What is a normal distribution?

Quantitative (continuous) variables are those whose values can, in theory, take any numerical value within a given range. Consider the SBP measurements of 4,000 subjects participating in a health survey. **Figure 4** shows the frequency distribution of these SBPs. In the left-hand histogram, the height of each vertical bar shows the proportion (or fraction) of subjects whose SBP corresponded to a value within the 5 mm Hg intervals plotted on the basal axis. If the heights of all the bars in the histogram are summed then they will total 1, because all the observed values are represented in the histogram.

In the right-hand image, we have rescaled the histogram by dividing the height of each vertical bar by the width of the bar (5 mm Hg), generating a density histogram. In this histogram, the sum of the areas within all the bars equals 1. Indeed, if a curve is superimposed joining the midpoints of each of the bars then it forms a bell shape (solid curve in the left panel of **Figure 4**) and is very close to an underlying 'normal distribution' (solid curve in the right panel of **Figure 4**).

Figure 5. Normal distributions for simulated systolic blood pressure (SBP), with different standard deviations (SDs) and means.

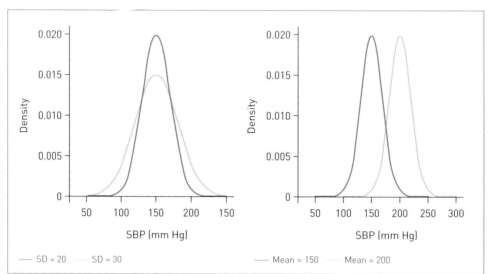

The normal distribution is the most important distribution in statistics. It is also known as the *Gaussian distribution* after the German mathematician Karl Friedrich Gauss who first gave the distribution its full description [3].

Properties of the (theoretical) normal distribution

The normal distribution is completely defined by two parameters: the *mean* (μ) or center point at which the curve peaks, and the *standard deviation* (σ) or a measure of the spread of each tail, expressed statistically as $N(\mu,\sigma^2)$. The value of the normal curve $N(\mu,\sigma^2)$ is:

$$f(x) = \frac{1}{\sigma\sqrt{2\pi}} \exp\left(\frac{-[x-\mu]^2}{2\sigma^2}\right)$$

$$\sigma > 0,\ -\infty < \mu < \infty,\ -\infty < x < \infty$$

Figure 5 gives examples of normal distributions for simulated SBP data. As μ changes, the normal distribution curve moves along the *x*-axis; as σ changes, the spread is closer or further away from μ. Distributions with different standard deviations have different spreads (**left panel**), whereas distributions with different means have different locations (**right panel**). However, whatever the shape of the distribution, the area under each curve is equal to 1, often expressed as 100%.

Some key properties of the normal distribution are as follows [2,3]:

- The curve has a single peak at the center; this peak occurs at the mean (μ).
- The curve is symmetrical about the mean (μ).
- The median is the value above and below which there is an equal number of values (or the mean of the two middle values if there is no middle number); hence, the median is equal to the mean.
- The total area under the curve is equal to 1.
- The spread of the curve is described by the standard deviation (σ) (the square of σ is the variance [σ^2]).
- 95% of the observations lie between $\mu - 1.96\sigma$ and $\mu + 1.96\sigma$.

Examples of random samples from normal distributions

For a variable measured from the population to be distributed normally, the above properties should be met. In clinical studies, we are usually interested in a set of values of a variable (or a sample) from a population with a certain disease. In this case, the distribution of the sample values might not exactly meet the above requirements. In fact, samples from a normal distribution will not necessarily seem to display a normal distribution themselves, especially if the sample size is small.

Figure 6 displays the histograms of samples of different sizes ($n = 20, 40, 100,$ and 400) drawn randomly from three normal distributions: $N(0,0.5^2)$, $N(0,1^2)$, and $N(0,5^2)$. The graphs show that few of the small samples display a normal distribution, but that closeness to a normal distribution increases with sample size.

Why is normal distribution important?

The normal distribution is statistically important for three reasons:

- Firstly, most biological, medical, and psychological variables such as height, weight, and SBP have approximately normal distributions.
- Secondly, many statistical tests assume that a quantitative outcome variable will have a normal distribution. Fortunately, these tests work very well even if the distribution is only approximately normally distributed.
- Thirdly, the sampling distribution of a mean is approximately normal even when the individual observations are not normally distributed, given a sufficiently large sample (such as >200) [3]. This particular notion is known as the *central limit theorem* [4].

Figure 6. Histograms for random samples from normal distributions.

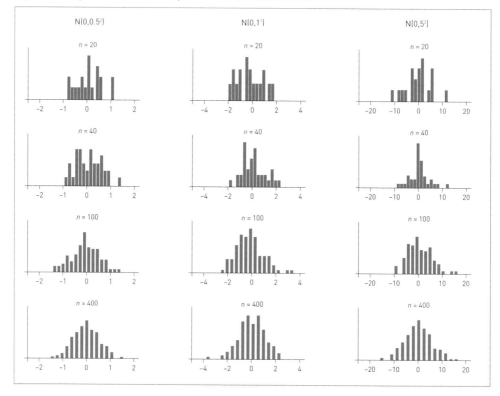

The sampling distribution is a distribution of a sample statistic (eg, the mean). The theorem says that if we draw N samples (each of size n) from a population and create a new variable, $\bar{X}$ (sampling distribution of mean), taking N values, the means for N samples will be $\bar{X}_1, \bar{X}_2, ..., \bar{X}_N$ and the distribution of $\bar{X}$ will be normal if the sample size n is large enough, regardless of whether the population distribution is normal. This theorem is fundamental to statistical inference [3,4].

What is a standard normal distribution?

The standard normal distribution is a special normal distribution with a mean of 0 and a standard deviation of 1 or N(0,1). This is a unique distribution whose distribution table is given in almost all statistical textbooks.

The standard normal distribution is important because any other normal distribution, N(μ,σ^2), can be converted to a standard normal distribution, N(0,1).

If a variable X follows N(μ,σ^2) then it can be mathematically transformed into a new variable Z with a standard normal distribution N(0,1) by the following formula:

$$Z = \frac{\overline{X} - \mu}{\sigma}$$

Z is sometimes called the *standard normal deviate* [2]. Take the SBP data as an example:

$$\text{as SBP follows N}(130,15^2), \text{ then } Z = \frac{SBP - 130}{15} \text{ follows the N(0,1)}$$

The transformation does not alter the shape of the distribution. All that happens is:

- The standardized mean takes the value 0 instead of 130 mm Hg, with lower values to the left and higher values to the right.
- The horizontal units are now standard deviations: +1 means one standard deviation away from the mean on the right.

Calculating the area under the curve

We can see from the last section that any normal distribution is linked to the standard normal distribution through a proper transformation. We can use this relationship to calculate some very useful statistics through the standard normal distribution table. **Table 3** gives areas in the tail of the standard normal distribution for some selected Z-values: the rows of the table refer to Z to one decimal place, and the columns to the second decimal place. The table shows the proportion of the area lying on the right (or upper tail) for each Z-value of the standard normal distribution. We will now use the SBP data (SBP follows N[130,15^2]) to demonstrate four common calculations performed on such data.

Area under the curve in the upper tail
Question 1: What proportion of subjects have an SBP above 160 mm Hg?
The above statistic can be computed in two steps:

Step 1: Obtain the standardized Z-value: Z = (160 – 130) / 15 = 2.00.

Step 2: Obtain a value of area corresponding to a Z-value of 2.00, by referring to **Table 3**, which states that the proportional area to the right of that Z-value is 0.0228.

Converting the proportion to a percentage, we can answer that about 2.28% of subjects will have an SBP above 160 mm Hg.

Table 3. Area in tail of the standard normal distribution.

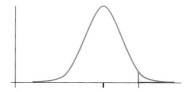

This table gives areas in the tail of the standard normal distribution for some selected Z-values: the rows of the table refer to Z to one decimal place, and the columns to the second decimal place. The table shows the proportion of the area lying on the right (or upper tail) for each Z-value of the standard normal distribution.

Z	Second decimal place of Z									
	0	0.01	0.02	0.03	0.04	0.05	0.06	0.07	0.08	0.09
0.0	0.5000	0.4960	0.4920	0.4880	0.4840	0.4801	0.4761	0.4721	0.4681	0.4641
0.1	0.4602	0.4562	0.4522	0.4483	0.4443	0.4404	0.4364	0.4325	0.4286	0.4247
0.2	0.4207	0.4168	0.4129	0.4090	0.4052	0.4013	0.3974	0.3936	0.3897	0.3859
0.3	0.3821	0.3783	0.3745	0.3707	0.3669	0.3632	0.3594	0.3557	0.3520	0.3483
0.4	0.3446	0.3409	0.3372	0.3336	0.3300	0.3264	0.3228	0.3192	0.3156	0.3121
0.5	0.3085	0.3050	0.3015	0.2981	0.2946	0.2912	0.2877	0.2843	0.2810	0.2776
0.6	0.2743	0.2709	0.2676	0.2643	0.2611	0.2578	0.2546	0.2514	0.2483	0.2451
0.7	0.2420	0.2389	0.2358	0.2327	0.2296	0.2266	0.2236	0.2206	0.2177	0.2148
0.8	0.2119	0.2090	0.2061	0.2033	0.2005	0.1977	0.1949	0.1922	0.1894	0.1867
0.9	0.1841	0.1814	0.1788	0.1762	0.1736	0.1711	0.1685	0.1660	0.1635	0.1611
1.0	0.1587	0.1562	0.1539	0.1515	0.1492	0.1469	0.1446	0.1423	0.1401	0.1379
1.1	0.1357	0.1335	0.1314	0.1292	0.1271	0.1251	0.1230	0.1210	0.1190	0.1170
1.2	0.1151	0.1131	0.1112	0.1093	0.1075	0.1056	0.1038	0.1020	0.1003	0.0985
1.3	0.0968	0.0951	0.0934	0.0918	0.0901	0.0885	0.0869	0.0853	0.0838	0.0823
1.4	0.0808	0.0793	0.0778	0.0764	0.0749	0.0735	0.0721	0.0708	0.0694	0.0681
1.5	0.0668	0.0655	0.0643	0.0630	0.0618	0.0606	0.0594	0.0582	0.0571	0.0559
1.6	0.0548	0.0537	0.0526	0.0516	0.0505	0.0495	0.0485	0.0475	0.0465	0.0455
1.7	0.0446	0.0436	0.0427	0.0418	0.0409	0.0401	0.0392	0.0384	0.0375	0.0367
1.8	0.0359	0.0351	0.0344	0.0336	0.0329	0.0322	0.0314	0.0307	0.0301	0.0294
1.9	0.0287	0.0281	0.0274	0.0268	0.0262	0.0256	0.0250	0.0244	0.0239	0.0233
2.0	0.0228	0.0222	0.0217	0.0212	0.0207	0.0202	0.0197	0.0192	0.0188	0.0183
2.1	0.0179	0.0174	0.0170	0.0166	0.0162	0.0158	0.0154	0.0150	0.0146	0.0143
2.2	0.0139	0.0136	0.0132	0.0129	0.0125	0.0122	0.0119	0.0116	0.0113	0.0110
2.3	0.0107	0.0104	0.0102	0.0099	0.0096	0.0094	0.0091	0.0089	0.0087	0.0084
2.4	0.0082	0.0080	0.0078	0.0075	0.0073	0.0071	0.0069	0.0068	0.0066	0.0064
2.5	0.0062	0.0060	0.0059	0.0057	0.0055	0.0054	0.0052	0.0051	0.0049	0.0048
2.6	0.0047	0.0045	0.0044	0.0043	0.0041	0.0040	0.0039	0.0038	0.0037	0.0036
2.7	0.0035	0.0034	0.0033	0.0032	0.0031	0.0030	0.0029	0.0028	0.0027	0.0026
2.8	0.0026	0.0025	0.0024	0.0023	0.0023	0.0022	0.0021	0.0021	0.0020	0.0019
2.9	0.0019	0.0018	0.0018	0.0017	0.0016	0.0016	0.0015	0.0015	0.0014	0.0014
3.0	0.0013	0.0013	0.0013	0.0012	0.0012	0.0011	0.0011	0.0011	0.0010	0.0010

Table 3 contd.

Z	Second decimal place of Z									
3.1	0.0010	0.0009	0.0009	0.0009	0.0008	0.0008	0.0008	0.0008	0.0007	0.0007
3.2	0.0007	0.0007	0.0006	0.0006	0.0006	0.0006	0.0006	0.0005	0.0005	0.0005
3.3	0.0005	0.0005	0.0005	0.0004	0.0004	0.0004	0.0004	0.0004	0.0004	0.0003
3.4	0.0003	0.0003	0.0003	0.0003	0.0003	0.0003	0.0003	0.0003	0.0003	0.0002
3.5	0.0002	0.0002	0.0002	0.0002	0.0002	0.0002	0.0002	0.0002	0.0002	0.0002
3.6	0.0002	0.0002	0.0001	0.0001	0.0001	0.0001	0.0001	0.0001	0.0001	0.0001
3.7	0.0001	0.0001	0.0001	0.0001	0.0001	0.0001	0.0001	0.0001	0.0001	0.0001
3.8	0.0001	0.0001	0.0001	0.0001	0.0001	0.0001	0.0001	0.0001	0.0001	0.0001
3.9	0.0000	0.0000	0.0000	0.0000	0.0000	0.0000	0.0000	0.0000	0.0000	0.0000
4.0	0.0000	0.0000	0.0000	0.0000	0.0000	0.0000	0.0000	0.0000	0.0000	0.0000

Area under the curve in the lower tail

Question 2: What percentage of subjects have an SBP below 110 mm Hg?
Similarly to in Question 1, we can calculate that $Z = -1.33$. As the standard normal distribution is symmetrical about zero, the area below -1.33 is equal to the area above 1.33; this area equals 0.0918. Thus, 9.18% of subjects have an SBP lower than 110 mm Hg.

The area under the curve within a certain range

Question 3: What proportion of subjects have an SBP between 110 and 160 mm Hg?
This can be calculated in three steps:

Step 1: The proportion above 160 mm Hg, as calculated in Question 1, is 2.28%.

Step 2: The proportion below 110 mm Hg, as calculated in Question 2, is 9.18%.

Step 3: The proportion of subjects with an SBP between 110 and 160 mm Hg:
= 1 – (proportion above 160 mm Hg + proportion below 110 mm Hg)
= 1 – (2.28% + 9.18%) = 88.54%

The area under the curve in two-sided symmetric tails

Question 4: What proportion of subjects have an SBP above 130 + 15 mm Hg and below 130 – 15 mm Hg?
The areas described here are known as two-sided percentages, as they cover the observations symmetrically in both the upper and lower tails. The proportions given in **Table 3** are one-sided areas in the each tail (α). To determine a two-sided proportion, we simply double the area (denoted as 2α).

The one-sided area above 130 + 15 mm Hg is 15.87% (calculated using the procedure set out in Question 1). Therefore, the two-sided area above 130 + 15 mm Hg or below 130 – 15 mm Hg is twice the one-sided area, ie, 2 × 15.87% = 31.74%.

This result suggests that, for any normal distribution, about 68% of all observations are bounded within one standard deviation distance either side of the mean (eg, for SBP data, 130 ± 15 mm Hg). It can be similarly calculated that about 95% of all observations fall within the mean ± 1.96 × standard deviations either side of the mean, which is often called the *95% reference range*.

How do we assess normality?

As mentioned, the normality assumption is a prerequisite for many statistical methods and models, such as *t*-tests, analyses of variance, and regression analysis. This assumption should be checked on a given dataset when conducting statistical analysis, especially with smaller sample sizes.

There are two ways of doing this:

- graphical inspection of the data to visualize differences between data distributions and theoretical normal distributions
- formal numeric statistical tests

Histograms are sometimes used for visual inspection, but are unreliable for small sample sizes (as demonstrated in **Figure 6**). The most common graphical approach is the *inverse normal plot*, or the *quantile–quantile plot* (Q-Q plot), which compares ordered values of a variable with corresponding quantiles of a specific theoretical normal distribution. If the data and the theoretical distributions match, the points on the plot form a linear pattern that passes through the origin and has a unit slope.

Figure 7 shows the inverse normal plots for the data represented in **Figure 6**. These demonstrate that the plots are almost linear and pass through the origin, suggesting that these samples represent a normal distribution. **Figure 8** displays a histogram and inverse normal plot for creatine kinase data for 2,668 patients with chronic heart failure from a clinical trial. The histogram indicates that the distribution of creatine kinase is not normal – it is positively skewed. The inverse normal plot shows marked departure from a linear pattern, especially at the lower and upper range of the data, indicating that a distribution other than the normal distribution would better fit these data.

Figure 7. Visual inspection of normality by inverse normal plot using data from Figure 6.

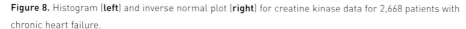

Figure 8. Histogram (**left**) and inverse normal plot (**right**) for creatine kinase data for 2,668 patients with chronic heart failure.

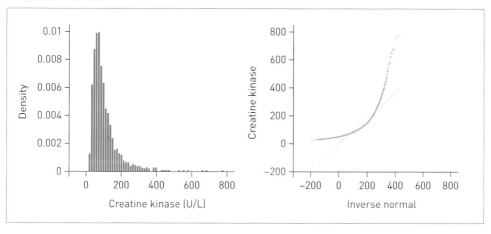

Although visually appealing, these graphical methods do not provide objective criteria to determine the normality of variables, and interpretations are a matter of judgment. Numerical methods, such as the Kolmogorov–Smirnov, Shapiro–Wilk, Anderson–Darling, and Cramer–von Mises tests, are more formal [4,5]. The most commonly performed test is the Shapiro–Wilk test, which produces an S-W statistic together with a *P*-value for testing the null hypothesis that the data are normally distributed [4,5].

Conclusion

In this chapter, we have described the different types of data and simple ways of summarizing and presenting them. Understanding these concepts and methods is important for using statistical methods properly. If you would like to understand more about these concepts, references [1] and [2] provide a useful discussion of the topics and issues discussed.

We have also provided an overview of the normal distribution. A normal distribution is characterized by a symmetrical bell curve defined by two parameters: mean (μ) and standard deviation (σ^2), expressed as $N(\mu,\sigma^2)$. The normal distribution is the fundamental basis of many statistical methods and models. The area under the normal distribution curve, which represents the proportion of subjects in a range, can be derived from the standard normal distribution $N(0,1)$ by transforming the given data distribution to the standard normal distribution.

The use of histograms for checking normality of a sample is limited when the sample size is small, and in this instance an inverse normal plot or numerical tests for normality should be performed. When the given data are not normally distributed then a more detailed transformation might be needed [1,2].

References

1. Altman DG. *Practical Statistics for Medical Research*. London: Chapman and Hall, 1999.
2. Kirkwood B, Sterne J. *Essential Medical Statistics*, 2nd edition. Oxford: Blackwell Publishing, 2003.
3. Armitage P, Colton T, editors. Encyclopaedia of Biostatistics: Statistical Theory and Methods. New York: John Wiley & Sons, 1998.
4. Cramér H. Random Variables and Probability Distributions (Cambridge Tracts in Mathematics), New edition. Cambridge: Cambridge University Press, 2004.
5. Shapiro SS, Wilk MB. An analysis of variance test for normality (complete samples). *Biometrika* 1965;**52**:591–611.

Chapter 18

Significance Tests and Confidence Intervals

Duolao Wang, Tim Clayton, and Hong Yan

The primary objective of a clinical trial is to provide a reliable estimate of the true treatment effect regarding the efficacy and/or safety of an investigational medicine or therapeutic procedure. Three major factors can influence the observed treatment difference away from the true treatment effect. These are bias, confounding, and chance/random error. Assuming no bias or confounding exists, statistical analysis deals with chance; by providing statistical estimation and testing (inference), it assesses whether random variation could reasonably explain the differences seen. While statistical estimates summarize the distribution of a measured outcome variable in terms of point estimate (eg, mean or proportion) and measure of precision (eg, confidence intervals), statistical testing involves an assessment of the probability of obtaining an observed treatment difference or more extreme difference in the outcome variable, assuming there is no difference in the population. In this chapter, we introduce the ideas underlying the principles of statistical inference and describe two statistical techniques (hypothesis testing and confidence intervals), with emphasis on their interpretation and application.

Sample, population, and statistical inference

Suppose that it is necessary to measure the average systolic blood pressure (SBP) level of all males aged ≥16 years in the UK in 2005. For practical and financial reasons, it is not possible to directly measure the SBP of every adult male in the UK; instead, we can conduct a survey among a subset (or 'sample') of 500 males within this population. Through statistical inference, we can measure the properties of the sample (such as the mean and standard deviation) and use these values to infer the properties of the entire UK adult male population [1,2]. This process is illustrated in **Figure 1**.

Population properties are usually determined by population parameters (numerical characteristics of a population) that are fixed and usually unknown quantities, such as the mean (μ) and standard deviation (σ) in a normal distribution $N(\mu,\sigma^2)$ (see **Chapter 17**). [3]. The statistical properties of the sample, such as the mean ($\bar{X}$) and standard deviation (S), can be used to provide estimates of the corresponding population parameters. Conventionally, Greek letters are used to refer to population parameters, while Roman letters refer to sample estimates.

Two strategies that are often used to make statistical inference are [2,3]:

- hypothesis testing
- confidence intervals (CIs)

These two methods are introduced below, illustrated with examples.

Hypothesis testing

Statistical inference can be made by performing a hypothesis (or significance) test, which involves a series of statistical calculations [3,4]. In the sample of 500 adult males, the mean SBP ($\bar{X}$) was 130 mm Hg, with a standard deviation (S) of 10 mm Hg. The empirical estimate for the mean SBP of this population from previous medical literature is reported as 129 mm Hg (denoted by μ_0). So, we want to know whether there is any evidence that the mean SBP value for all adult males in the UK in 2005 (μ) is different from 129 mm Hg (μ_0).

Step 1: Null and alternative hypotheses
We start by stating a hypothesis that the population mean SBP for all adult men in 2005 is 129 mm Hg, or $\mu = \mu_0$ (ie, no different to that reported in the medical literature). This is referred to as the null hypothesis and is usually written as H_0,

Figure 1. Making statistical inferences about a population from a sample by means of a significance test and confidence intervals.

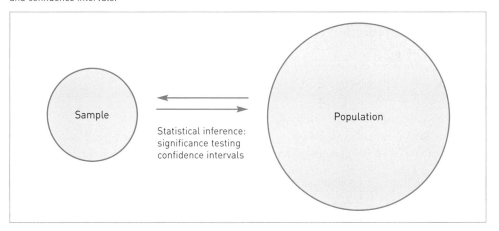

representing a theory that has been put forward as a basis for argument [2–4]. The hypothesis test is a means to assess the strength of evidence against this null hypothesis of no difference.

The alternative hypothesis, usually written as H_a, is that the mean SBP for the study population is not equal to the specified value, ie, $\mu \neq \mu_0$. Note that under the alternative hypothesis, the 2005 population mean could be higher or lower than the reference mean. The statistical test for the above hypotheses is usually referred to as a two-sided test.

Step 2: Choose an appropriate statistical method and calculate a test statistic

Once the null hypothesis has been chosen we need to calculate the probability that, if the null hypothesis is true, the observed data (or data that were more extreme) could have been obtained [2,3]. To reach this probability, we need to calculate a test statistic from the sample data (eg, $\bar{X}$, S, and n for quantitative outcomes) using an appropriate statistical method. This test statistic is then compared to the distribution (eg, the normal distribution) implied by the null hypothesis to obtain the probability of observing our data or more extreme data.

For the SBP data, given the relatively large sample size, we can use the Z-test to calculate the value of the test statistic Z. The Z-test is expressed by the following formula [2,3]:

$$Z = \frac{\bar{X} - \mu_0}{S / \sqrt{n}}.$$

This statistic follows a normal standard distribution under the null hypothesis [2,3]. For the SBP data:

- $\overline{X} = 130$ mm Hg
- $S = 10$ mm Hg
- $n = 500$
- $\mu_0 = 129$ mm Hg

Replacing the values in the formula generates $Z = 2.24$.

A variety of statistical methods can be used to address different study questions (eg, comparing treatment difference in means and proportions), and we will introduce a number of standard statistical methods in later chapters. The choice of statistical test will depend on the types of data and hypotheses under question [2,3].

Step 3: Specify a significance level and determine its critical values according to the distribution of the test statistic

Having obtained the appropriate test statistic (in our example, the Z-value), the next step is to specify a significance level. This is a fixed probability of wrongly rejecting the null hypothesis, H_0, if it is in fact true. This probability is chosen by the investigators, taking into account the consequences of such an error [2,3]. That is, the significance level is kept low in order to reduce the chance of inadvertently making a false claim. The significance level, denoted by α, is usually chosen to be 0.05 (5%), but can sometimes be set at 0.01.

Figure 2 graphically displays the α of a two-sided Z-test under the null hypothesis, ie, the area under the normal distribution curve below $-Z_{\alpha/2}$ and above $Z_{\alpha/2}$. The corresponding $Z_{\alpha/2}$ is called the critical value of the Z-test. The critical value for a hypothesis test is a threshold with which the value of the test statistic calculated from a sample is compared in order to determine the P-value to be introduced in the next step.

From **Figure 2**, we see that a two-sided Z-test has an equal chance of showing that μ (mean SBP of adult males in our sample) is bigger than μ_0 on one side (above $Z_{\alpha/2}$) or smaller than μ_0 (below $-Z_{\alpha/2}$) on the other side if the null hypothesis is true. The area under the curve below $-Z_{\alpha/2}$ and above $Z_{\alpha/2}$ is known as the *null hypothesis rejection region*. If the Z-value falls within this region then the null hypothesis is rejected at the α level.

- If $\alpha = 0.05$, we have $Z_{0.05/2} = 1.96$.
- If $\alpha = 0.01$, we have $Z_{0.01/2} = 2.58$.

Figure 2. Null hypothesis rejection regions (shaded areas) of two-sided Z-test.

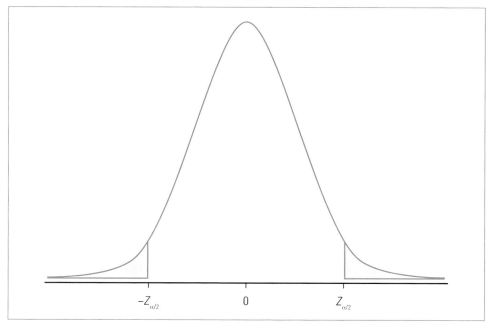

Step 4: Determine a P-value by comparing the value of the test statistic with the critical value

A P-value is the probability of our result ($Z = 2.24$ for the SBP data) or a more extreme result ($Z \leq -2.24$ or $Z > 2.24$) being observed, assuming that the null hypothesis is true. The exact P-value in the Z-test is the probability of $Z \leq -Z_{\alpha/2}$ or $Z \geq Z_{\alpha/2}$, which can always be determined by calculating the area under the curve in two-sided symmetric tails from a statistical table, specifically of a normal distribution (see **Chapter 17**) [3]. For the SBP data, the exact P-value is 0.025.

In a practical application, we often need to determine whether the P-value is smaller than a specified significance level, α. This is done by comparing the value of the test statistic with the critical value. It can be seen from **Figure 2** that $P \leq \alpha$ if, and only if:

- $Z \leq -Z_{\alpha/2}$; or
- $Z \geq Z_{\alpha/2}$

For the SBP data, since $Z = 2.24 > Z_{0.05/2} = 1.96$, we can conclude that $P < 0.05$. It can be seen from **Figure 2** that a smaller P-value indicates that Z is further away from the center (ie, the null value $\mu - \mu_0 = 0$), and consequently provides stronger evidence to support the alternative hypothesis of a difference.

Although the P-value measures the strength of evidence for a difference, which is largely dependent on the sample size, it does not provide the size and direction of that difference. Therefore, in a statistical report, P-values should be provided together with CIs (described in detail later) for the main outcomes [3].

Step 5: Make a statistical inference

We are now in a position to interpret the P-value in relation to our data and decide whether there is sufficient evidence to reject the null hypothesis. Essentially, if $P \leq \alpha$, the prespecified significance level, then there is evidence against the null hypothesis and we accept the alternative hypothesis and say that there *is* a statistically significant difference. The smaller the P-value, the lower the chance of obtaining a difference as big as the one observed if the null hypothesis were true, and, therefore, the stronger the evidence against the null hypothesis. Otherwise, if $P > \alpha$, there is insufficient evidence to reject the null hypothesis, or there is *no* statistically significant difference.

For our SBP data, since $P < 0.05$, we can state that there is some evidence to reject the null hypothesis of no difference at the 5% significance level, and, therefore, that the mean SBP for the adult male population is statistically significantly different from 129 mm Hg. Furthermore, the actual P-value equals 0.025, which suggests that the probability of falsely rejecting the null hypothesis is 1 in 40 if the null hypothesis is indeed true. On the other hand, $Z_{0.005} = 2.58 > Z = 2.24$, calculating $P > 0.01$. Now we say that there is no evidence to reject the null hypothesis of no difference if the significance level α is chosen as 0.01.

The implementation of the above procedures for hypothesis testing with the SBP data is summarized in **Table 1**.

Type I (alpha) and Type II (beta) errors

When performing a hypothesis test, two types of error can occur. To explain these two types of error, we will use the example of a randomized, double-blind, placebo-controlled clinical trial on a cholesterol-lowering drug 'A' in middle-aged men and women considered to be at high risk for a heart attack. The primary endpoint is the reduction in the total cholesterol level at 6 months from randomization.

The null hypothesis is that there is no difference in mean cholesterol reduction at 6 months following randomization between patients receiving drug A (μ_1) and patients receiving placebo (μ_2) (H$_0$: $\mu_1 = \mu_2$); the alternative hypothesis is that there is a difference (H$_a$: $\mu_1 \neq \mu_2$). If the null hypothesis is rejected when it is in fact true, then a Type I error (or false-positive result) occurs. For example, a Type I error is made if the trial result suggests that drug A reduced cholesterol levels when in fact there is no difference between drug A and placebo. The chosen

Table 1. Practical procedures for hypothesis testing.

Step	Procedure	Illustration with SBP data
1	Set up a null hypothesis and alternative hypothesis that is of particular interest to study	H_0: $\mu = \mu_0$ (= 129), ie, population mean SBP is equal to 129 mm Hg H_a: $\mu \neq \mu_0$, ie, population mean SBP is different from 129 mm Hg
2	Choose a statistical method according to data type and distribution, and calculate its test statistic from the data collected	$Z = \dfrac{\bar{X} - \mu_0}{S / \sqrt{n}} = 2.24$ $\bar{X} = 130$ mm Hg $S = 10$ mm Hg $n = 500$
3	Define a significance level α and its corresponding critical value	$\alpha = 0.05$ and $Z_{\alpha/2} = 1.96$ $\alpha = 0.01$ and $Z_{\alpha/2} = 2.58$
4	Determine the P-value by comparing the test statistic and the critical value, or calculate the exact P-value	Since $Z = 2.24 > 1.96$, $P < 0.05$ Since $Z = 2.24 < 2.58$, $P > 0.01$ Exact P-value = 0.025
5	Make your conclusion according to the P-value	As $0.01 < P < 0.05$, there is evidence to reject the null hypothesis of no difference at the 5% level of significance, but there is no evidence to reject the null hypothesis at the 1% level. The P-value of 0.025 means that the probability of falsely rejecting the null hypothesis is 1 in 40 if the null hypothesis is true

SBP = systolic blood pressure.

probability of committing a Type I error is known as the significance level [1–4]. As in Step 3 above, the level of significance is denoted by α. In practice, α represents the *consumer's risk* [5], which is often chosen to be 5% (1 in 20).

On the other hand, if the null hypothesis is not rejected when it is actually false, then a Type II error (or false-negative result) occurs [1–4]. For example, a Type II error is made if the trial result suggests that there is no difference between drug A and placebo in lowering the cholesterol level when in fact drug A does reduce the total cholesterol. The probability of committing a Type II error, denoted by β, is sometimes referred to as the *manufacturer's risk* [5]. The power of the test is given by $1 - \beta$, representing the probability of correctly rejecting the null hypothesis when it is in fact false. It relates to detecting a prespecified difference (see **Chapter 8** for more). Type I and II errors are summarized in **Table 2**.

Confidence intervals

The second strategy for making statistical inference is through the use of CIs. In making inference about a population, we might want to know the likely value of the unknown population mean (μ). This is estimated from the sample mean ($\bar{X}$), and we call $\bar{X}$ a point estimate of μ.

Table 2. Type I and II errors in hypothesis testing.

	If $H_0 : \mu_1 = \mu_2$ is:	
Statistical inference	**True**	**False**
Reject H_0: significant difference	Type I error (α) 'Consumer's risk'	Correct
Retain H_0: nonsignificant difference	Correct	Type II error (β) 'Manufacturer's risk'

In addition, we might want to provide some measure of our uncertainty as to how close the sample mean is to the true population mean. This is done by calculating a CI (or interval estimate) – a range of values that has a specified probability of containing the true population parameter being estimated. For example, a 95% CI for the mean is usually interpreted as a range of values containing the true population mean with a probability of 0.95 [2]. The formula for the $(1 - \alpha)\%$ CI around the sample mean ($\bar{X}$) corresponding to the Z-test, is given by:

$$\bar{X} \pm Z_{\alpha/2} SE(\bar{X})$$

where $SE(\bar{X})$ is the standard error of $\bar{X}$, calculated by $S / \sqrt{n}$. This is a measure of the uncertainty of a single sample mean ($\bar{X}$) as an estimate of the population mean [2]. This uncertainty decreases as the sample size increases. The larger the sample size, the smaller the standard error – therefore the narrower the interval, the more precise the point estimate.

For our SBP example, the 95% CI for the population mean (μ) can be calculated with the following formula:

$$\bar{X} \pm 1.96S / \sqrt{n} = 129.1 \text{ to } 130.9 \text{ mm Hg}$$

This means that the interval between 129.1 and 130.9 mm Hg has a 0.95 probability of containing the population mean μ. In other words, we are 95% confident that the true population mean is between 129.1 and 130.9 mm Hg, with the best estimate being 130 mm Hg.

CIs can be calculated not just for a mean, but also for any estimated parameter depending on the data types and statistical methods used (see references [2,3] for more). For example, you could estimate the proportion of people who smoke in a population, or the difference between the mean SBP in subjects taking an antihypertensive drug and those taking a placebo.

Relationship between significant testing and CIs

When comparing, for example, two treatments, the purpose of significance testing is to assess the evidence for a difference in some outcome between the two groups, while the CI provides a range of values around the estimated treatment effect within which the unknown population parameter is expected to be with a given level of confidence.

There is a close relationship between the results of significance testing and CIs. This can be illustrated using the previously described Z-test for the SBP data analysis. If $H_0: \mu = \mu_0$ is rejected at the $\alpha\%$ significance level, the corresponding $(1 - \alpha)\%$ CI will not include μ_0. On the other hand, if $H_0: \mu = \mu_0$ is not rejected at the $\alpha\%$ significance level, then $(1 - \alpha)\%$ CI will include μ_0.

For the SBP data of adult males, the significance test shows that μ is significantly different from μ_0 (= 129 mm Hg) at the 5% level, and the 95% CI (= 129.1 to 130.9 mm Hg) did not include 129 mm Hg. On the other hand, the difference between μ and μ_0 is not significant at the 1% level; the 99% CI ($129 \pm [2.58 \times 10] / \sqrt{500} = 128.8$ to 131.2 mm Hg) for μ does indeed contain μ_0. Further information about the proper use of the above two statistical methods can be found in [6].

Further examples

Let us assume that four randomized, double-blind, placebo-controlled trials are conducted to establish the efficacy of two weight-loss drugs (A and B) against placebo, with all subjects, whether on a drug or placebo, receiving similar instructions as to diet, exercise, behavior modification, and other lifestyle changes. The primary endpoint is the weight change (kg) at 2 months from baseline. The difference in the mean weight change between active drug and placebo groups can be considered as weight reduction for the active drug against placebo. **Table 3** presents the results of hypothesis tests and CIs for the four hypothetical trials. The null hypothesis for each trial is that there is no difference between the active drug treatment and placebo in mean weight change.

In trial 1 of drug A, the reduction of drug A over placebo was 6 kg, with only 40 subjects in each group. The P-value of 0.074 suggests that there is no evidence against the null hypothesis of no effect of drug A at the 5% significance level. The 95% CI shows that the results of the trial are consistent with a difference ranging from a large reduction of 12.6 kg in favor of drug A to a reduction of 0.6 kg in favor of placebo.

Table 3. Point estimate and 95% CI for the difference in mean weight change from baseline between the active drug and placebo groups in four hypothetical trials of two weight-reduction drugs.

Trial	Drug	No. of patients per group	Difference in mean weight change from baseline (kg) between the active drug and placebo groups	Standard deviation of difference	Standard error of difference	95% CI for difference		P-value
1	A	40	-6	15	3.4	-12.6	0.6	0.074
2	A	400	-6	15	1.1	-8.1	-3.9	<0.001
3	B	40	-4	15	3.4	-10.6	2.6	0.233
4	B	800	-2	15	0.8	-3.5	-0.5	0.008

The results for trial 2 among 400 patients, again for drug A, suggest that mean weight was again reduced by 6 kg. This trial was much larger, and the P-value ($P < 0.001$) shows strong evidence against the null hypothesis of no drug effect. The 95% CI suggests that the effect of drug A is a greater reduction in mean weight over placebo of between 3.9 and 8.1 kg. Because this trial was large, the 95% CI was narrow and the treatment effect was therefore measured more precisely.

In trial 3, for drug B, the reduction in weight was 4 kg. Since the P-value was 0.233, there was no evidence against the null hypothesis that drug B has no statistically significant benefit effect over placebo. Again, this was a small trial with a wide 95% CI, ranging from a reduction of 10.6 kg to an increase of 2.6 kg for drug B against placebo.

The fourth trial on drug B was a large trial in which a relatively small, 2-kg reduction in mean weight was observed in the active treatment group compared with the placebo group. The P-value (0.008) suggests that there is strong evidence against the null hypothesis of no drug effect. However, the 95% CI shows that the reduction is as little as 0.5 kg and as high as 3.5 kg. Even though this is convincing statistically, any recommendation for its use should consider the small reduction achieved alongside other benefits, disadvantages, and costs of this treatment. This is an important concept since even a clinically small benefit can be made to be statistically significant with enough patients. This may not, however, be a cost-effective change in practice.

Key points from the four trials are summarized in **Table 4**.

Table 4. Summary of the key points from the results described in Table 3.

Key points from significance test and CI	Examples
In a small study, a large *P*-value does not mean that the null hypothesis is true – 'absence of evidence is not evidence of absence'	Trials 1 and 3
A large study has a better chance of detecting a given treatment effect than a small study, and is therefore more powerful	Trials 2 and 4
A small study usually produces a CI for the treatment effect that is too wide to allow any useful conclusion	Trials 1 and 3
A large study usually produces a narrow CI, and therefore a precise estimate of treatment effect	Trials 2 and 4
The smaller the *P*-value, the lower the chance of falsely rejecting the null hypothesis, and the stronger the evidence for rejecting the null hypothesis	Trials 2 and 4
Even if the *P*-value shows a statistically significant result, it does not mean that the treatment effect is clinically significant. The clinical importance of the estimated effects should always be assessed	Trial 4

Conclusion

Based on the assumption of no bias or confounding in an ideal clinical trial, statistical inference assesses whether an observed treatment difference is real or due to chance.

The most common type of inference involves comparing different parameters, such as means and proportions, by performing a hypothesis test and estimating a CI. The former indicates the strength of the evidence against the null hypothesis, while the latter gives us a point estimate of the population difference, together with the range of values within which we are reasonably confident that the true population difference lies.

Both *P*-values and CIs for the main outcomes should be reported in an analysis report. Any statistical inferential results are subject to two types of errors: Type I (false positive) and Type II (false negative). Finally, it should be stated that a statistically significant difference is not always the same as a clinically significant difference, and both should be considered when interpreting trial results.

References

1. Zelen M. Inference. In: *Encyclopedia of Biostatistics*. Armitage P, Colton T, editors. New York: John Wiley & Sons, 1998:2035–46.
2. Altman DG. *Practical Statistics for Medical Research*. London: Chapman & Hall, 1999.
3. Kirkwood B, Sterne J. *Essential Medical Statistics*, 2nd edition. Oxford: Blackwell Publishing, 2003.

4. Salsburg D. Hypothesis testing. In: *Encyclopedia of Biostatistics*. Armitage P, Colton T, editors. New York: John Wiley & Sons, 1998:1969–76.

5. Chow SC, Liu JP. *Design and Analysis of Clinical Trials. Concept and Methodologies*. New York: John Wiley & Sons, 1998.

6. Sterne JA, Davey Smith G. Sifting the evidence – what's wrong with significance tests? *BMJ* 2001;**322**:226–31.

Chapter 19

Comparison of Means

Duolao Wang, Felicity Clemens,
and Tim Clayton

Data on efficacy and safety in clinical trials often take the form of continuous (or quantitative or numerical) variables. They are usually summarized descriptively by statistics such as number of observations, mean or median, and standard deviation or range by treatment groups, and by graphics such as histograms, box plots, and dot plots. In this chapter, we describe statistical methods for evaluating treatment effects for a quantitatively measured outcome using hypothesis testing and confidence intervals, and demonstrate their uses and interpretations through examples.

Introduction

In the previous chapter, we described how to use the information from a sample (eg, sample size, mean, standard deviation) to make inferences about the corresponding population parameters (eg, mean) by performing a hypothesis test and calculating a confidence interval (CI). We now extend the idea to situations where we want to compare the mean outcomes in two treatment groups.

Example: Chronic airways limitation trial

Consider 24 patients with chronic airways limitation (CAL) participating in a randomized placebo-controlled clinical trial to evaluate the efficacy of a bronchodilator drug (denoted by treatment A) against placebo (denoted by treatment B). The primary endpoint of this study is forced expiratory volume in 1 second (FEV_1) at 6 months. The secondary endpoint is the relative change in FEV_1 from baseline (pretreatment) to 6 months (posttreatment). **Table 1** lists the raw data of FEV_1 on these patients.

Table 2 gives some summary statistics of the primary and secondary endpoints (FEV_1 and percentage change in FEV_1, respectively) for these patients. These results suggest a possible difference between active treatment and placebo in terms of 6-month FEV_1 values. However, the observed difference could be due to bias (systematic errors), confounding (differences in some predictors of FEV_1 between treatments at baseline), or random (chance) variation (see **Chapter 1**) [1]. In the absence of bias and confounding, we are able to assess whether chance variation could reasonably explain the observed difference using significance testing or the CI methods we illustrated in the previous chapter. Various questions can be raised regarding the data in **Table 2**. Three frequently asked questions are as follows.

Question 1
At the start and end of the study, are the mean FEV_1 values seen in both treatment groups as expected from the overall population of similar subjects?

Question 2
Is there any evidence of a significant change in mean FEV_1 from baseline in either treatment group?

Question 3
Is the posttreatment mean FEV_1 or mean FEV1 change within the active treatment group significantly different from that in the control treatment?

Table 1. FEV$_1$ measured at pre- and posttreatment and relative change from baseline in 24 patients.

Subject	Treatment	Pretreatment FEV$_1$ (mL)	Posttreatment FEV$_1$ (mL)	Relative change (%)
1	B	2188	2461	12.5
2	B	1719	1641	−4.5
3	B	1875	1641	−12.5
4	A	1797	2215	23.3
5	B	1563	1559	−0.3
6	A	2344	3117	33.0
7	A	1719	2051	19.3
8	B	1875	2215	18.1
9	B	2031	1805	−11.2
10	A	1719	1969	14.5
11	A	2016	2264	12.3
12	A	2188	3117	42.5
13	B	1875	2051	9.4
14	B	1797	1969	9.6
15	B	2500	3035	21.4
16	A	2266	2953	30.3
17	B	2422	2625	8.4
18	A	2031	2379	17.1
19	A	2500	3035	21.4
20	B	1875	1723	−8.1
21	B	2188	2297	5.0
22	A	1797	2215	23.3
23	A	1875	2264	20.8
24	A	1875	2215	18.1

Table 2. Summary statistics for pre- and posttreatment FEV$_1$ and relative change by treatment group.

	Treatment A (active)			Treatment B (placebo)		
	Pretreatment FEV$_1$ (mL)	Posttreatment FEV$_1$ (mL)	Relative change (%)	Pretreatment FEV$_1$ (mL)	Posttreatment FEV$_1$ (mL)	Relative change (%)
Patients	12	12	12	12	12	12
Mean	2010.6	2482.8	23.0	1992.3	2085.2	4.0
Standard deviation	260.4	437.2	8.5	281.7	456.5	11.3
Median	1945.5	2264.0	21.1	1875.0	2010.0	6.7

To address these questions, we can perform the statistical significant tests introduced below [2–4]. As described in **Chapter 18**, statistical inference concerns the problem of generalizing findings from a sample to the population from which it was drawn.

One-sample *t*-test

To address Question 1, we need to perform a one-sample *t*-test. This tests the null hypothesis that the mean of a population (μ) from which the sample is drawn is equal to a constant (μ_0). Therefore, the hypotheses are expressed as:

$$H_0 : \mu = \mu_0$$

$$\text{vs} \qquad\qquad (1)$$

$$H_a : \mu \neq \mu_0$$

The statistic (*t*) for testing the above hypotheses is given by:

$$t = \frac{\bar{X} - \mu_0}{SE(\bar{X})} \qquad\qquad (2)$$

$$SE(\bar{X}) = S / \sqrt{n}$$

where:

- $\bar{X}$ is the sample mean
- S is the standard deviation
- n is the sample size
- $SE(\bar{X})$ is the standard error of the sample mean ($\bar{X}$)

Under the null hypothesis, the test statistic in equation (2) is distributed as the *t*-distribution (or Student distribution) with $n - 1$ degrees of freedom [5].

Degrees of freedom

Note that there is a different *t*-distribution for each sample size, and we have to specify the degrees of freedom for each distribution (see reference [4] for more about degrees of freedom).

The *t*-density distribution curves are symmetric and bell-shaped, like the standard normal distribution, and peak at 0. However, the spread is wider than that of the

Figure 1. Three *t*-distributions and their relationship with a standard normal distribution.

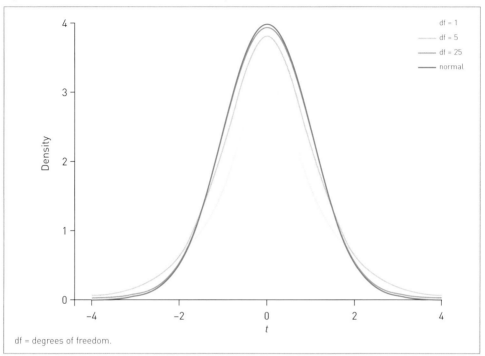

df = degrees of freedom.

standard normal distribution. **Figure 1** displays three *t*-distributions with degrees of freedom of 1, 5, and 25, and the standard normal distribution. We can see that as the number of degrees of freedom increases, the *t*-distribution approaches the standard normal distribution. Therefore, as the degrees of freedom increases, the *t*-distribution moves towards the normal distribution and the Z-test introduced in **Chapter 18** can be used for hypothesis testing, rather than the *t*-test.

Critical values

The principles for a significance test are as described in **Chapter 18**. For the one-sample *t*-test, if:

$$|t| \geq t_{\alpha/2, n-1}$$

where $t_{\alpha/2, n-1}$ is a critical value of a *t*-distribution with $n - 1$ degrees of freedom, we would have evidence against the null hypothesis that $\mu = \mu_0$, ie, the population mean (μ) is statistically significantly different from the constant μ_0 at the α level of significance.

Table 3 displays some selected critical values for *t*-distributions with different degrees of freedom. This table contains the significance levels for one- and two-tailed (sided) *t*-tests (a tail is either end of a *t*-distribution curve) (see references [3] and [4] for more about one- and two-sided tests). For the alternative hypothesis currently under examination, we use a two-sided test because the true population mean could be larger or smaller than the hypothesized mean FEV_1.

The corresponding $100(1 - \alpha)\%$ CI for a population mean (μ) can be calculated from the following equation:

$$\bar{X} \pm t_{\alpha/2, n-1} \times SE(\bar{X}) \qquad (3)$$

Example

The *t*-test can be illustrated using the CAL trial data. Suppose, from the literature, the mean FEV_1 for patients with CAL is 2000 mL ($= \mu_0$). Hence, it might be of clinical interest to know whether the mean FEV_1 for the CAL patient population treated with test drug A is different from 2000 mL.

From **Table 2**, we have $\bar{X} = 2482.8$, $S = 437.2$, and $n = 12$ for FEV_1 at posttreatment. Placing those values in equation (2), we have:

$$SE(\bar{X}) = 437.2 / \sqrt{12} = 126.2$$

$$t = \frac{2482 - 2000}{126.2} = 3.83$$

From **Table 3**, we can see that the critical *t*-values corresponding to 11 degrees of freedom are $t_{0.01/2,11} = 3.11$ and $t_{0.001/2,11} = 4.44$ for $\alpha = 0.01$ and 0.001, respectively. Since $t_{0.01/2,11} < 3.83 < t_{0.001/2,11}$, then $0.001 < P\text{-value} < 0.01$. Therefore, we conclude that the data provide evidence that the population mean for FEV_1 after active treatment A is (statistically) significantly different from 2000 mL at the 5% significance level. The corresponding 95% CI, as calculated from equation (3), is (2205.1, 2760.6), suggesting that we estimate that the true posttreatment FEV_1 mean for patients in group A is 95% likely to fall between 2205.1 and 2760.6 mL.

Similarly, we can perform *t*-tests ($H_0: \mu = 2000$) for FEV_1 and estimate the 95% CIs for the population mean of FEV_1 for patients in group A at baseline, and for patients in group B at baseline and posttreatment. These corresponding results are presented in **Table 4**. The results show that there is insufficient evidence to suggest that population means for the three outcomes are significantly different from 2000 mL.

Table 3. Critical t-values by degrees of freedom.

Degrees of freedom	Level of significance		
	One-tailed test		
	0.025	0.005	0.0005
	Two-tailed test		
	0.05	0.01	0.001
1	12.71	63.66	636.58
2	4.30	9.92	31.60
3	3.18	5.84	12.92
4	2.78	4.60	8.61
5	2.57	4.03	6.87
6	2.45	3.71	5.96
7	2.36	3.50	5.41
8	2.31	3.36	5.04
9	2.26	3.25	4.78
10	2.23	3.17	4.59
11	2.20	3.11	4.44
12	2.18	3.05	4.32
13	2.16	3.01	4.22
14	2.14	2.98	4.14
15	2.13	2.95	4.07
16	2.12	2.92	4.01
17	2.11	2.90	3.97
18	2.10	2.88	3.92
19	2.09	2.86	3.88
20	2.09	2.85	3.85
21	2.08	2.83	3.82
22	2.07	2.82	3.79
23	2.07	2.81	3.77
24	2.06	2.80	3.75
25	2.06	2.79	3.73
30	2.04	2.75	3.65
40	2.02	2.70	3.55
50	2.01	2.68	3.50
60	2.00	2.66	3.46
120	1.98	2.62	3.37
∞	1.96	2.58	3.30

Table 4. The results from *t*-testing the $H_0 : \mu = 2000$ together with 95% CIs for FEV_1 at pre-and posttreatment.

Treatment	Time	Point estimate	*t*-value	*P*-value	95% CI	
A	Pretreatment	2010.6	0.14	0.891	1845.1	2176.0
	Posttreatment	2482.8	3.83	0.003	2205.1	2760.6
B	Pretreatment	1992.3	−0.09	0.927	1813.4	2171.3
	Posttreatment	2085.2	0.65	0.531	1795.1	2375.2

These results imply that the posttreatment mean FEV_1 in the population on treatment A is significantly different from the reference value of 2000 mL, but baseline measurements and the posttreatment mean in the placebo group are not. The interpretation of this finding depends on what the value of 2000 mL represents; if it is the mean FEV_1 expected of a 'typical' group of patients suffering from severe CAL, we could conclude that there is evidence to suggest that patients who had taken drug A were significantly improved compared to the 'typical' group following standard treatment.

By implication, the one-sample *t*-test is based on the assumption that the outcome variable is normally distributed, and it is the mean of a normal distribution that is tested. We can check for this assumption using an inverse normal plot (Q-Q plot) (see **Chapter 17**) [6]. **Figure 2** shows the inverse normal plots for the four outcome variables displayed in **Table 1**. As these plots are close to linear patterns, the implication is that these samples are approximately normally distributed [6].

Paired *t*-test

For some uncontrolled open-label clinical trials, the main objective is to evaluate the drug effect before and after the treatment based on changes from baseline. This generates 'paired' data. The key feature of paired data is that the two samples to be compared are not independent. Alternatively, there might be two separate samples that have been selected in pairs to resemble each other. Statistical analysis assesses whether the data provide evidence that there is a statistically significant difference in the outcome variable before and after treatment within a treatment group, in this case group A (Question 2). We can now address this question by performing a paired *t*-test.

The null hypothesis can be expressed as:

$$H_0 : \mu_d = \mu_{pre} - \mu_{post} = 0$$

Figure 2. Inverse normal plots for the four outcome variables given in Table 1.

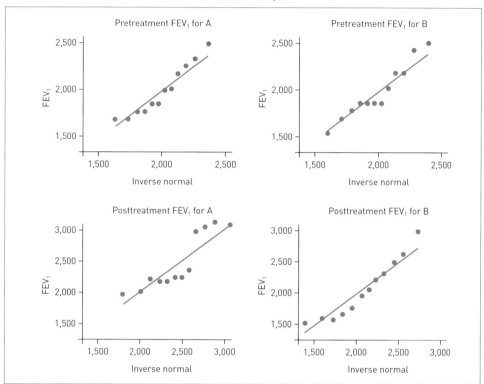

meaning that there is no difference in pre- and posttreatment population means of FEV_1 in group A. The alternative hypothesis is:

$$H_a : \mu_d = \mu_{pre} - \mu_{post} \neq 0.$$

The test statistic for testing the above hypotheses is given by:

$$t = \frac{\overline{X}_d}{SE(\overline{X}_d)} \qquad (4)$$

$$SE(\overline{X}_d) = S_d / \sqrt{n}$$

where:

- $\overline{X}_d$ is the sample mean of the paired FEV_1 difference
- S_d is the standard deviation of the paired FEV_1 difference
- n is the number of pairs of observations (in this case, the number of patients)
- $SE(\overline{X}_d)$ is the standard error of $\overline{X}_d$

Table 5. The individual differences in FEV_1 between pre- and posttreatment in group A, together with summary statistics for the paired t-test.

Subject	Treatment	Pretreatment FEV$_1$ (mL)	Posttreatment FEV$_1$ (mL)	Difference
4	A	1797	2215	418
6	A	2344	3117	773
7	A	1719	2051	332
10	A	1719	1969	250
11	A	2016	2264	248
12	A	2188	3117	930
16	A	2266	2953	688
18	A	2031	2379	348
19	A	2500	3035	535
22	A	1797	2215	418
23	A	1875	2264	389
24	A	1875	2215	340
n				12
$\overline{X}_d$				472.4
S				216.4
SE				62.5

S = standard deviation; SE = standard error.

Under the null hypothesis, the test statistic in equation (4) is distributed as the t-distribution with $n - 1$ degrees of freedom [2,5]. Therefore, there is evidence against the null hypothesis of H_0 at the α level of significance if $|t| \geq t_{\alpha/2,n-1}$. The corresponding $100(1 - \alpha)\%$ CI can be calculated from the following equation:

$$\overline{X}_d \pm t_{\alpha/2,n-1} \times SE(\overline{X}_d) \qquad (5)$$

Table 5 displays the individual differences in FEV_1 between pre- and posttreatment in group A, together with some summary statistics required for the paired t-test. Using these statistics, the paired t-test statistic is given by:

$$t = \frac{\overline{X}_d}{SE(\overline{X}_d)} = \frac{472.4}{62.5} = 7.56$$

The two-sided critical *t*-value for α = 0.001 ($t_{0.001/2,11}$), according to **Table 3**, is 4.44. Since |*t*| is greater than $t_{0.001/2,11}$, the *P*-value is <0.001. Therefore, we can say that there is very strong evidence against the null hypothesis, and state that FEV_1 is significantly increased from baseline within the population who received active treatment group A. The 95% CI of $μ_d$ calculated from equation (5) is (334.9, 609.8) mL.

The inference of strong evidence of a difference between baseline and posttreatment FEV_1 in the treatment group does not necessarily imply that the treatment is effective at increasing FEV_1. The observed significant difference could be due to the effects of time of day, the placebo effect, the practice effect of having used a spirometer previously when taking the follow-up reading, or a number of other variables, rather than due to having taken drug A. To establish whether drug A is effective, we need to compare its effect on FEV_1 with that observed in the placebo group.

It is clear from equations (2) and (4) that the two-sample paired *t*-test is equivalent to performing a one-sample *t*-test on the paired differences with a null hypothesis of 0 difference. The assumption for the paired *t*-test is therefore that the paired differences are normally distributed.

Two-sample *t*-test

In a comparative clinical trial, the primary objective is to evaluate the efficacy and safety of a study drug compared to a control (a placebo control or an active control). For this purpose, a parallel design is usually employed and the two treatment groups are compared for some outcome.

Suppose that some continuous outcome is measured in a two-way parallel clinical study, and the two populations (to be treated with drug A and placebo) to which the two treatment groups are randomized are distributed normally with means $μ_1$ and $μ_2$ and standard deviations $σ_1$ and $σ_2$, respectively. The efficacy of the test drug, against the control, can be examined by testing the following hypotheses:

$$H_0 : μ_1 = μ_2$$

$$\text{vs} \qquad (6)$$

$$H_a : μ_1 ≠ μ_2$$

The above hypotheses address Question 3 and can be tested using a t-test statistic, as defined in the following equation:

$$t = \frac{\overline{X}_1 - \overline{X}_2}{SE(\overline{X}_1 - \overline{X}_2)} \qquad (7)$$

$$SE(\overline{X}_1 - \overline{X}_2) = \left(\frac{[n_1 - 1]S_1^2 + [n_2 - 1]S_2^2}{n_1 + n_2 - 2} \left[\frac{1}{n_1} + \frac{1}{n_2} \right] \right)^{1/2}$$

where:

- $\overline{X}_1, \overline{X}_2$ are the sample means of the two treatment groups
- S_1, S_2 are the sample standard deviations of the two treatment groups
- n_1, n_2 are the number of patients in each group
- $SE(\overline{X}_1 - \overline{X}_2)$ is the standard error of difference in two sample means

Hence, if $|t| \geq t_{\alpha/2,n_1+n_2-2}$, we can say that there is evidence against the null hypothesis of no treatment difference ($H_0 : \mu_1 = \mu_2$) and state that the treatment difference is significant at the α level, where $t_{\alpha/2,n_1+n_2-2}$ is the critical t-value of a t-distribution with $n_1 + n_2 - 2$ degrees of freedom. Based on this test, a $100(1 - \alpha)\%$ CI for $\mu_1 - \mu_2$ is given by:

$$(\overline{X}_1 - \overline{X}_2) \pm t_{\alpha/2,n_1+n_2-2} \times SE(\overline{X}_1 - \overline{X}_2)$$

Example

We can again consider the CAL data to illustrate the use of a two-sample t-test. The posttreatment FEV_1 concerns two independent samples. Therefore, we can use the t-test described in equation (7) to test the null hypothesis of no treatment difference, as described in (6). Using the summary statistics provided in **Table 2**, we can calculate the t-value as 2.18. From **Table 3**, we have $t_{0.05/2,22}$ = 2.07 and $t_{0.01/2,22}$ = 2.82. Since $t_{0.05/2,22}$ < 2.18 < $t_{0.01/2,22}$, then $0.05 > P > 0.01$, meaning the treatment difference between the two posttreatment FEV_1 means is significant at the 5% level, but not at the 1% level. The corresponding 95% and 99% CIs for $\mu_1 - \mu_2$ are (19.2, 776.1) (mL) and (–116.7, 912.0) (mL), respectively. Since the 95% CI does not contain 0 but the 99% CI does contain 0, we reach the same conclusion as the t-test – ie, the treatment difference in posttreatment FEV_1 between the two groups is statistically significant at the 5% level, but not at the 1% level.

For most purposes where the significance level is 5%, the inference here is that CAL patients on drug A have a better FEV_1 value. In some situations, rather than comparing drug A with placebo, the trial design might compare drug A with a known efficacious drug in order to look for evidence of drug A's superiority over an established standard therapy.

Assumptions

Four key assumptions are required in the two-sample t-test. Firstly, we assume that the two treatment group populations from which the samples are drawn are distributed normally [2–4].

Secondly, we assume that the variances (or standard deviations) of the two populations are equal [2–4], ie, $\sigma_1^2 = \sigma_2^2 = \sigma^2$. The equality of variances assumption can be formally verified with an F-test [2–4]. We can also do an informal check by looking at the relative magnitude of the two-sample variances S_1^2 and S_2^2. For example, if S_1^2 / S_2^2 is considerably different from 1 then the assumption that $\sigma_1^2 = \sigma_2^2 = \sigma^2$ will be in doubt. In cases where $\sigma_1^2 \neq \sigma_2^2$, we need to use a modified t-test or nonparametric method [3–5].

Thirdly, we assume that the observations in the two treatment groups are independent of each other, ie, no observation in one group is influenced by another observation in the second group [3–5]. Taking the posttreatment FEV_1 as an example, the value of posttreatment FEV_1 in the active treatment group is not affected by that in the placebo group. Therefore, the values of the two sets of posttreatment FEV_1 measurements constitute two independent samples.

Finally, we assume that the two populations are homogeneous in terms of the observed and unobserved characteristics of patients (ie, free from confounding). These characteristics might be demographics (eg, age), prognosis (eg, clinical history, disease severity), or baseline measurements of outcome variables (eg, pretreatment FEV_1 in the CAL trial).

Although we might never know the unobservable heterogeneity (differences) between two populations, we can assess whether the two populations are comparable by looking at the observed summary statistics, such as means or proportions at baseline by treatment. This is why a table that summarizes the baseline information in a clinical trial by treatment group is always provided in a clinical report. If the two treatment groups are not balanced with regard to some of the predictors of outcome, covariate adjustment by means of stratification or regression modeling can be employed (see **Chapters 24–26**) [1,4,5].

Two-sample Z-test

If the sample sizes n_1 and n_2 are large (say n_1 and $n_2 > 50$) [2–4], we can use a Z-statistic to test the null hypothesis in equation (6), as discussed earlier:

$$Z = \frac{\overline{X}_1 - \overline{X}_2}{SE(\overline{X}_1 - \overline{X}_2)}$$

$$\text{where } SE(\overline{X}_1 - \overline{X}_2) = \left(\frac{S_1^2}{n_1} + \frac{S_2^2}{n_2} \right)^{1/2}$$

According to statistical theory (central limit theorem), Z is approximately normally distributed with mean 0 and standard deviation 1 when n_1 and n_2 are large [2]. Therefore, the treatment difference will be significant at the α level of significance if:

$$|Z| \geq Z_{\alpha/2}$$

where $Z_{\alpha/2}$ is the critical value of the standard normal distribution (see **Chapter 17**) [6]. The corresponding $100(1 - \alpha)\%$ CI for $\mu_1 - \mu_2$ is given by:

$$(\overline{X}_1 - \overline{X}_2) + Z_{\alpha/2} \times SE(\overline{X}_1 - \overline{X}_2)$$

Unlike the two-sample t-test, the two-sample Z-test does not require the standard deviations to be similar (ie, $\sigma_1 = \sigma_2 = \sigma$), although there are still assumptions of normality, independence, and homogeneity [2–4].

Two-sample Wilcoxon rank-sum (Mann–Whitney) test

In previous sections, statistical inferences have been primarily based on the assumption that the outcome under evaluation follows a normal distribution. In practice, this 'normality' might not be present. For example, consider that the outcome is length of stay in hospital – this outcome usually has a skewed distribution, with most people staying a short duration. We now need different statistical methods using nonparametric methods that do not require normality to draw statistical conclusions. Corresponding to the one-sample t-test, paired t-test, and two-sample t-test to address Questions 1, 2, and 3, three nonparametric (or distribution-free) methods are available [7–9]:

- Wilcoxon signed rank test
- Wilcoxon matched pairs signed rank-sum test
- Wilcoxon rank-sum (Mann–Whitney) test

For illustrative purposes, we will focus on the Wilcoxon rank-sum test for comparing two independent treatment groups.

The null hypothesis in the Wilcoxon rank-sum test is that the two samples are drawn from a single population. The test involves the calculation of a statistic, usually called T, whose distribution under the null hypothesis is unknown. The Wilcoxon method requires all the observations to be ranked as if they were from a single population. If the data are tied or equal, then averaged ranks across tied values are used (see **Table 6**). Wilcoxon's test statistic is the sum of the ranks for the observations in the first sample [7–9]:

$$T_1 = \sum_{i = 1}^{n_1} R_1$$

With this Wilcoxon's test statistic, we can find the corresponding exact P-value from a statistical table [7–9]. However, we will illustrate how the P-value can be obtained from an alternative approximate Z-test, whose working can be readily examined.

When the sample size in each group is large, the statistic T_1 has an approximately normal distribution with:

$$\text{mean } \mu_T = \sqrt{n_1(n_1 + n_2 + 2) / 2}$$

$$\text{standard deviation } \sigma_T = n_1 n_2(n_1 + n_2 + 1) / 12$$

From these, we can calculate the test statistic Z as $(T_1 - \mu_T) / \sigma_T$ and refer to the standard normal distribution table for determining the P-value.

Table 5 shows the data of relative change in FEV_1 treated in this way. The sums of the ranks in the two treatment groups are 211 and 89, respectively. So we have $T_1 = 211$. The mean and standard deviation of the test statistic under the null hypothesis are given by:

$$\mu_T = 12 * (12 + 12 + 1) / 2 = 150$$

and

$$\sigma_T = \sqrt{12 * 12(12 + 12 + 1) / 12} = 17.32$$

yielding:

$$Z = \frac{211 - 150}{17.32} = 3.52$$

Table 6. Calculation of ranks of relative changes for the Wilcoxon rank-sum test.

Subject	Treatment	Relative change (%)	Rank of relative change Treatment A	Rank of relative change Treatment B
1	B	12.5		11
2	B	−4.5		4
3	B	−12.5		1
4	A	23.3	20.5	
5	B	−0.3		5
6	A	33.0	23	
7	A	19.3	16	
8	B	18.1		14.5
9	B	−11.2		2
10	A	14.5	12	
11	A	12.3	10	
12	A	42.5	24	
13	B	9.4		8
14	B	9.6		9
15	B	21.4		18.5
16	A	30.3	22	
17	B	8.4		7
18	A	17.1	13	
19	A	21.4	18.5	
20	B	−8.1		3
21	B	5.0		6
22	A	23.3	20.5	
23	A	20.8	17	
24	A	18.1	14.5	
Sum of ranks			$T_1 = 211$	$T_2 = 89$

which, from the standard normal distribution table, corresponds to $P = 0.0004$. Since $P < 0.05$, there is evidence against the null hypothesis that the two samples are drawn from a single population at the 5% significance level. As the median relative change in FEV_1 for the active treatment group is 21.1%, much higher than 6.7% in the placebo group, we can conclude that there is strong evidence to suggest that the active drug increases FEV_1.

Thus, we can see that using ranking to assess whether the changes are really equal in both groups allows us to determine whether the two groups are drawn from the same population.

How to report *t*-test results

It is preferable to report the *P*-value itself and not to report, for example, '*P* < 0.05' or '*P* = not significant' as this does not give the reader an idea of the magnitude of the statistical significance. The treatment effect and CI should be reported (where possible) in order to give the reader an idea of the uncertainty surrounding the estimate of the difference(s) and the clinical significance of the difference(s).

Furthermore, if performing a two-sample *t*-test for a difference in means, it is desirable to quote summary statistics for each sample (number of observations, mean, and standard deviation or standard error), rather than just quoting the *P*-value. Equally, for a paired *t*-test, summary statistics for the differences between pairs should be presented.

How to make multiple group comparisons

It often happens in research practice that we need to compare more than two groups (eg, drug 1, drug 2, and placebo). In these cases, we need to analyze the data using regression modeling techniques (see **Chapter 24**). These include analysis of variance (ANOVA), which can be considered a generalization of the *t*-test [1,3,4]. In fact, for two-group comparisons, regression analysis will give results identical to a *t*-test [1]. However, when the study design is more complex, regression modeling offers advantages over the *t*-test and can avoid the problem of conducting multiple statistical tests (see **Chapter 29**).

Conclusion

In this chapter, we have introduced significance test methods and corresponding CI calculations for the analysis of continuous data (summarized in **Table 7**). Of those methods, the *t*-test has been widely used in data analysis and has two important applications in clinical research:

- to assess if there is a statistically significant change after treatment in an endpoint from baseline within a treatment group
- to assess if there is a significant difference between two treatment groups

For both forms of the *t*-test, the test statistic is calculated by comparing the ratio of the mean difference (or difference in means) to its standard error with a critical *t*-value from a *t*-distribution with an appropriate number of degrees of freedom. For large samples, the Z-test can be used to replace the *t*-test.

Table 7. Summary of statistical test methods described in this article.

Type of tests	Null hypothesis	Test statistics and confidence interval	Assumptions
One-sample t-test	$H_0 : \mu = \mu_0$	$t = \dfrac{\bar{X} - \mu_0}{SE(\bar{X})}, df = n - 1$ $SE(\bar{X}) = S / \sqrt{n}$ CI: $\bar{X} \pm t_{\alpha/2, n-1} \times SE(\bar{X})$	Sample is from a normal distribution
Paired t-test	$H_0 : \mu_d = \mu_{pre} - \mu_{post} = 0$	$t = \dfrac{\bar{X}_d}{SE(\bar{X}_d)}, df = n - 1$ $SE(\bar{X}_d) = S_d / \sqrt{n}$ CI: $\bar{X}_d \pm t_{\alpha/2, n-1} \times SE(\bar{X}_d)$	The paired population differences are normally distributed
Two-sample t-test	$H_0 : \mu_1 = \mu_2$	$t = \dfrac{\bar{X}_1 - \bar{X}_2}{SE(\bar{X}_1 - \bar{X}_2)}, df = n_1 + n_2 - 2$ $SE(\bar{X}_1 - \bar{X}_2) =$ $\left(\dfrac{[n_1 - 1]S_1^2 + [n_2 - 1]S_2^2}{n_1 + n_2 - 2} \left[\dfrac{1}{n_1} + \dfrac{1}{n_2} \right] \right)^{1/2}$ CI: $(\bar{X}_1 - \bar{X}_2) \pm t_{\alpha/2, n_1+n_2-2} \times SE(\bar{X}_1 - \bar{X}_2)$	For the two populations (eg, all patients to receive treatment A and B): • the two samples are independent • the two samples are from two normal populations • the variances of the two populations are equal • the two populations are homogeneous in terms of observed and unobserved characteristics at baseline
Two-sample Z-test	$H_0 : \mu_1 = \mu_2$	$Z = \dfrac{\bar{X}_1 - \bar{X}_2}{SE(\bar{X}_1 - \bar{X}_2)}$ $SE(\bar{X}_1 - \bar{X}_2) = \left(\dfrac{S_1^2}{n_1} + \dfrac{S_2^2}{n_2} \right)^{1/2}$ CI: $(\bar{X}_1 - \bar{X}_2) \pm Z_{\alpha/2} \times SE(\bar{X}_1 - \bar{X}_2)$	• The two samples are independent • The two samples are from two normal populations • The samples have large sizes • The two populations are homogeneous in terms of observed and unobserved characteristics at baseline
Wilcoxon rank-sum (Mann–Whitney) test	The two samples are drawn from a single population	$T = \sum_{i=1}^{n_1} R_{1i}$ $\mu_T = n_1(n_1 + n_2 + 1) / 2$ $\sigma_T = \sqrt{n_1 n_2 (n_1 + n_2 + 1) / 12}$ $Z = (T - \mu_T) / \sigma_T$	The two samples are independent

When assessing the treatment effect in a two-arm parallel design using t-test, the assumptions of approximate normality of distribution, approximate equality of variance, independence of observations, and comparability of two treatment groups at baseline should be borne in mind. When such assumptions are not reasonable, alternative methods such as a nonparametric approach or regression modeling should be considered.

References

1.   Pocock SJ. *Clinical Trials: A Practical Approach*. Chichester: John Wiley & Sons, 1983.

2.   Hoel PG. *Introduction to Mathematical Statistics*, 2nd edition. New York: John Wiley & Sons, 1954.

3.   Altman DG. *Practical Statistics for Medical Research*. London: Chapman & Hall, 1999.

4.   Kirkwood B, Sterne J. *Essential Medical Statistics*, 2nd edition. Oxford: Blackwell Publishing, 2003.

5.   Lee AFS. Student's *t* distribution and student's *t* statistics. In: *Encyclopedia of Biostatistics*. Armitage P, Colton T, editors. New York: John Wiley & Sons, 1998:4396–7.

6.   Tong YL. Normal distribution. In: *Encyclopedia of Biostatistics*. Armitage P, Colton T, editors. New York: John Wiley & Sons, 1998:3064–7.

7.   Wilcoxon, F. Individual comparisons by ranking methods. *Biometrics* 1945;**1**:80–3.

8.   Mann H, Whitney D. On a test of whether one of two random variables is stochastically larger than the other. *Ann Math Stat* 1947;**18**:50–60.

9.   Conover, WJ. *Practical Nonparametric Statistics*, 3rd edition. New York: John Wiley & Sons, 1999.

Chapter 20

Comparison of Proportions

Duolao Wang, Tim Clayton, and Felicity Clemens

In clinical trials, patients' responses to treatments are often recorded according to the occurrence of some meaningful and well-defined event such as death, cure, or reduction in severity of disease. These records generate efficacy and safety endpoints in the form of categorical data on either a nominal (specific named outcome) or ordinal scale, which are often summarized by proportions or percentages by treatment groups (or frequency tables) and displayed graphically using bar or pie charts. In this chapter, we introduce some fundamental concepts and methods for the analysis of categorical data, and illustrate their uses and interpretations through examples.

Introduction

Categorical data are common in clinical research, arising when outcomes are categorized into one of two or more mutually exclusive groups. The first step for a categorical data analysis is to produce a frequency table of each outcome, and calculate relevant proportions or percentages of patients with each outcome within each treatment group. The second step is to compare these proportions using significance tests and confidence intervals (CIs). In this chapter, we describe the methods for such comparisons and illustrate these with examples.

Example: myocardial infarction trial

Let us assume that a multicenter, randomized, placebo-controlled clinical trial is conducted to determine whether a new drug, compared to placebo, reduces all-cause mortality in 4,067 patients following myocardial infarction (MI), who otherwise receive optimal treatment. The primary endpoint is the occurrence of death from any cause at 30 days following randomization. This generates a binary variable (died or survived), which is often summarized as the proportion of patients who have died.

The numbers of patients who died or survived at 30 days in each of the two treatment groups form a *2 × 2* contingency table, as shown in **Table 1**. This also shows the notations representing the number of patients in each group in brackets. For example, we use the letters *a* and *b* to denote the number of patients who died, *c* and *d* to denote the number of patients who survived, and n_1 and n_2 to denote the number of patients randomized in the active drug and placebo groups, respectively. The total number of patients is n $(= n_1 + n_2)$.

Following the above notations, the proportion of deaths in the active drug and placebo groups are denoted by $p_1 = a / n_1$ and $p_2 = b / n_2$, respectively. From **Table 1**, we can see that the proportion of deaths was lower in the active drug group ($p_1 = [110 / 2045] \times 100 = 5.38\%$) than in the placebo group ($p_2 = [165 / 2022] \times 100 = 8.16\%$). Overall, 6.76% ($p = [\{a + b\} / n] \times 100 = [\{110 + 165\} / \{2045 + 2022\}] \times 100$) of MI patients died within the first 30 days after randomization. In this chapter, the proportion and percentage are interchangeably used in the text, but distinguished in the formulas.

Although the observed difference in mortality from the above data is in favor of the active drug treatment, we are not certain whether this is a real drug effect or caused by random error, confounding, or bias (see also **Chapters 1**, **18**, and **19**) [1]. Assuming the study has no systematic bias or confounding, we can use significance testing or CI methods to assess whether chance variation could reasonably explain

Table 1. A 2 × 2 contingency table (notation) for the myocardial infarction trial.

Death	Treatment		Total
	Active drug	**Placebo**	
Yes	110 (a)	165 (b)	275 (a + b)
No	1935 (c)	1857 (d)	3792 (c + d)
Total	2045 (n_1)	2022 (n_2)	4067 ($n_1 + n_2$)
Proportion of deaths	5.38% ($p_1 = \frac{a}{n_1} \times 100$)	8.16% ($p_2 = \frac{b}{n_2} \times 100$)	6.76% ($p = \frac{a + b}{n} \times 100$)

the observed difference. In other words, we need to assess whether there is statistical evidence against the null hypothesis that there is no difference between the active drug and placebo in terms of mortality at 30 days.

In the following sections, we describe some basic methods for reporting and analyzing this type of data and illustrate these methods with the MI trial data. In addition, we discuss dealing with analyses of outcomes with more than two categories.

Making statistical inferences for one treatment group

Consider that the true population proportions of patients who die on the active drug or placebo are π_1 and π_2, respectively. We aim to estimate the two population parameters and make statistical inferences using the two respective sample proportions, p_1 and p_2. While the main focus of the analysis will be a comparison of proportions in the two treatment groups, it might also be clinically useful to know whether, within a treatment group, the proportion of patients who died is equal to some expected value.

For example, suppose that, from other observational studies, we know that about 8% of such MI patients who are not treated with the new drug will die within 30 days. It may be of clinical interest to know whether the proportion of MI patients treated with the test drug is (statistically) significantly different from 8%. The following hypotheses can be constructed to address this question:

$$H_0 : \pi_1 = \pi_0 = 8\%$$

$$\text{vs} \qquad\qquad (1)$$

$$H_a : \pi_1 \neq \pi_0$$

We can perform a Z-test to test this hypothesis. Under the null hypothesis, a Z-statistic approximation can be generated as follows:

$$Z = \frac{p_1 - \pi_0}{SE(p_1)}$$

$$SE(p_1) = \sqrt{\frac{p_1(1-p_1)}{n_1}}$$

(2)

where $SE(p_1)$ stands for the standard error of p_1.

At a prespecified level of significance α, we have evidence against the null hypothesis in equation (1) and conclude that the proportion of MI patients who died in the test drug group is statistically significantly different from 8% if:

$$|Z| \geq Z_{\alpha/2}$$

where $Z_{\alpha/2}$ is the critical value from the standard normal distribution.

The exact P-value in the Z-test is the probability that $Z \leq -Z_{\alpha/2}$ or $Z \geq Z_{\alpha/2}$. This can be determined by calculating the area under the curve in two-sided symmetric tails from a standard normal distribution table.

Using the data in **Table 1**:

$$p_1 = 5.38\%$$

$$SE(p_1) = \sqrt{\frac{5.38/100 \times (1 - 5.38/100)}{2045}} = 0.005 \text{ or } 0.50\%$$

$$Z = \frac{5.38\% - 8\%}{0.50\%} = -5.24$$

As a result, since the absolute value of observed Z is $>Z_{0.05/2} = 1.96$, the P-value is <0.05, and, in fact, the actual P-value is <0.0001. Therefore, we reject the null hypothesis at the 5% level of significance, and conclude that the proportion of MI patients who died in the treatment group is statistically significantly different (lower) than 8%.

Similarly, we can test whether the proportion of patients who died in the placebo group is different from 8%. The calculated Z-value is 0.26, with an associated P-value of 0.798. As this P-value is >0.05, there is insufficient evidence to suggest

Table 2. Summary statistics for one-sample statistical inference by treatment for the myocardial infarction trial.

Statistics	Treatment	
	Active drug	Placebo
Null hypothesis (π_0 = 8.00%)	$H_0 : \pi_1 = \pi_0$	$H_0 : \pi_2 = \pi_0$
Proportion of death (number of patients)	5.38% (2045)	8.16% (2022)
Standard error	0.50%	0.61%
Z-statistic	−5.25	0.26
P-value	$P < 0.001$	$P = 0.792$
95% CI	(4.40%, 6.36%)	(6.97%, 9.35%)

that the population proportion of MI patients who died (π_2) in the placebo group is statistically significantly different from 8% (π_0) at the 5% significance level. The detailed summary results for one-sample inference based on the **Table 1** data are presented in **Table 2** for the active treatment and placebo groups, respectively.

The statistical inference for one sample can also be made by calculating a CI. Based on equation (2), a 100 (1 − α) % CI for the population proportion in the active treatment group (π_1) can be obtained as:

$$p_1 \pm Z_{\alpha/2} \, SE(p_1)$$

Thus the 95% CI is:

$$5.38\% \pm 1.96 \times 0.50\% = 4.40\% \text{ to } 6.36\%$$

Based on the 95% CIs, we can reach the same conclusion as the Z-test. The 95% CI (4.40%, 6.36%) does not contain 8% in the active drug group, and we therefore conclude that it is significantly lower than 8%. For the placebo group, the 95% CI includes 8% (6.97%, 9.35%), so we therefore conclude that the proportion of MI patients who died is not significantly different from 8%, as revealed in the Z-test.

In this example, death has been used as the outcome. However, the significance testing and CI used in this example can apply to any binary outcome, such as whether or not a patient shows improvement after treatment, whether or not there is recurrence of disease, whether or not the patient has an admission to hospital, and so on.

Comparing proportions between two groups

The primary objective of the MI trial is to directly compare the proportion of MI patients who died on the active drug with that of patients on placebo, within the time period of the trial follow-up (30 days). The efficacy of the active drug, against the control, can be examined by testing the null hypothesis that the proportions of deaths in both populations are equal:

$$H_0 : \pi_1 = \pi_2$$

vs (3)

$$H_a : \pi_1 \neq \pi_2$$

This section will describe three methods for testing the above hypotheses: the chi-squared (χ^2) test, Fisher's exact test, and the Z-test [2,3].

Chi-squared (χ^2) test

The most common approach for comparing two proportions is the chi-squared test. The chi-squared test involves comparing the *observed* numbers in each of the four categories in the contingency table with the numbers *expected* if there was no difference in proportions between the active drug and placebo groups.

Overall, 275 / 4067 (6.76%) patients died during the trial. If the active drug and placebo were equally effective, one would expect the same proportion of deaths in each of the two groups: that is, 275 / 4067 × 2045 = 138.3 in the drug group and 275 / 4067 × 2022 = 136.7 in the placebo group. Similarly, 3792 / 4067 × 2045 = 1906.7 patients in the active drug group and 3792 / 4067 × 2022 = 1885.3 patients in the placebo group would be expected to survive to 30 days after randomization.

The expected numbers are shown in **Table 3**. They add up to the same row and column totals as the observed numbers. The chi-squared value used to assess the difference in the proportions under the null hypothesis (3) can be expressed as:

$$\chi^2 = \sum \frac{(O - E)^2}{E} \qquad (4)$$

where:

- *O* represents the observed numbers in each cell of the *2 × 2* table
- *E* represents the expected numbers in each cell of the *2 × 2* table

as shown in **Table 3**.

Table 3. Calculation of chi-squared statistics using the *2 × 2* contingency table in Table 1.

Death	Treatment		Total
	Active drug	Placebo	
Observed numbers			
Yes	110	165	275
No	1935	1857	3792
Total	2045	2022	4067
Expected numbers			
Yes	138.3	136.7	275
No	1906.7	1885.3	3792
Total	2045	2022	4067

Hence, the further the observed values are from the expected, the larger χ^2 will be. Using the data in **Table 3** and formula (4), we have:

$$\chi^2 = \frac{(110 - 138.3)^2}{138.3} + \frac{(1935 - 1906.7)^2}{1906.7} + \frac{(165 - 136.7)^2}{136.7} + \frac{(1857 - 1885.3)^2}{1885.3}$$

$$= 12.48$$

Under the null hypothesis of no difference in the proportion of deaths between the two groups, χ^2 should follow a chi-squared distribution with 1 degree of freedom (*df*) (see reference [3] for more about degrees of freedom). Like the *t*-distribution, the shape of the chi-squared distribution depends on the number of degrees of freedom.

Table 4 shows some selected critical values of the chi-squared distribution ($\chi^2_{\alpha,df}$) with different degrees of freedom and significance levels (α). For example, when $df = 1$ and $\alpha = 0.05$, $\chi^2_{0.05,1} = 3.84$. To determine the probability that the observed result or more extreme results would be observed if the null hypothesis were true, we need to compare χ^2 with $\chi^2_{\alpha,df}$. For an observed χ^2, $P \leq \alpha$ if, and only if, $\chi^2 \geq \chi^2_{\alpha,df}$. Therefore, using the principles described in **Chapter 18**, with the chi-squared test, we would have evidence against the null hypothesis in equation (3) and state that the treatment difference is significant at the α level if $\chi^2 \geq \chi^2_{\alpha,df}$.

For the MI trial data, since χ^2 (12.48) > $\chi^2_{0.001,1}$ (10.83), $P < 0.001$. We can therefore say that the treatment difference in the proportion of deaths between the two treatment groups is highly significant at the $\alpha = 0.1\%$ level.

Table 4. Selected critical values of the chi-squared distribution.

Degrees of freedom	Significance level		
	0.05	0.01	0.001
1	3.84	6.63	10.83
2	5.99	9.21	13.82
3	7.81	11.34	16.27
4	9.49	13.28	18.47
5	11.07	15.09	20.51
6	12.59	16.81	22.46
7	14.07	18.48	24.32
8	15.51	20.09	26.12
9	16.92	21.67	27.88
10	18.31	23.21	29.59
11	19.68	24.73	31.26
12	21.03	26.22	32.91
13	22.36	27.69	34.53
14	23.68	29.14	36.12
15	25.00	30.58	37.70
16	26.30	32.00	39.25
17	27.59	33.41	40.79
18	28.87	34.81	42.31
19	30.14	36.19	43.82
20	31.41	37.57	45.31

Assumptions

There are two important assumptions when using the chi-squared test. The first assumption is that the two treatment groups are homogeneous in terms of the patients' characteristics (eg, demographic information, disease-related risk factors, medical histories, concurrent medical treatments). We can check whether the two groups are comparable by looking at observed baseline summary statistics. If the two treatment groups are not balanced with regard to some predictor(s) of outcome, logistic regression modeling can be used to adjust for these potential confounding factors [1–3].

The second assumption is that the sample sizes in the two treatment arms are large, say >50 [2,3]. If the sample size is small, we need to use the Fisher's exact test, which follows [2,3].

Fisher's exact test

When the overall sample size is small or the expected frequency in any cell is <5, an approximation using a procedure such as the chi-squared test might be inadequate. This is because the smaller the number of patients in each cell, the more likely the influence of chance on the number of outcomes seen. In this situation, we can consider Fisher's exact method for comparing two proportions in a 2 × 2 contingency table. This method consists of evaluating the sum of probabilities associated with the observed frequency table and all possible 2 × 2 tables that have the same row and column totals as the observed data, but exhibit more extreme departure from the null hypothesis of no difference [2,3]. Technical details about calculating Fisher's exact test are not covered here, but most statistical packages can be used to compute this statistic very easily.

For the MI trial data, the Fisher's exact test gives a two-sided P-value of <0.001, leading to the same conclusion as that of the chi-squared test.

Two-sample Z-test

A chi-squared test provides a P-value, but not the point estimate of a treatment difference and its CI. The Z-test [2,3], however, has the advantage that the point estimate and CI can easily be calculated.

The Z-test is defined as:

$$Z = \frac{p_1 - p_2}{SE(p_1 - p_2)}$$

$$SE(p_1 - p_2) = \sqrt{(p\,[1 - p][1/n_1 + 1/n_2])}$$

where:

- $p = \dfrac{a + b}{n}$

- $SE(p_1 - p_2)$ is the standard error of $p_1 - p_2$

According to statistical theory (central limit theorem), Z has an approximately standard normal distribution when n_1 and n_2 are large. Therefore, we can apply the Z-test to the null hypothesis in equation (3) and state that there is a significant difference at the α level of significance if $|Z| \geq Z_{\alpha/2}$, where $Z_{\alpha/2}$ is the critical value from the standard normal distribution. The corresponding $100\,(1 - \alpha)\,\%$ CI for the difference in the proportion between two treatments $(\pi_1 - \pi_2)$ can be calculated from the following formula:

$$(p_1 - p_2) \pm Z_{\alpha/2} SE(p_1 - p_2)$$

In the case of the MI trial data, the calculated $Z = -3.55$, which corresponds to a probability of $P < 0.001$. The estimated difference in proportions is -2.78% with a 95% CI of $(-4.32\%, -1.24\%)$. Since the absolute Z-value is $> Z_{0.05/2} = 1.96$ with an associated P-value of <0.001, there is very strong evidence against the null hypothesis. It can therefore be concluded that patients in the treatment group have a significantly lower risk of death within 30 days than patients in the placebo group at the 5% level. One can reach the same conclusion by noting that the 95% CI $(-4.32\%, -1.24\%)$ does not contain 0%.

Assessing the size of the treatment effect in a two-arm trial

In the previous sections, we have introduced different methods for assessing whether there is any evidence against the null hypothesis of no difference. In this section, we describe three commonly used measurements for assessing the size of any treatment effect.

Risk difference

The difference in the proportion of the outcomes between two groups, $p_1 - p_2$, is called the *risk difference*. In the case of the MI trial data, the risk difference is the risk of death between the active drug and placebo, ie, $5.38\% - 8.16\% = -2.78\%$. This means that the estimated absolute risk of death is 2.78% lower (about three in 100 MI patients) in the active drug group compared to the placebo group. Statistical inferences about the risk difference, such as point estimate and CIs can be made by means of a Z-test, as described in the last section.

Risk ratio

The *risk ratio* is the ratio of the risks in the active drug treatment group compared to the placebo group. The risk ratio is often abbreviated to *RR*, and is also sometimes called the relative risk:

$$RR = \frac{p_1}{p_2} = \frac{a/n_1}{b/n_2} = \frac{a/(a+c)}{b/(b+d)}$$

For the MI trial, the $RR = 0.66$ ($5.38\% / 8.16\%$), meaning that the risk of death for the patients in the active drug treatment group is only 66% of the risk in the placebo group. Equivalently, we could say that the drug treatment is associated with a 34% ($100\% - 66\%$) reduction in mortality at 30 days.

We can make statistical inferences about risk ratio using the Z-test or CI for the *RR*. If the null hypothesis of no difference between the risks in the two groups is true, $RR = 1$ and hence $\log(RR) = 0$ ('log' stands for natural logarithm). We can use log (RR) and its standard error to derive a Z-statistic and test the null hypothesis using the following formula:

$$Z = \frac{\log RR}{SE(\log RR)}$$

$$SE(\log RR) = \sqrt{1/a - 1/n_1 + 1/b - 1/n_2}$$

where $SE(\log RR)$ is the standard error of log RR [3].

In the MI trial example:

$$SE(\log RR) = \sqrt{1/110 - 1/2045 + 1/165 - 1/2022} = 0.12$$

$$Z = \frac{\log RR}{SE(\log RR)} = \frac{\log(0.66)}{0.12} = -3.46$$

This corresponds to a P-value of <0.001. Therefore, there is strong evidence against the null hypothesis that $RR = 1$.

To calculate the 95% CI for RR, we need to follow the following steps:

Step 1: Calculate the standard error of log RR.

Step 2: Calculate the error factor (EF) as follows:

$$EF = \exp(1.96 \times SE[\log RR])$$

Step 3: 95% CI = RR / EF to $RR \times EF$

Considering the MI trial data in **Table 1**, EF is given by:

$$EF = \exp(1.96 \times 0.12) = 1.26$$

The 95% CI for RR is therefore:

$$95\% \text{ CI} = 0.66 / 1.26 \text{ to } 0.66 \times 1.26 = 0.52 \text{ to } 0.83$$

Once more, we are able to conclude that RR is significantly different from 1 at the 5% significance level.

Odds ratio

A third measure of treatment effect is the *odds ratio* (*OR*). The odds of an outcome event are calculated as the number of events divided by the number of nonevents. For example, in the active treatment arm in the MI trial, the number of deaths is 110 and the number of survivals is 1,935, so the odds of death are 110 / 1935 = 0.057. If the odds of an event are >1, the event is more likely to happen than not. In particular, the odds of an event that is certain to happen are infinite, and the odds of an impossible event are zero. The *OR* is calculated by dividing the odds in the active treatment group (*a* / *c*) by the odds in the placebo group (*b* / *d*):

$$OR = \frac{a/c}{b/d} = \frac{ad}{bc}$$

For the MI trial data, the *OR* is calculated as (110 × 1857) / (1936 × 165) = 0.64, meaning that the odds of deaths after MI in the drug group are 64% of the odds in the placebo group. Clinical trials typically look at treatments that reduce the proportion of patients with an event or, equivalently, have an *OR* of <1. In these cases, a percentage reduction in the *OR* is often quoted instead of the *OR* itself. For the preceding *OR*, we can say that there is a 36% (100% − 64%) reduction in the odds of deaths in the active treatment group.

As for the *RR*, we can also carry out statistical inference about the *OR* in the population. We can test the null hypothesis that the *OR* = 1; hence, that the odds of death are equal in both treatment groups. The following formula can be used for performing a hypothesis test:

$$Z = \frac{\log OR}{SE(\log OR)}$$

$$SE(\log RR) = \sqrt{1/a + 1/b + 1/c + 1/d}$$

where *SE*(log *OR*) is the standard error of logarithmic odds ratio.

Considering the data from the MI trial in **Table 1**, we have the standard error of the log *OR* as:

$$SE(\log OR) = \sqrt{1/a + 1/b + 1/c + 1/d} = \sqrt{1/110 + 1/165 + 1/1935 + 1/1875} = 0.13$$

so, *Z* = log(0.64) / 0.13 = −3.43

Table 5. Three measurements for comparing a binary outcome between two treatment groups, together with the results for the myocardial infarction trial data in Table 1.

Measure of comparison	Formula	Value	95% CI	Z-statistics	P-value
Risk difference	$p_1 - p_2$	-2.78%	(-4.32%, -0.24%)	-3.53	<0.001
Risk ratio (relative risk)	p_1 / p_2	0.66	(0.52, 0.83)	-3.46	<0.001
Odds ratio	$\dfrac{a/c}{b/d} = \dfrac{ad}{bc}$	0.64	(0.50, 0.82)	-3.43	<0.001

p_1 = 5.38% for active drug; p_2 = 8.16% for placebo.

This corresponds to a *P*-value <0.001. Therefore, there is strong evidence against the null hypothesis that the *OR* = 1. CIs for *OR*s are calculated in a similar fashion as for *RR*s. The results are shown in **Table 5**.

Relationships between risk ratio and odds ratio

As discussed in the last section, the risk ratio and odds ratio are two different measurements of treatment effects in clinical research. The risk ratio has immediate intuitive interpretation. It is relatively easy to explain that, for example, if the *RR* = 0.50, patients in the active treatment group have half the risk of having an event than patients in the placebo group (*RR* = 1/2). By contrast, interpretation of the odds ratio is more difficult.

In clinical papers, it is common to mistake the odds ratio for a risk ratio; indeed, when events are rare, the odds ratio and risk ratio are very similar. For example, in the MI trial, the risk ratio of death is 0.66, very close to the odds ratio of 0.64, because the mortality rate is small (6.76% in total). This close approximation holds only when events are rare. For common outcomes, the odds ratio and risk ratio can be markedly different. **Figure 1** shows the relationship between the odds ratio and risk ratio for hypothetical studies assessing the active treatment effect on improving cure rate (synonymous with risk) of a disease. Each line on the graph relates to a different risk in the placebo group. We can use this graph to get a grasp of how misleading it could be to interpret an odds ratio as if it were a risk ratio.

It is clear from **Figure 1** that when the risk in the placebo group is low, say 1%, the odds ratio is a good approximation of the risk ratio. For example, when *RR* = 4.8, *OR* = 5. However, when the risk is 50%, *RR* = 1.7 is equivalent to *OR* = 5.

Figure 1. Relationship between odds ratio and risk ratio.

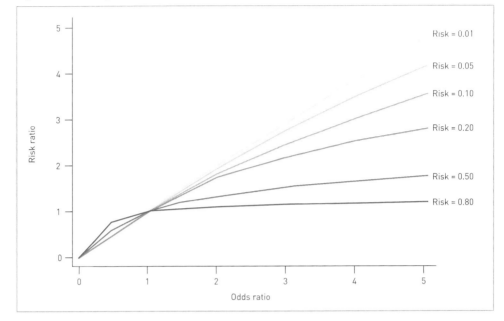

Why use odds ratios?

If odds ratios are difficult to interpret, why do we not always use risk ratios instead? There are several reasons for this, most of which are related to the superior mathematical properties of odds ratios. Firstly, odds ratios can always take values between zero and infinity, which is not the case for risk ratios. For example, if the risk of death is 0.60, it is not possible to double it. Odds ratios also possess symmetry: if the outcomes in the analysis are reversed, the relationships will have reciprocal odds ratios. In case of the MI trial data, we have:

$$OR(\text{death}) = 1 \,/\, OR(\text{survival})$$

However, no such relationship exists for risk ratios. In addition, if we need to make adjustments for confounding factors using regression, odds ratios can be modeled very easily by a logistic regression model, whereas a regression model for risk ratios cannot always be fitted. Furthermore, while a risk ratio is only accurate with complete subject follow-up, an odds ratio is a useful measure of association for a variety of study designs, such as a case-control study.

Table 6. Number (%) of patients in NYHA classes by treatment in a cardiovascular trial.

NYHA	Treatment	
	Active drug	Placebo
Class I	276 (7.6)	267 (7.5)
Class II	1946 (53.8)	1932 (54.4)
Class III	1334 (36.9)	1280 (36.0)
Class IV	58 (1.6)	74 (2.1)
Total	3614 (100.0)	3553 (100.0)

Comparing endpoints with more than two categories by treatment groups

In some clinical trials, a discrete efficacy or safety point has more than two categories (ordered or unordered). For example, in cardiovascular trials dealing with patients with heart failure, the New York Heart Association (NYHA) classification (four classes: I, II, III, and IV) is often used as a measure of a patient's functional capacity with respect to heart failure. We might also need to compare more than two groups (eg, drug 1, drug 2, and placebo), which gives a $r \times c$ contingency table (r = rows and c = columns). This can be analyzed by a chi-squared test in a similar way to a 2×2 contingency table [2,3].

Table 6 presents some data on NYHA class, measured at the end of a cardiovascular trial. This is a 4×2 contingency table with four rows standing for the four NYHA classes and two columns representing the two treatments. For this table, the chi-squared test can be used to assess whether the percentage distributions in NYHA class are statistically significantly different between the two treatments. Following the procedures described above for a 2×2 contingency table, we obtained $\chi^2 = 2.74$. For an $r \times c$ contingency table, the number of the degrees of freedom is $(r - 1) \times (c - 1) = (4 - 1) \times (2 - 1) = 3$. From **Table 4**, we have $\chi^2_{0.05,3} = 7.81$. Since $\chi^2 < \chi^2_{0.05,3}$, $P > 0.05$. We can therefore conclude that there is insufficient evidence to suggest that the two population percentage distributions of NYHA class are significantly different.

It should be noted that the chi-squared test compares the distribution of four NYHA classes, not taking into account the ordinal nature of NYHA class. For an $r \times c$ contingency table with an ordered categorical variable like NYHA class, we can also use the nonparametric Wilcoxon rank sum (Mann–Whitney) test to assess whether there is a statistically significant difference in the outcome distribution between treatment groups (see **Chapter 19**). In the case of the NYHA data in **Table 6**, the Wilcoxon rank sum test yields a P-value of >0.05, suggesting

Table 7. Summary of the statistical test methods described in this chapter.

Statistical issues	Tests or measurements	Null hypothesis	Test statistics	Confidence intervals
Estimate of the population proportion	One-sample Z-test	$H_0 : \pi_1 = \pi_0$, π_1 is the population proportion for the drug group and π_0 is a fixed proportion	$Z = \dfrac{p_1 - \pi_0}{SE[p_1]}$, $SE[p_1 - p_2] = \sqrt{p_1(1-p_1)/n_2}$	$p_1 \pm Z_{\alpha/2} SE[p_1]$
Comparison of two proportions	Chi-squared test	$H_0 : \pi_1 = \pi_2$, π_1 and π_2 are the population proportions for the active drug and placebo groups, respectively	$\chi^2 = \sum \dfrac{(O - E)^2}{E}$, $df = 1$	Not available
	Z-test	$H_0 : \pi_1 = \pi_2$	$Z = \dfrac{p_1 - p_2}{SE[p_1 - p_2]}$, $SE[p_1 - p_2] = \sqrt{p[1-p][1/n_1 + 1/n_2]}$, $p = \dfrac{(a+b)}{(n_1 + n_2)}$	$(p_1 - p_2) \pm Z_{\alpha/2} SE[p_1 - p_2]$
Assessment of the size of treatment effect	Risk difference	$H_0 : \pi_1 = \pi_2$	The same as in the Z-test, above	The same as in the Z-test, above
	Risk ratio (RR)	$H_0 : RR = 1$	$Z = \dfrac{\log RR}{SE(\log RR)}$, $RR = \dfrac{p_1}{p_2}$, $SE(\log RR) = \sqrt{1/a - 1/n_1 + 1/b - 1/n_2}$	$95\%\ CI(RR) = RR/EF$ to $RR \times EF$, $EF = \exp[1.96 \times SE(\log RR)]$
	Odds ratio (OR)	$H_0 : OR = 1$	$Z = \dfrac{\log OR}{SE(\log OR)}$, $OR = \dfrac{a/c}{b/d}$, $SE(\log OR) = \sqrt{1/a + 1/b + 1/c + 1/d}$	$95\%\ CI(OR) = OR/EF$ to $RR \times EF$, $EF = \exp[1.96 \times SE(\log OR)]$
Comparison of $r \times c$ table	Chi-squared test	H_0: percentage distributions are the same among different groups	$\chi^2 = \sum \dfrac{(O - E)^2}{E}$, $df = (r - 1)(c - 1)$	Not available

that the NYHA distribution in the active treatment group is not significantly different from that in the placebo group.

Conclusion

In this chapter, we have described statistical methods for the analysis of categorical data, focusing mainly on the analysis of *2 × 2* tables (see **Table 7**). Generally, a chi-squared test can be used to analyze any *r × c* contingency table, involving the calculation of the expected numbers of frequencies in each cell and then comparing these to the observed numbers. The purpose of the chi-squared test is to assess whether the percentage distributions differ among different groups. The limitation of a chi-squared test is that it does not produce a point estimate or CI for the treatment effect.

To quantify the treatment effect in a clinical trial, the risk difference, risk ratio, or odds ratio for a binary endpoint can be used to address different research questions. It should be noted that the latter two are different measures, except when the outcome event is rare.

It is important to appreciate how proportions or percentages of outcomes are compared in a trial so that we can be clear about when to use terms such as 'odds ratios' and 'risk ratios'. These statistical tools are appropriate in specific situations: an odds ratio is useful for summarizing treatment effects in systematic reviews and determining the epidemiology risk of a particular exposure, while a risk ratio is useful in a balanced trial to represent the benefit of a treatment exposure.

References

1. Pocock SJ. *Clinical Trials: A Practical Approach.* New York: John Wiley & Sons, 1983.
2. Altman DG. *Practical Statistics for Medical Research*. London: Chapman & Hall, 1999.
3. Kirkwood B, Sterne J. *Essential Medical Statistics*, 2nd edition. Oxford: Blackwell Publishing, 2003.

Chapter 21

Analysis of Survival Data

Duolao Wang, Tim Clayton, and Ameet Bakhai

In clinical research, an endpoint is often the time to the occurrence of some particular event, such as the death of a patient. These types of data are known as time-to-event data or survival data. However, the event of interest need not be death, but could be some other well-defined event, such as the first episode of malaria in a vaccine trial or the end of a period spent in remission from a disease. The outcome could also be a positive event, such as relief from symptoms. In this chapter, we introduce some fundamental methods for the analysis of such survival data and illustrate their applications through examples.

Introduction

In many clinical trials, the outcome is not just whether an event occurs, but also the time it takes for the event to occur. For example, in a cancer study comparing the relative merits of surgery and chemotherapy treatments, the outcome measured could be the time from the start of therapy to the death of the subject. In this case the event of interest is death, but in other situations it might be the end of a period spent in remission from cancer spread, relief of symptoms, or a further admission to hospital. These types of data are generally referred to as *time-to-event* data or *survival* data, even when the endpoint or the event being studied is something other than the death of a subject. The term *survival analysis* encompasses the methods and models for analyzing such data representing time free from events of interest.

Example: pancreatic cancer trial

The death rate from pancreatic cancer is amongst the highest of all cancers. A randomized controlled clinical trial was conducted on 36 patients diagnosed with pancreatic cancer. The aim of this trial was to assess whether the use of a new treatment A could increase the survival of patients compared to the standard treatment B. Patients were followed-up for 48 months and the primary endpoint was the time, in months, from randomization to death. **Table 1** displays the survival data for the 36 patients. We will use this example to illustrate some fundamental survival analysis methods and their applications.

Basic concepts in survival analysis

Censoring

In survival analysis, not all subjects are involved in the study for the same length of time due to *censoring*. This term denotes when information on the outcome status of a subject stops being available. This can be because the patient is lost to follow-up (eg, they have moved away) or stops participating in the study, or because the end of the study observation period is reached without the subject having an event. Censoring is a nearly universal feature of survival data. **Table 2** summarizes the main reasons for censoring that can occur in a clinical trial. Survival analysis takes into account censored data and, therefore, utilizes the information available from a clinical trial more fully.

Table 1. Survival data for 36 patients with pancreatic cancer in a trial of a new treatment versus the standard treatment.

New treatment		Standard treatment	
Survival time (months)	Survival status (0 = survival, 1 = dead)	Survival time (months)	Survival status (0 = survival, 1 = dead)
2	0	3	0
5	0	5	1
10	1	6	0
12	1	7	1
15	0	8	1
27	1	10	1
36	0	11	0
36	0	12	1
37	1	13	0
38	0	15	1
39	0	16	0
41	0	23	1
42	0	30	1
44	0	39	1
45	1	40	1
46	0	45	1
48	0	48	0
48	0	48	0

Table 2. Reasons for censoring observations in clinical trials.

Reason	Example
Lost to follow-up	Patient moved away or did not wish to continue participation
Patient withdrawn	Patient withdraws from the study due to side-effects
Patient has an outcome that prevents the possibility of the primary endpoint (competing risk)	Death from cancer where death from cardiac causes is the primary endpoint
Study termination	All patients who have not died are considered censored at the end of the study

Table 3. Kaplan–Meier estimate of survival function for patients receiving treatment A in the pancreatic cancer trial.

Survival time (months) t_j	Number at risk at t_j n_j	Number of events at t_j d_j	Survival function at t_j $S(t_j)$
2	18	0	1.000
5	17	0	1.000
10	16	1	0.938
12	15	1	0.875
15	14	0	0.875
27	13	1	0.808
36	12	0	0.808
37	10	1	0.727
38	9	0	0.727
39	8	0	0.727
41	7	0	0.727
42	6	0	0.727
44	5	0	0.727
45	4	1	0.545
46	3	0	0.545
48	2	0	0.545

Step 2: Determine the number of individuals at risk and the number of events at each time. At each time t_j, there are n_j individuals who are said to be at risk of an event. 'At risk' means that they have not experienced an event, nor have they been censored prior to time t_j. Cases that are censored at exactly time t_j are also considered to be at risk at t_j. Let d_j be the number of individuals who have an event at time t_j.

Step 3: Calculate the KM estimator using the following formula:

$$\hat{S}(t_1) = \left(1 - \frac{d_1}{n_1}\right)$$

$$\hat{S}(t_2) = \hat{S}(t_1) \times \left(\frac{1 - d_2}{n_2}\right)$$

$$...$$

$$\hat{S}(t_j) = \hat{S}(t_{j-1}) \times \left(\frac{1 - d_j}{n_j}\right)$$

Figure 1. Kaplan–Meier survival functions by treatment group for the pancreatic cancer trial data.

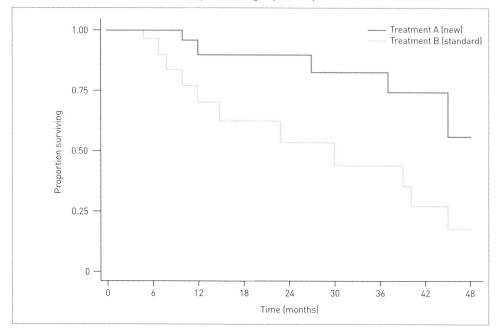

Number of patients at risk.

Time (months)	0	6	12	18	24	30	36	42	48
Treatment A	18	17	15	14	14	13	12	6	2
Treatment B	18	16	11	8	7	6	6	4	2

In other words,

$$\hat{S}(t_j) = \left(\frac{1 - d_1}{n_1}\right) \times \left(\frac{1 - d_2}{n_2}\right) \times \dots \times \left(\frac{1 - d_j}{n_j}\right)$$

where $t_1 \leq t_j \leq t_k$.

Table 3 displays the derivation of the KM estimate of survival function for patients receiving treatment A from the pancreatic cancer trial. The table estimates that the proportion of surviving patients is 87.5% at 12 months, 80.8% at 36 months, and 54.5% by the end of the study.

Kaplan–Meier survival curves
The KM estimates of the survival curves by the two treatment groups for the pancreatic cancer trial data are displayed in **Figure 1**. The survival curve is shown

in a step function: the curve is horizontal at all times at which there is no event, with a vertical drop corresponding to the change in the survival function at each time, t_j, when an event occurs.

In reports, KM curves are usually displayed in one of two ways. The curves can decrease with time from 1 (or 100%), denoting how many people survive (or remain event-free). However, in general it is recommended that the increase in event rates is shown starting from 0 (or 0%) subjects with an increasing curve $(1 - \hat{S}[t])$, unless the event rate is high [3]. Placing the curves for different treatment groups on the same graph allows us to graphically review any treatment differences.

Limitations of the Kaplan–Meier method

The KM method has some limitations, however. As survival rates are calculated throughout the study, a decreasing number of subjects will be available for follow-up as the curve progresses with time. Therefore, near the end of the study, when we have a relatively small number of subjects who have survived and are still at risk, the data are less representative of the overall effect and some sensible cut-off is needed in order to represent the data.

For this reason, a well-presented chart will also include a table to show the number of people available to the study and event-free at each point in time, as shown in **Figure 1**, which allows an appreciation of the censored data [3]. In addition, the KM method is a descriptive statistical approach and therefore does not estimate the treatment effect. To establish whether there is any significant statistical difference in the survival rates between the treatment groups, a statistical test is required.

Log-rank test

For the two KM curves by treatment group shown in **Figure 1**, the obvious question to ask is: "Did the new treatment make a difference in the survival experience of the two groups?" A natural approach to answering this question is to test the null hypothesis that the survival function is the same in the two groups: that is $H_0 : S_1(t) = S_2(t)$ for all t, where 1 and 2 represent the new treatment and the standard treatment, respectively.

The above hypothesis can be assessed by performing a log-rank test [1,2,4]. The main purpose of this test is to calculate the number of events expected in each treatment group, and to compare this expected number of events with the observed number of events in each treatment group if the null hypothesis is true. The log-rank statistic can be computed by the following steps:

Step 1: Pool the two groups and sort the event times in ascending order. Suppose there are r distinct event times, $t_1 < t_2 < \ldots < t_r$.

Step 2: Determine the number of individuals at risk and the number of events at each time in each group, as well as in the two groups combined. At each time t_j ($t_1 \le t_j \le t_r$), we assume there are n_{1j}, n_{2j}, and n_j individuals at risk of the event and d_{1j}, d_{2j}, and d_j individuals who have had an event in groups 1, 2, and the two groups combined, respectively.

Step 3: Calculate the expected number of events and the variance of v_{1j} in group 1 at each time t_j. The expected number of events is given by:

$$e_{1j} = \frac{n_{1j} - d_j}{n_j}$$

and the variance of v_{1j} is given by:

$$v_{1j} = \frac{n_{1j}\, n_{2j}\, d_j\, (n_j - d_j)}{n_j^2\, (n_j - 1)}$$

Step 4: Calculate the log-rank statistic using the following formula:

$$U_L = \sum_{j=1}^{r} (d_{1j} - e_{1j})$$

$$V_L = \sum_{j=1}^{r} (v_{1j})$$

$$\chi^2 = \frac{U_L^2}{V_L}$$

where χ^2 is a chi-squared statistic that follows chi-squared distribution with one degree of freedom (see **Chapter 20** for more about the chi-squared [χ^2] test).

The detailed calculation for the pancreatic cancer trial data is displayed in **Table 4**: $U_L = -4.4776$, $V_L = 3.6967$, so:

$$\chi^2 = \frac{(-4.4776)^2}{3.6967} = 5.42$$

This χ^2 value is converted to a P-value of 0.020. As $P < 0.05$, the log-rank test has shown a significant survival difference between the new treatment A and standard treatment B. This test readily generalizes to three or more groups, with the null hypothesis that all groups have the same survival function. If the null hypothesis is true, the test statistic has a chi-squared distribution with the degrees of freedom equal to the number of groups minus 1.

Table 4. Calculation of the log-rank statistic for the pancreatic cancer trial data.

Time (months)	Treatment A		Treatment B		Total		Treatment A	
	d_{1j}	n_{1j}	d_{2j}	n_{2j}	d_j	n_j	e_{1j}	v_{1j}
5	0	17	1	17	1	34	0.5000	0.2500
7	0	16	1	15	1	31	0.5161	0.2497
8	0	16	1	14	1	30	0.5333	0.2489
10	1	16	1	13	2	29	1.1034	0.4770
12	1	15	1	11	2	26	1.1538	0.4686
15	0	14	1	9	1	23	0.6087	0.2382
23	0	13	1	7	1	20	0.6500	0.2275
27	1	13	0	6	1	19	0.6842	0.2161
30	0	12	1	6	1	18	0.6667	0.2222
37	1	10	0	5	1	15	0.6667	0.2222
39	0	8	1	5	1	13	0.6154	0.2367
40	0	7	1	4	1	11	0.6364	0.2314
45	1	4	1	3	2	7	1.1429	0.4082
Total	**5**						**9.4776**	**3.6967**

A = new treatment; B = standard treatment.

Limitations to the log-rank test

There are three major limitations to the log-rank test.

- It does not provide a direct estimate of the magnitude of treatment effect.
- It is mainly used to compare groups on the basis of a single variable, such as treatment.
- It is more likely to detect a difference between groups when the risk of an event is consistently higher for one group than another, but it is unlikely to detect the difference when survival curves cross [1,2].

KM survival curves should always be plotted before making group comparisons. In addition, all of the above shortcomings can be overcome by the application of a hazards regression model, such as the Cox proportional hazards model, introduced in the next section [1,2].

Proportional hazards model

Model description

As described earlier, the hazard function $h(t)$ is the risk that a subject experiences an event at time t given that the subject has not experienced the event up to t. The proportional hazards model relates the hazard function to a number of covariates (such as the patient's characteristics at randomization and the treatment received in a clinical trial) as follows [1,2,5]:

$$h_i(t) = h_0(t)\exp(b_1 x_{1i} + b_2 x_{2i} + \ldots + b_p x_{pi}) \qquad (1)$$

where x_{ki} is the value of the covariate x_k $(k=1, 2,\ldots, p)$ for an individual i $(i=1, 2,\ldots, n)$.

The equation shows that the hazard for individual i at time t is the product of two factors:

- A baseline hazard function $h_0(t)$ that is left unspecified, except that it cannot be negative.
- A linear function of a set of p fixed covariates, which is then exponentiated.

The baseline hazard function can be regarded as the hazard function for individuals whose covariates all have value 0 and changes according to time t.

Two basic types of model are available for us to use, depending on whether we specify $h_0(t)$. In general, if we specify a parametric function for $h_0(t)$ in equation (1), we will have a *parametric* hazards regression model. So, if we specify $h_0(t) = \lambda t^\alpha$, we get the *Weibull* hazards regression model. The most widely used hazards regression model, however, is the *Cox* regression model, in which such choices of $h_0(t)$ are unnecessary [1,2]. In the Cox model, the baseline hazard function $h_0(t)$ can take any form. Therefore, the Cox regression model is sometimes called a semi-parametric hazards regression model and is commonly referred to as the Cox proportional hazards regression model.

Proportional hazards assumption

Why is this called a proportional hazards model? The reason is that while the baseline hazard can constantly change over time, the hazard for any individual is assumed to be proportional to the hazard for any other individual for all times t, and will depend on the covariate values. To illustrate this, let us assume that the model has only one covariate (treatment, x_{1i}, $x_{1i} = 0$ for standard treatment and 1 for new treatment). We first calculate the hazards for two individuals *1* and *2* according to equation (1) and then take the ratio of the two hazards:

Figure 2. Proportional hazards assumption: equal distance between two hazards functions for two individuals.

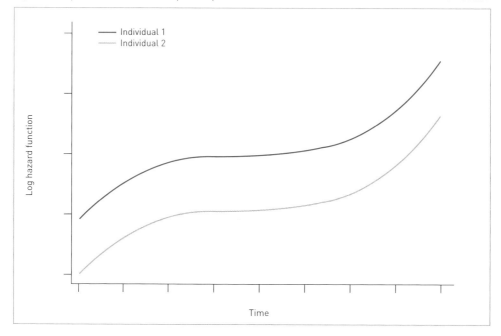

$$h_1(t) = h_0(t)\exp(b_1 x_{11})$$

$$h_2(t) = h_0(t)\exp(b_1 x_{12})$$

$$\frac{h_1(t)}{h_2(t)} = \exp(b_1[x_{11} - x_{12}]) \qquad (2)$$

What is important about equation (2) is that $h_0(t)$ is canceled out of the numerator and denominator. As a result, the ratio of hazards, $\exp(b_1[x_{11} - x_{12}])$, is constant over time. In this example, $\exp(b_1[x_{11} - x_{12}]) = \exp(0) = 1$ if the two individuals have the same treatment, or $\exp(b_1[x_{11} - x_{12}]) = \exp(b_1)$ (or $\exp[-b_1]$) if they have different treatments. After performing a logarithmic transformation to both sides of equation (2), we have the following equation:

$$\log(h_1[t]) - \log(h_2[t]) = b_1(x_{11} - x_{12})$$

If we plot the log hazards for the two individuals, the proportional hazards property implies that the hazard functions should strictly have the same distance at any time during the study as shown in **Figure 2**. If these curves cross each other or diverge, then the proportional hazards (sometimes called proportionality) assumption may not be met.

However, the graphical method to assess proportionality is still a subjective approach and does not provide a statistical test for assessing the proportional assumption for a group of covariates. The proportionality can be formally assessed using a chi-squared test with the two hazard functions proportional in the null hypothesis, ie:

$$H_0 : \frac{h_1(t)}{h_2(t)} = \gamma$$

where γ is a constant [1,2].

If nonproportionality is found in an analysis, the proportional hazards model (1) is no longer suitable and more complex modeling may be necessary, for example by incorporating some sort of interaction between treatment and time into the model [1,2].

Interpretation of regression results

Table 5 displays the extracted results from the Cox proportional model analysis of primary endpoint in the CHARM (Candesartan in Heart failure Assessment of Reduction in Morbidity and mortality) trial [6]. In this trial, the primary endpoint was the time to first occurrence of cardiovascular death or hospitalization due to chronic heart failure (CHF). **Table 5** gives the coefficient estimate (b_k) and associated statistics. The column labeled hazard ratio is e^{b_k}.

For a binary (dummy) variable with values of 1 and 0, the hazard ratio can be interpreted as the ratio of the estimated hazard for those with a value of 1 to the estimated hazard for those with a value of 0 (controlling for other covariates). For example, the estimated hazard ratio for the variable 'female' is 0.83. This means that the hazard of having a cardiovascular death or CHF hospitalization for females is estimated to be 83% (95% confidence interval [CI] 76%, 91%) of the hazard for males (controlling for other covariates).

For a quantitative covariate, a more helpful statistic is obtained by subtracting 1 from the hazard ratio and multiplying by 100. This gives the estimated percent change in the hazard for each 1-unit increase in the covariate. For the variable 'age' in **Table 5**, the hazard ratio is 1.04, yielding $(1.04 - 1) \times 100 = 4$. Therefore, for each 1-year increase in the age of the patient at randomization, the hazard of having a primary endpoint goes up by an estimated 4% (95% CI 3%, 5%).

For a categorical covariate, the hazard ratio can be interpreted as the ratio of hazard for those in a group compared with that of the reference group. For example, the covariate 'diabetes' has three categories:

Table 5. Selected predictors of cardiovascular death or hospitalization due to chronic heart failure (CHF) in the CHARM trial (7,599 patients) [5].

Variables	Coefficient	Hazard ratio	95% CI		P-value
Age (years)	0.04	1.04	1.03	1.05	<0.0001
Diabetes					
Insulin treated (vs none)	0.71	2.03	1.80	2.29	<0.0001
Non-insulin-dependent (vs none)	0.46	1.58	1.43	1.74	<0.0001
Ejection fraction (per 5%)	−0.12	0.88	0.87	0.90	<0.0001
Prior CHF					
Prior CHF hosp within 6 months (vs no prior CHF)	0.55	1.73	1.55	1.93	<0.0001
Prior CHF hosp, but not within 6 months (vs no prior CHF)	0.20	1.22	1.09	1.37	<0.001
Cardiomegaly (vs none)	0.30	1.35	1.23	1.47	<0.0001
NYHA					
Class III (vs class II)	0.28	1.32	1.20	1.45	<0.0001
Class IV (vs class II)	0.43	1.54	1.25	1.89	<0.0001
DBP (10 mm Hg)	−0.11	0.9	0.86	0.93	<0.0001
Heart rate (10 beats/min)	0.08	1.08	1.05	1.11	<0.0001
Candesartan (vs placebo)	−0.20	0.82	0.76	0.89	<0.0001
Dependent edema (vs none)	0.21	1.23	1.12	1.35	<0.0001
Female (vs male)	−0.18	0.83	0.76	0.91	<0.0001

CI = confidence interval; DBP = diastolic blood pressure; hosp = hospitalization; NYHA = New York Heart Association.

- no diabetes
- insulin-treated diabetes
- non-insulin-dependent diabetes

In the **Table 5** analysis, the group with no diabetes was chosen as the reference group. The estimated hazard ratios for patients with insulin- and non-insulin-dependent diabetes at baseline are 2.03 and 1.58, respectively. Therefore, for diabetic patients on insulin there is a doubling in hazard compared with nondiabetics, whereas non-insulin-dependent diabetics have a 58% increase in hazard.

Assessing the size of treatment effect in a two-arm trial for survival data

In this section, we introduce some measurements of treatment effect in a two-arm trial and discuss their advantages and disadvantages.

Risk difference, risk ratio, and odds ratio

Risk is simply measured as the proportion of subjects who have an event of interest by a specific time point. The odds are the ratio of patients with an event compared to those without the event [5]. The risk difference or ratio and the odds ratio are sometimes used to measure the treatment effect at a specific point in follow-up when an endpoint is time to the occurrence of an event. However, these measurements may be biased for the following reasons:

- They are based on the assumption that all patients were followed-up to the end of the study if they had not died. In our example, not all patients who had not died reached 48 months of follow-up due to censoring.
- Patients with censored events might not be balanced between the two groups.
- No distinction is made between patients who die at 1 month and those who die at 48 months.

Incidence rate difference and ratio

To take different follow-up times into account, we can calculate an incidence rate, ie, the number of events divided by the number of units of time [5]. By comparing the incidence rates between treatment groups, we can derive the incidence rate difference and ratios following the procedures described by Kirkwood and Sterne [5]. For the pancreatic cancer trial data, the incidence rates are calculated as 0.9 and 2.9 deaths per 100 person-months for the new treatment group and the standard treatment group, respectively. The estimates of incidence rate difference and rate ratio, together with their 95% CI and P-value, are as follows:

- incidence rate difference: -2.0, 95% CI (-3.9, -0.1), $P = 0.034$
- incidence rate ratio: 0.30, 95% CI (0.08, 0.94), $P = 0.026$

The above results suggest that the new treatment reduces deaths by two per 100 person-months, with a 95% CI of 0.1, 3.9 per 100 person-months, and that the incidence rate for patients in the new treatment group is only about 30% of the incidence rate for those in the standard treatment group.

Although the incidence rate uses the information on censored observations, it is based on the assumption that the hazard of an event is constant during the study period or has an exponential distribution. In the case of the pancreatic cancer trial, it means that the hazard of death is constant over the 48-month period. However, the risk of an event can change with time. To overcome this problem, the Cox model, which does not require such assumptions, can be used to derive a better measurement for the treatment effect.

Hazard ratio

The treatment can be simply measured as a binary covariate (1 for new treatment A and 0 for standard treatment B in the pancreatic cancer trial) and introduced into a Cox proportional hazards model. In the pancreatic cancer trial, the estimated hazard ratio of death for patients who received treatment A to those who received standard treatment B is 0.31, with 95% CI (0.11, 0.89), $P = 0.030$. This means that the new treatment is estimated to reduce the hazard of death by 69%, with 95% CI (11%, 89%), and the reduction in hazard is statistically significant at the 5% significance level. As there is only one covariate (treatment) in the Cox model, the estimated hazard ratio is called a *crude* or *unadjusted treatment effect*. The adjusted hazard ratio for the treatment will be generated if other baseline patient characteristics are introduced into the model.

The assumption of the Cox proportional hazards model is that the hazard ratio between two treatment groups is constant over the entire time interval. As direct estimates of a hazard function are difficult, especially when the sample size is small, the proportionality is often checked visually by plotting two log–log survival curves [1,2]. A log–log survival curve or log (–log [survival rate]) is a logarithmic transformation of negative logarithmically transformed survival function. According to statistical theory, if two hazard functions are proportional, the two log–log survival curves differ by a constant amount [1,2].

Figure 3 displays the estimated log–log survival curves for the two treatment groups in the pancreatic cancer trial. We see that the two curves are approximately the same shape and are nearly parallel over the study period, so the proportional hazards assumption does not seem to be seriously violated. A formal statistical test of proportional hazards assumption yields a chi-squared value of 0.20 with a *P*-value of 0.655. Since $P = 0.655$, we accept that the proportional hazards assumption holds true since there is no evidence against the null hypothesis.

Figure 3. Examination of proportionality assumption: log–log survival plots for the two treatment groups in the pancreatic cancer trial data.

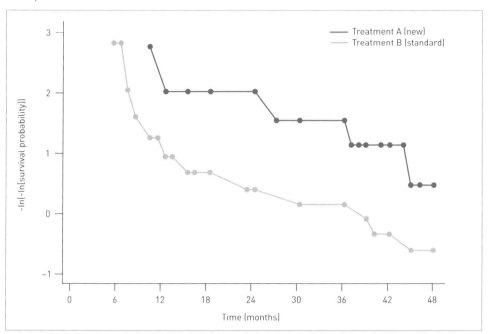

Conclusion

Survival analysis is the study of the duration of time to the occurrence of event outcomes, and is a means of determining the influence of covariates on the occurrence and timing of events. It is a set of techniques that utilize all of the information on survival time, including censored (or incomplete) data. KM curves are a powerful way of showing data and visually displaying differences between the study groups.

We can test the data by looking at the event history of subjects, with respect to treatment, by using the log-rank test, and then extend the analysis further to estimate treatment effects by using the Cox proportional hazards model. When analyzing and reporting clinical trials with time-to-event outcomes, it is recommended that the treatment effect is given as the hazard ratio estimated by the Cox proportional hazards model, unless the proportionality assumption is clearly violated, where alternative approaches may be necessary.

References

1. Collett D. *Modelling Survival Data in Medical Research*, 2nd edition. London: Chapman and Hall, 2003.
2. Cox DR, Oakes D. *Analysis of Survival Data*. London: Chapman and Hall, 1984.
3. Pocock SJ, Clayton TC, Altman DG. Survival plots of time-to-event outcomes in clinical trials: good practice and pitfalls. *Lancet* 2002;**359**:1686–9.
4. Bland JM, Altman DG. Survival probabilities (the Kaplan–Meier method). *BMJ* 1998;**317**:1572.
5. Kirkwood B, Sterne J. *Essential Medical Statistics*, 2nd edition. Oxford: Blackwell Publishing, 2003.
6. Pocock SJ, Wang D, Pfeffer MA, et al. Predictiors of mortality and morbidity in patients with chronic heart failure. *Eur Heart J* 2006;**27**:65–75.

Part IV

Special Trial Issues in Data Analysis

Chapter 22

Intention-to-Treat Analysis

Duolao Wang and Ameet Bakhai

In a clinical trial, the presentation of the results is a key event that can have many implications. Therefore, it is of critical importance to know whether these results have been generated using data from all subjects (intention-to-treat [ITT] analysis) or only from the subjects who adhered fully to their assigned treatment protocol (per-protocol analysis). Between randomization and completion of the trial, subjects may stop being compliant, switch treatments unexpectedly, or withdraw from the study. Excluding data from such subjects (even if these data are incomplete) can result in bias. Therefore, an ITT analysis is more informative and gives results that are closer to those that would be seen if the treatments were given to the population as a whole. In this chapter, we review the advantages and limitations of an ITT strategy for compiling clinical trial results.

Figure 1. Trial profile for the preeclampsia study described in Example 1 [3].

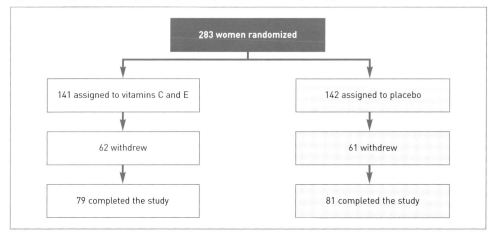

What is an intention-to-treat analysis?

An intention-to-treat (ITT) analysis is a specific strategy for generating the results of a randomized controlled trial. Using this method, all subjects are compared in the treatment groups to which they were originally randomized, regardless of any treatment that they subsequently received [1,2]. When analyzing the results of a study, the ITT method accepts that some subjects might not have complied fully with their treatment protocol, but assumes that if the subjects are randomized adequately then noncompliant subjects will be balanced across all the treatment groups.

An alternative method of analysis is to exclude subjects who were not fully compliant with the study protocol. This form of analysis is known as a per-protocol (PP) analysis, efficacy analysis, or analysis by treatment administered. By focusing only on the fully compliant subjects, one can determine the maximal efficacy of a treatment.

Example 1
We can illustrate these two methods of analysis (ITT and PP) through the following study on preeclampsia. Preeclampsia is a condition of pregnancy where women have raised blood pressure, fluid retention, and excessive protein in the urine, and may go on to develop seizures. Since an excessive build-up of oxidative chemicals might be responsible, a randomized trial was conducted to see whether supplementing women at high risk with vitamins C and E (known to have antioxidant properties) could reduce the frequency of preeclampsia [3]. This study

Table 1. Summary and analysis of the preeclampsia treatment described in Example 1 [3].

Numbers	Study groups		Results
	Vitamins C and E	Placebo	Odds ratio (95% CI); P-value
Women randomized	141	142	
Women who withdrew from the study	62	61	
Women developing preeclampsia	11	24	
Analysis. Percentage of women developing preeclampsia according to:			
Intention-to-treat analysis	8% (11/141)	17% (24/142)	0.42 (0.18, 0.93); P = 0.020
Per-protocol analysis	8% (6/79)	26% (21/81)	0.23 (0.07, 0.66); P = 0.002

identified 283 women as being at increased risk and randomly assigned them to treatment with either a combination of vitamin C (1,000 mg/day) and vitamin E (400 IU/day) or placebo during weeks 16–22 of gestation.

Of the 141 women randomized to vitamins C and E, 62 women withdrew from the study, 79 completed it, and 11 (of whom six were fully compliant) developed preeclampsia. Among the 142 women randomized to the placebo group, 61 withdrew from the study, 81 participated until delivery, and 24 women (of whom 21 were fully compliant) developed preeclampsia (**Figure 1**).

The results, as calculated by both methods of analysis, are presented in **Table 1**. In the ITT analysis, the risk of women developing preeclampsia differed significantly between groups, with 11 of 141 (8%) women in the vitamin group developing preeclampsia versus 24 of 142 (17%) women in the placebo group (odds ratio 0.42; 95% confidence interval [CI] 0.18, 0.93; $P = 0.020$). Using the PP method, which considers only the women who completed the entire study, the difference in the frequency of preeclampsia was more pronounced, with 6 of 79 (8%) women on vitamin therapy developing preeclampsia versus 21 of 81 (26%) women on placebo (odds ratio 0.23; 95% CI 0.07, 0.66; $P = 0.002$). The results from both the ITT and PP analyses suggest that supplementation with vitamins C and E may be beneficial in the prevention of preeclampsia in women at increased risk of the disease, with vitamins shown to be more effective by the PP analysis than the ITT analysis.

What is the justification for an ITT analysis?

It might initially appear from the example that the ITT method is not optimal since it might not capture the full potential benefit of a therapy. However, an ITT analysis actually has several specific advantages:

- From a statistical point of view, an ITT analysis aims to preserve the strengths of randomization [1,2], ie, to minimize bias. An ITT analysis assumes that the rates of noncompliance or withdrawal are equal in both groups. If bias is introduced into such a model, an ITT analysis is more likely to identify this bias. For example, if a large number of subjects withdraw from the new treatment arm compared with the standard treatment arm, the trial will either show no difference in outcomes (since these subjects might switch to standard treatment) or, if the withdrawing subjects take no treatment until the end of the study, may show improved outcomes in the standard treatment arm.
- An ITT analysis captures what happens in real-life more closely than the method that uses data only from subjects with perfect compliance, making it a particularly relevant method for treatments that are difficult to tolerate (ie, drugs with lots of side-effects, such as chemotherapeutics).
- An ITT analysis uses the information from all the subjects in a trial at any given time point in the study, which enables an interim analysis to be performed, while the PP method is best applied when the study is over and all noncompliant patients can be identified and excluded.
- ITT analysis provides practical information on the administration of a treatment. If, for example, subjects are allocated to a surgical treatment for coronary artery disease instead of a less invasive percutaneous coronary intervention and these subjects have to wait 3 months before surgery, during which time some die, an ITT analysis would correctly assign this mortality rate (possibly due to the delay in surgery) to the surgical group, rather than excluding these data as a PP analysis might do.

Therefore, an ITT analysis gives a pragmatic estimate of the effect of a treatment strategy rather than just the specific efficacy of the treatment itself, as given by the PP method [4,5].

What are the limitations of the ITT method?

The main limitation of an ITT analysis is that it includes data from both compliant and noncompliant subjects, and also those who might switch treatment groups unexpectedly during the study. It does not aim to determine the maximum potential effectiveness of a treatment as a PP method would [1,2,4,5]. Therefore, in some studies, the ITT method might not show a statistically significant benefit, or might show the benefit to be smaller than that generated by a PP analysis [2]. Consequently, a routine ITT analysis might find an efficacious treatment to be no more effective than placebo.

When using the ITT method, the issue of how to classify subjects who drop out of the study – ie, stop attending for follow-up – must be dealt with before a study starts. In the worst-case scenario, one could assume that all subjects who withdraw count as deaths or as 'no events', but in reality these subjects will suffer a mixture of events. In some studies it may be assumed that the event rate in the missing subjects is the same as in the group of subjects with data available (a method known as *imputing event rates*). This imputation method should only be used if it proves impossible to get outcome data from a large proportion of subjects, and the results should be presented with and without imputation.

How do the results of ITT and PP analyses compare?

When performed on data from the same study, either or both of the results from the ITT and PP analyses might reach significance. The following are suggestions for how these combinations of results can be interpreted:

- In most trials reaching significance – ie, where the results from an ITT analysis support rejecting the null hypothesis (no significant difference between treatment groups) – if the results of the PP method are slightly more significant, this suggests that while some subjects were noncompliant, they were equally distributed between groups.
- If the PP results are much more significant than the ITT results, this might suggest a high rate of noncompliance in the study.
- If the PP results are not significant but the ITT results are significant, there might be a confounding reason for the difference in outcomes other than it being due to treatment differences. For example, in a trial comparing medicine and surgery, a significant number of subjects may die before having surgery.
- If the result from an ITT analysis is not significant, while that from a PP analysis is significant, this might be due to a considerable proportion of subjects switching treatments (crossover) in one direction (eg, from placebo to new treatment).

Are there analysis strategies beyond the ITT and PP methods?

Given the limitations of an ITT analysis, occasionally we may feel that an explanatory PP analysis is more suitable since it attempts to remove the effects of variable compliance patterns. However, the PP method can lead to a biased comparison if compliance itself is associated with the effectiveness of a treatment or the risk of outcome events [4]. For example, elderly subjects are more likely to have side-effects

Figure 2. Trial profile for the vitamin A supplementation trial described in Example 2 [5].

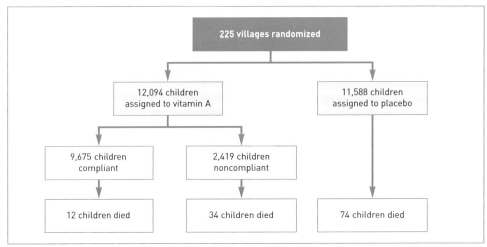

and subsequently withdraw from a study, so excluding such patients will result in a greater treatment effect being shown than that likely to be seen in the general population. In both ITT and PP analyses, a judgment call may need to be made about how to deal with subjects for whom data are incomplete, and by doing this there is a risk of biasing the effectiveness of a drug. Therefore, when it is inappropriate to use either method alone, statistical methods beyond both ITT and PP can add essential insight. This point is illustrated in the following example.

Example 2

Subjects with vitamin A deficiency are more susceptible to infections due to impaired immunity. Therefore, a community-based randomized trial was conducted in rural Indonesia, where infant mortality due to infections is high. The aim of the study was to estimate whether two high doses of vitamin A given twice over an 8-month period would reduce mortality among preschool children. In total, 23,682 children were randomized to vitamin A or placebo. During the study, 20% of children in the treatment group did not receive vitamin A because distribution to their villages was a significant problem. **Figure 2** plots the trial profile and **Table 2** summarizes the results of the trial and analyses.

On completion of the study, there were 46 deaths out of the 12,094 children (0.38%) who were randomized to vitamin A supplementation, and 74 out of 11,588 (0.64%) in the no-supplementation group. Using an ITT analysis, the odds ratio for death was estimated to be 0.59 (95% CI 0.40, 0.87; $P = 0.005$), suggesting a 41% lower rate of death in the group who were supposed to receive vitamin A. The PP analysis calculated an odds ratio of 0.19 (95% CI 0.10, 0.36; $P = 0.001$),

Table 2. Summary and analysis of the vitamin A trial described in Example 2 [5].

Numbers	Study groups		Results
	Vitamins A	Placebo	Odds ratio (95% CI); P-value
Children randomized	12,094	11,588	
Compliant subjects	9,675		
Noncompliant subjects	2,419		
Deaths among randomized subjects	46	74	
Deaths among compliant subjects	12		
Deaths among noncompliant subjects	34		
Analysis			
Mortality rates in:			
Randomized subjects	0.38%	0.64%	
Compliant subjects	0.12%		
Noncompliant subjects	1.41%		
Mortality rates according to:			
Intention-to-treat analysis	0.38% (46/12,094)	0.64% (74/11,588)	0.59 (0.40, 0.87); P = 0.005
Per-protocol analysis	0.12% (12/9,675)	0.64% (74/11,588)	0.19 (0.10, 0.36); P = 0.001

suggesting an 81% reduction in mortality in children who actually received vitamin A as part of the supplementation program.

The information on compliance in **Table 2** shows that, of the 2,419 children in the supplementation group who did not receive vitamin A, 34 (1.41%) died. This rate was twice that of the no-supplementation group (0.64%), despite theoretically having similar treatments (no supplementation). The reason for this was that the same issues responsible for noncompliance – transportation and distribution difficulties – were also responsible for other healthcare deficiencies in the same villages, leading to a higher rate of infant mortality. In the trial, mortality was associated with the bias of whether the child came from a village that could or could not receive delivery of vitamin A. In this situation, comparing only the compliant children (PP analysis) would overestimate the efficacy.

To achieve an unbiased result, the risk of mortality among compliant children in the supplementation group should be compared with the risk of mortality of a comparable subgroup in the no-supplementation group. This comparison would be more appropriate if it can be assumed that randomization led to an equal proportion of noncompliant children in both groups. For further results and an explanation of the methodology used to analyze the data in **Table 2**, see [5].

How should the ITT strategy be implemented in clinical trials?

An ITT strategy should be considered to be both a method of analysis and a way of conducting an entire research study, including trial design [6,7]. When designing a trial, it should be specified whether the study aim is pragmatic (to determine the practical impact of a treatment strategy in a trial setting) or explanatory (using a trial to determine the maximal effectiveness of a treatment strategy). For pragmatic trials the ITT method is optimal, while for an explanatory trial a combination of PP and ITT methods will provide insights. The distinction between these methods is relevant only when a significant number of subjects withdraw, have missing data, or are noncompliant. If these aspects are minimal then the results of both the ITT and PP analyses are likely to be similar.

In addition, more complex statistical methods beyond ITT can be explored to take into account the issue of noncompliers or crossovers. It might also be possible to determine factors that influence compliance, such as genetics. For example, tamoxifen – a treatment for breast cancer – is targeted at subjects in whom a particular type of receptor is present, and some asthma therapies work better in subjects who are also susceptible to hay fever.

What considerations are there when reporting trial results?

When reporting a trial, it should be stated that an ITT strategy has been used to conduct the trial and compile the results. The handling of missing values, noncompliant subjects, and those deviating from the treatment allocated to them at randomization should be clearly described. Lastly, while the main conclusions of the study should be drawn from the results of the ITT analysis, supplemental results using other strategies, such as the PP method, can be shown in addition.

Conclusion

The ITT approach is used to provide an unbiased assessment of a treatment strategy and is usually the optimal method for analyzing the results of a trial. In essence, the ITT method provides the basis for designing, conducting, and reporting an entire clinical trial and comparing treatment strategies. It accounts for treatment effects, difficulties in administering the drug, and compliance issues. Meanwhile, a PP analysis evaluates the maximum benefit possible from a treatment, given perfect compliance. When noncompliance is considerable, the results of both ITT and PP analyses might be unreliable and other statistical methods should be explored.

References

1. Ellenberg JH. Intention-to-treat analysis versus as-treated analysis. *Drug Inf J* 1996;**30**:535–44.
2. Senn S. Intention to treat. Section 11. In: *Statistical Issues in Drug Development*. Chichester: John Wiley and Sons, 1997:153–60.
3. Chappell LC, Seed PT, Briley AL, et al. Effect of antioxidants on the occurrence of preeclampsia in women at increased risk: a randomised trial. *Lancet* 1999;**354**:810–16.
4. Goetghebeur EJT, Pocock SJ. Statistical issues in allowing for noncompliance and withdrawal. *Drug Inf J* 1993;**27**:837–45.
5. Sommer A, Zeger SL. On estimating efficacy from clinical trials. *Stat Med* 1991;**10**:45–52.
6. Hollis S, Campbell F. What is meant by intention to treat analysis? Survey of published randomized controlled trials. *BMJ* 1999;**319**:670–4.
7. Lewis JA, Machin A. Intention to treat—who should use ITT? *Br J Cancer* 1993;**68**:647–50.

Chapter 23

Subgroup Analysis

Ameet Bakhai, Zoe Fox, and Duolao Wang

Subgroup analyses in a clinical trial explore whether there is a relationship between the specific characteristics of subjects and their responses to treatments. Although subgroup analyses are reported in most clinical trials, considerable controversy exists about the best means of performing these investigations. Statisticians are wary of performing multiple subgroup analyses – 'data dredging' – since this increases the risk of finding a false-positive result (a Type I error). Meanwhile, clinicians try to justify 'torturing the data' with the notion that such analyses might identify the patients who benefit the most from specific treatment strategies. In this chapter, we discuss appropriate uses and common abuses of subgroup analyses, and how to interpret the results generated by them.

What is a subgroup analysis?

A clinical study is usually concerned with the overall impact of a treatment on an entire trial population. However, individuals within this population can differ in many ways with respect to their age, gender, other medical problems, and risk of side-effects. These factors can influence their response to treatments. By understanding the relationship between these characteristics and the treatment effect, clinicians can make more accurate treatment decisions for specific patients using knowledge gained through subgroup analyses.

Subgroups can be identified on the basis of patients having specific features not shared by the whole trial population. These features might be patient characteristics (eg, male gender or age >75 years), risk factors (eg, high blood pressure for heart disease, asbestos exposure for lung cancer), specific procedures (eg, keyhole surgery rather than a traditional procedure) or specific tests (eg, a new assay test to measure amylase). Subgroups can also be defined by the level of compliance in the trial (eg, fully compliant) or by the occurrence of a specific outcome (eg, the occurrence of a stroke or survival to 5 years).

Example 1

For example, in a trial of adjuvant chemotherapy for breast cancer, survival was assessed according to nodal status (two categories) and by age group (two categories). Ascertaining survival according to these subgroups provided four survival curves and, consequently, better estimates of survival for individual patients [1]. Using these data, physicians and patients were able to have a more informed discussion about whether chemotherapy would be likely to have benefits or disadvantages in their specific situation.

What is an appropriate subgroup?

An appropriate subgroup consists of subjects with one or more characteristics that have rational relationships to the disease or treatment. For example, consider a trial where patients are being prescribed a novel beta-blocker to reduce high blood pressure. Within this population, examining the treatment effect in subgroups of patients with and without heart failure or minor cardiac rhythm disturbances would be appropriate. Raised blood pressure can lead to heart failure and may therefore be associated with a greater benefit from beta-blockers. However, beta-blockers also reduce the rate at which the heart contracts and may make some patients with slow heart rhythm disturbances worse, thereby decreasing the treatment effect. It would be rational to examine both of these example subgroups in the above trial. Subgroups of subjects recruited on a

Table 1. Potential pitfalls of subgroup analyses.

• Over-interpreting positive results as evidence of cause and effect
• Not supporting the results of subgroup analyses with a strong biological rationale
• Not increasing the significance threshold for multiple analyses
• Having an inadequate number of subjects in the subgroups to be able to give a good estimate of the treatment effect
• Selecting subgroups *post hoc*, which can be biased by the treatment effect itself
• Not considering supporting evidence from other studies

Wednesday or born only in the year 1940 are much less likely to have a rational biological association with a disease process, and so would usually form inappropriate subgroups.

What are the uses of subgroup analyses?

Subgroup analyses are used in many ways. The most common applications are:

- to examine whether the treatment effect or side-effects of treatments are the same or greater in patients with a specific feature or risk factor so that more specific treatment decisions can be made
- to generate hypotheses for future studies such as novel associations (eg, patients with asthma and rheumatoid arthritis had more joint pains in a trial of patients using a new formulation of salbutamol; might rheumatoid arthritis and asthma therapies be linked?)
- in rare situations, to review whether the randomization process worked evenly (eg, in a large multinational trial, were the 100 patients from country X equally distributed to new and control treatments? If not, did the imbalance change the size of the treatment effect for that country's patients?)

What are the problems with subgroup analyses?

A number of pitfalls of subgroup analyses are listed in **Table 1**. The immediate problem with subgroup analyses is that the individual subgroups of interest are usually small compared with the trial population, which can therefore reduce the statistical power for determining an estimate of the true treatment effect within the subgroup. Although the beneficial effect of the treatment might increase if the treatment is restricted to subjects at higher risk of trial endpoints, the confidence interval for the size of the true treatment effect will widen [2].

Table 2. The effect of multiple statistical tests on the overall Type I error rate.

Number of tests with a 5% significance level	Overall chance of a Type I error (%)
1	5.00
2	9.75
3	14.26
4	18.55
5	22.62
10	40.13
20	64.15

Secondly, when many subgroup analyses are undertaken in a clinical trial, the chance of finding a false-positive result (Type I error) by random chance alone increases if the significance level or threshold is kept the same (traditionally a *P*-value of 0.05; ie, a 1 in 20 chance). **Table 2** shows results from a model using treatments of equal efficacy. As the number of subgroup analyses increases, so does the probability of finding at least one result meeting the 5% threshold, even though the treatments are of equal effect. For five subgroup analyses, the overall chance of a Type I error inflates to 22.62% instead of the expected 5%. In other words, the odds of at least one false-positive result increases from 1 in 20 to about 1 in 5, using a 0.05 level. **Chapter 9** contains more on sample size and power.

This method of multiple subgroup analyses has been termed 'torturing the data until it confesses to something', 'a fishing expedition' or 'data dredging' [3,4].

Example 2
A classic demonstration of a 'fishing expedition' was published by Yusuf and colleagues, who looked at the results of the ISIS-2 (Second International Study of Infarct Survival) trial [5,6]. The aim of this study was to determine whether the use of aspirin for patients after a heart attack was associated with a reduction in the risk of further heart attacks. While the overall study results found that aspirin reduced the risk of further heart attacks by 50%, which was a highly significant observation ($P < 0.0001$), one subgroup analysis showed that aspirin was beneficial for all astrological signs except Gemini and Libra. Such an association with birth signs is likely to have arisen due to chance rather than have a plausible pathological association with the risk of heart disease.

Patient imbalance
A further problem for subgroup analyses is that the balance created by randomization might not be maintained in smaller subgroups. For example, while in the overall study men and women might be equally balanced by design,

in a small subgroup of patients >80 years of age, there might be more women since women generally live longer than men. The way to avoid both these limitations is for investigators to calculate an appropriate sample size for the study with well-informed predictions of the likely size of the subgroups in mind.

Are there solutions to deal with the problems of subgroup analyses?

A number of solutions have been devised to overcome the problems stated above.

1. Adjusting the threshold of significance for subgroup analyses

One option would be to adjust the significance level (usually a 1 in 20 chance, or $P < 0.05$) by the number of planned comparisons. For example, if the overall treatment effect was significant at the 5% level and the aim was to investigate the subgroup effect over 20 categories (such as by study sites), then one could divide the original significance level (0.05) by the total number of categories, meaning that a P-value of < 0.0025 is required to declare significance for any one subgroup analysis. This significance adjustment is sometimes called a *Bonferroni correction*.

2. Using an interaction test

In addition to adjusting the significance level, a subgroup analysis should be supported by some sort of interaction test to see whether the association between the treatment effect and the specific characteristic of the subset is significant. For example, let us say that a traditional subgroup analysis found a higher treatment effect in women. We could then ask the question: "Was the treatment effect seen in women significantly different from that seen in men?" If so, this implies that female gender influences treatment response.

In a study of 35 trials where subgroup analyses were performed, only 15 trials used such statistical tests of interaction to confirm the subgroup effect [7]. The limitation of interaction tests, as with other tests, is that with smaller populations to compare they have less statistical power either to capture or to rule out an association.

3. Avoiding bias arising from *post hoc* analysis

Subgroup analyses are often defined after a study is complete; therefore, they are not prespecified or predefined. The method is termed retrospective or '*post hoc*' analysis. Such an analysis should be used mainly to form ideas or propose associations – ie, hypothesis generating – but a large number of researchers use the results of such analyses to support conclusions or explain results, leading to over-interpretation of the positive result. The reason that this may not be a valid strategy is that the treatment itself can influence how the subgroup is formed. An example of this effect is given below.

Example 3

Consider a study that shows a new treatment to be beneficial overall, and that the results are even stronger in younger patients. The trial coordinators state that the treatments work even more effectively in younger patients. However, the reason that these results may occur is because older patients may not be able to tolerate the side-effects of the drug and therefore might withdraw early from the study, making it appear that the benefits are greater in young patients. The statement that the treatment is not beneficial in older patients may also be made. In truth, the effect is not dependent on age but rather the ability of patients to tolerate side-effects. Therefore, neither statement about the young or old subgroups is entirely correct. If we had predefined that we would review the effect of treatments in older and younger patients, we would have aimed to balance the groups during recruitment and would soon have spotted that the groups do not remain balanced after randomization. We would, therefore, have seen the effect of drug side-effects on compliance from older patients.

4. Reviewing existing data to seek support for the subgroup results

More credibility is given to subgroup analysis results if they are supported by similar results from previous independent trials or systematic reviews such as meta-analyses (see **Chapter 38**).

What factors should be considered when planning a subgroup analysis?

If the primary outcome of the trial is related to factors other than the treatment strategies, such as age and gender, then these and other subgroups of interest from previous studies should be prespecified in the protocol with some biological rationale to support their choice. Stratifying randomization and analysis will help reduce imbalance between the subgroups, thereby improving the accuracy of subsequent observations. However, if the size of the study is fixed, it might only be possible to stratify randomization by a small number of characteristics, which limits the number of subgroups that can be predefined. The analysis should examine the relationship between the primary outcome and only these few prespecified subgroups. Subgroup analyses with outcomes occurring with a high frequency in the study will also be more reliable than those investigating rare events.

Conclusion

Clinical trials are conducted to identify whether the use of a specific treatment would be beneficial for populations of patients with a specific disease. In addition, it is important to consider how, within this group, patients with specific characteristics will respond to the treatment. Subgroup analyses allow us to explore the relationship of characteristics to treatment effect. There are, however, a variety of pitfalls and limitations with such analyses, and their results should not be over-interpreted, particularly without rational biological explanations. Interaction tests should also be performed, rather than simple comparisons alone. With these reservations, well-conducted and predefined analyses provide insights to allow better-informed treatment decisions for individual patients.

References

1. Fisher B, Redmond C, Brown A, et al. Influence of tumour estrogen and progesterone receptor levels on the response to tamoxifen and chemotherapy in primary breast cancer. *J Clin Oncol* 1983;**1**:227–41.

2. Bakhai A. Practical issues in trial design. Part 3: confidence intervals. *Clinical Researcher* 2001;**1**(6):46–7.

3. Mills JL. Data torturing. *N Engl J Med* 1993;**329**:1196–9.

4. Cerrito PB. Subgroup analysis. In: Chow SC. *Encyclopedia of Biopharmaceutical Statistics*. New York: Marcel Dekker, 2000;497–507.

5. Randomised trial of intravenous streptokinase, oral aspirin, both, or neither among 17,187 cases of suspected acute myocardial infarction. ISIS-2 (Second International Study of Infarct Survival) Collaborative Group. *Lancet* 1988;**2**;349–60.

6. Yusuf S, Wittes J, Probstfield J, et al. Analysis and interpretation of treatment effects in subgroups of patients in randomized clinical trials. *JAMA* 1991;**266**:93–8.

7. Assmann SF, Pocock SJ, Enos LE, et al. Subgroup analysis and other (mis)uses of baseline data in clinical trials. *Lancet* 2000;**355**:1064–9.

Chapter 24

Regression Analysis

Fiona Steele and Duolao Wang

Most medical events have multiple causes, and these causes are often related. Multiple regression analysis is a statistical tool that has become increasingly important for medical research. It is used to determine the relationship between a single event or outcome and its different causes. These causes can then be established as risk factors for the occurrence of events or protective factors for the prevention of events. In this chapter, we introduce three commonly used types of regression analysis – linear, logistic, and hazards regression – and focus on practical issues, such as when to apply each method and how to interpret the results.

Introduction

The purpose of a clinical trial analysis is to obtain an accurate estimate of any treatment effect. This is often measured as the difference between treatment groups in the primary outcome, based on the assumption of perfect balance among baseline characteristics. If important imbalances are found among some variables, covariate (or a variable related to the outcome) adjustment analysis is sometimes employed to estimate adjusted treatment effects with an aim to take imbalances into account. Furthermore, we might want to assess the associations between patient characteristics measured at baseline (before randomization) and the primary outcome measured during the follow-up. By doing this, we can identify factors that have increased or decreased the likelihood of events occurring. These tasks can often be achieved with multiple regression methods.

In statistical terminology, the outcome variable in regression analysis is often called the *dependent* or *response* variable, and the baseline characteristics of patients are referred to as *independent*, *explanatory*, or *predictor* variables or covariates. The most simple form of regression analysis, looking at the relationship between one outcome variable and only one predictor variable, is called a *univariate analysis* (or more accurately *bivariate analysis*).

Suppose that we are interested in estimating the effect of smoking behavior (the predictor) on the occurrence of death among patients with heart failure. We know that, in reality, a number of other variables are potential predictors of death. Even if we are interested only in the effect of smoking behavior, we need to control for the effects of variables such as age, gender, body mass index, cardiac function, systolic blood pressure (SBP), and history of previous heart failure or heart attacks. These variables are associated not only with the risk of death, but also with smoking behavior.

In order to assess the contribution of smoking status to risk of death, we could simply do a univariate analysis and look at the rates of death in smokers and nonsmokers. This would be crude and would not allow us to determine what the exact contribution of smoking was. To answer this more complex question we must compare like with like, ie, control for differences in the characteristics of smokers and nonsmokers that might be related to death. For example, if death rates are higher among obese patients and this group also has a higher proportion of smokers than other groups, a simple comparison of smokers and nonsmokers across all weight groups would distort the true effect of smoking.

One approach to the problem would be to split the sample into different weight groups (eg, lean, normal, obese) and to compare smokers and nonsmokers within each. In practice, however, there will be many control variables and repeatedly splitting the sample can lead to a large number of small subgroups. A more efficient method is to perform a multivariate (multiple) regression analysis. This assesses the effect of smoking status on the risk of death, while simultaneously taking into account the influence of the other variables chosen to be in the analysis.

Classification of regression methods

Regression methods can be classified according to the measurement of the response variable. While several methods exist, the three usual methods used are as follows:

- If the response is continuous (eg, blood pressure, or total cholesterol level) then linear regression can be used.
- If the response is binary (eg, whether or not an individual has been diagnosed with lung cancer) then logistic regression is applied.
- If the response is time to the occurrence of an event (eg, the time from randomization to patient death in a cancer trial) then hazards regression is an appropriate method.

All regression models can handle both continuous and categorical predictor variables.

Multiple linear regression

The first step of any regression analysis is to examine the distribution of each variable and the bivariate distributions of each pair of variables, particularly the response (or outcome) variable paired with each of the predictors. If the response is a continuous variable with a symmetrical (normal) distribution, multiple linear regression can be used. However, a response with a skewed distribution might first need to be transformed. For example, a log transformation can remove a positive skew. Scatterplots of the response variable versus continuous predictors should be inspected to check that the relationship is linear; a non-linear relationship can be handled by fitting a curve rather than a line, or by categorizing the predictor. Graphical checks of the data can also reveal unusual observations or outliers, which should be investigated further before being retained in the analysis.

Let y_i denote the value of individual i on the continuous outcome variable, where i indexes the individuals in the sample ($i = 1, 2, ..., n$). Suppose that there are p predictor variables, which we denote by $x_1, x_2, ..., x_p$ (they can be continuous, binary, or categorical). Again, we use an i subscript to denote the value taken by the ith individual on each variable. The multiple linear regression model can be written:

$$y_i = a + b_1 x_{1i} + b_2 x_{2i} + ... + b_p x_{pi} + e_i \quad (1)$$

where e_i is called a *residual*, and represents variables other than the p predictors that affect y. Various assumptions are made about the residuals, namely that they follow a normal distribution and have constant variance across different values of the predictor variables (the assumption of homoskedasticity). The adequacy of these assumptions should be checked by examining plots of the estimated residuals.

a is called the *intercept* and is interpreted as the mean of y when all the xs equal 0. Of more interest are the bs, referred to as the *regression coefficients*; b_k ($k = 1, 2, ..., p$). Regression coefficients are interpreted as either the predicted change in y for a one unit increase in x_k if it is a continuous variable, or the difference between two groups if it is a binary variable, adjusting for the effects of the other predictor variables in the model. *P*-values and confidence intervals (CIs) can be obtained for each regression coefficient to assess whether the associated predictors have statistically significant effects on the response.

Example

To illustrate the use of multiple linear regression, let us consider a randomized controlled trial on 220 depressed residents aged ≥65 without severe cognitive impairment, conducted by Llewellyn-Jones et al [1]. The primary endpoint (response variable) was the geriatric depression scale score at follow-up: a higher depression score meant more depression features. They used multiple linear regression analysis to evaluate the effect of intervention on the depression scale score at follow-up, while controlling for the other independent variables measured. **Table 1** presents the estimates of the regression coefficients, their 95% CIs, and associated *P*-values for the intervention variable and some significant predictors from this study. Multiple linear regression analysis found a significant intervention effect after controlling for possible confounders, with the intervention group showing an average improvement of 1.87 points on the geriatric depression scale compared with the control group (95% CI 0.76, 2.97; $P = 0.0011$). The regression coefficients also tell us that geriatric depression scale score at follow-up increases by 0.73 points for every geriatric depression scale score at baseline, by 0.55 points for neuroticism score, and 0.10 points for every year of age, but decreases by 0.54 points for every score of basic functional ability at baseline.

Table 1. Factors affecting geriatric depression scale score at follow-up, determined by multiple linear regression analysis: extracted results from [1].

Variable	Regression coefficient (95% CI)	P-value
Intervention group vs control	−1.87 (−2.97, −0.76)	0.0011
Baseline geriatric depression scale score	0.73 (0.56, 0.91)	<0.0001
Neuroticism score[a]	0.55 (0.20, 0.90)	0.0021
Physical maintenance scale score[b]	−0.54 (−0.99, −0.09)	0.0202
Age (years)	0.10 (0.00, 0.19)	0.0395

[a]Neuroticism scored 0–8: higher score indicates higher neuroticism.

[b]Measure of basic functional ability, for example, to dress or feed oneself independently (scored 0–8: higher score indicates higher independence).

Logistic regression

Logistic regression is used when the response variable, y, is binary, ie, a variable that takes the value 0 or 1. For example, if death is the endpoint of a study, then $y = 1$ if the patient dies and $y = 0$ if the patient is alive at the end of the study. There are two main problems with applying a multiple linear regression model to binary responses. Firstly, the normality assumption does not hold (binary variables follow a Bernoulli distribution). Secondly, the model might give meaningless predictions. A fitted regression equation can be used to predict the mean response for given values of the predictor variables, which for a binary response is equal to the probability that $y = 1$. Although probabilities must theoretically lie between 0 and 1, a multiple regression model can yield predicted probabilities that are outside this range.

The probability that individual i has a response of 1 is denoted by p_i. In logistic regression, we replace the left-hand side of the multiple linear regression model (1) with a transformation of the odds that $y_i = 1$, leading to the following model:

$$\log \left(\frac{p_i}{1 - p_i} \right) = a + b_1 x_{1i} + b_2 x_{2i} + \dots + b_p x_{pi} \quad (2)$$

where $p_i / (1 - p_i)$ is the odds that the response variable takes the value of 1. The right-hand side of a logistic regression model in (2) is a linear function of the predictor variables, as in the multiple linear regression model. The coefficient b_k of x_k is interpreted as the predicted change in the log odds for a one unit increase in x_k, if x_k is a continuous variable.

Table 2. Results from a logistic regression analysis of a lack of reperfusion therapy in patients with ST-segment elevation myocardial infarction [2].

Predictor	Odds ratio (95% CI)	P-value
Age ≥75 years vs <75 years	2.63 (2.04, 3.38)	<0.0001
Female vs male	1.52 (1.21, 1.91)	0.0003
Presented without chest pain vs with chest pain	3.57 (2.42, 5.28)	<0.0001
Diabetes mellitus vs none	1.55 (1.19, 2.00)	0.001
Previous congestive heart failure vs none	3.88 (2.53, 5.96)	<0.0001
Previous myocardial infarction vs none	2.11 (1.63, 2.72)	<0.0001
Previous coronary artery bypass grafting vs none	2.38 (1.47, 3.87)	0.0004

The magnitude of an effect on the log odds scale is difficult to interpret, but if we take the exponential (anti-log) of b_k then we obtain something more meaningful; e^{b_k} is interpreted as the multiplicative effect of a one-unit increase in x_k on the odds. The quantity is called an *odds ratio* because it compares the odds of having a response of 1 for individuals with values of x_k that are one unit apart. If x_k is binary, e^{b_k} compares the odds that $y = 1$ for individuals with $x_k = 1$, relative to those with $x_k = 0$.

Example

We can illustrate the use of logistic regression in medical research with an example from the GRACE (Global Registry of Acute Coronary Events) study [2]. This study assessed current practices in relation to reperfusion therapy of ST-segment elevation myocardial infarction (MI) from data collected in a multinational, prospective registration study. One purpose of this study was to assess the characteristics that would identify patients who did not receive reperfusion therapy. The response variable was a binary indicator of not receiving reperfusion therapy (coded 1 if not given reperfusion therapy and 0 otherwise). The predictors included age, gender, history of diabetes, history of congestive heart failure, previous coronary bypass surgery, history of MI, presentation without chest pain, teaching status of the admitting hospital, presence of a catheterization laboratory on site, and geographic region.

Table 2 shows the odds ratios of not receiving reperfusion therapy. These values were obtained from a model where only statistically significant effects (at the 1% level) were retained. Also shown are 95% CIs for the odds ratios and P-values. All effects are significant at the 5% level, as indicated by both the P-values and the fact that none of the 95% CIs contain 1 (the value of the odds ratio if a predictor has no effect). The results show that patients aged ≥75 years, patients presenting without chest pain but with another symptom such as dyspnea, patients with diabetes, patients with a history of congestive heart failure or MI, and patients who had previously undergone coronary bypass surgery had higher odds of not receiving reperfusion therapy, and were therefore less likely to receive reperfusion therapy than their counterparts. For example, the odds for a patient aged ≥75 years is 2.63 times that for a patient <75 years, of not having therapy.

Hazards regression

Hazards regression is used when the response variable is the time until the occurrence of an event. Such responses are commonly called *survival times*, which is particularly appropriate in medical research where the event of concern is often death. A special feature of survival data is that there are usually some individuals in the sample who have not experienced the event by the end of the study period, but who may do so in the future. For these individuals, survival times are incompletely observed or 'right censored'. Since excluding censored cases will lead to bias, hazards regression has been developed to allow censored survival times to be included in the analysis.

The left-hand side of a hazards regression model is a transformation, usually the logarithm, of the *hazard function*. The hazard, denoted as $h(t)$, is the instantaneous risk of having the event at time t, given that the event did not occur before time t. A useful quantity that can be derived from the hazard is the *survivor function*, which is the probability of having the event after time t, ie, 'surviving' beyond time t. As in the multiple linear and logistic regression models, the right-hand side of a hazards model is a linear function of the predictor variables:

$$h_i(t) = h_0(t)\exp(b_1 x_{1i} + b_2 x_{2i} + \ldots + b_p x_{pi})$$

or

$$\log(h_i[t]) = \log(h_0[t]) + b_1 x_{1i} + b_2 x_{2i} + \ldots + b_p x_{pi} \qquad (3)$$

where $h_0(t)$ is the hazard function for an individual whose covariates (x_k, $k = 1, 2, \ldots, p$) all have values of 0.

Different specifications of this function in equation (3) lead to different hazards regression models. For example, if $h_0(t)$ is assumed to be constant over time, this leads to an exponential hazards regression model. The most commonly used hazards model is the Cox proportional hazards model, where $h_0(t)$ is unspecified.

Table 3. Hazard ratios and 95% confidence intervals (CIs) for the effects of baseline characteristics on mortality in the long-term PRAIS (Prospective Registry of Acute Ischaemic Syndromes in the UK) follow-up study (653 patients): Cox regression analysis [3].

Variable	Hazard ratio	95% CI	P-value
Age			
<60 years	1.00		
60–70 years	2.29	1.18, 4.44	0.014
>70 years	4.88	2.62, 9.06	<0.001
ECG changes			
Normal	1.00		
ST-depression or BBB	3.44	1.62, 7.29	<0.001
Other changes[a]	1.94	0.92, 4.07	0.081
Male vs female	1.78	1.22, 2.59	0.003
Smoker vs nonsmoker	1.18	0.74, 1.87	0.480
Diabetes vs none	1.01	0.64, 1.58	0.977
SBP (per 10 mm Hg increase)	0.94	0.88, 1.00	0.048
Heart rate (per 5 bpm increase)	1.06	1.01, 1.10	0.008
Prior heart failure vs none	2.41	1.60, 3.63	<0.001
Prior MI vs none	1.41	0.95, 2.08	0.088
Prior angina vs none	0.83	0.52, 1.33	0.444
Prior PCI/stent or CABG vs none	0.69	0.43, 1.11	0.123
Prior stroke vs none	2.39	1.44, 3.97	<0.001

[a]Other changes include T-wave inversion, Q-waves, and other ST- and T-wave changes.
BBB = bundle branch block; CABG = coronary artery bypass graft; ECG = electrocardiogram; MI = myocardial infarction; PCI = percutaneous coronary intervention; SBP = systolic blood pressure.

In a hazards model, the coefficient of a continuous predictor variable represents the additive effect of a one-unit change in that variable on the log hazard. It is more usual, however, to present the exponential of the coefficients, which are interpreted as the multiplicative effects of predictors on the hazard. The exponentiated coefficients are called *hazards ratios* or *relative risks*.

Example

The PRAIS-UK (Prospective Registry of Acute Ischaemic Syndromes in the UK) long-term follow-up study was a registry study identifying risk factors following hospital admission in patients with non-ST-elevation acute coronary syndrome [3]. A cohort of 653 patients was followed for mortality over 4 years. A Cox proportional hazards model was used to identify the prognostic factors, and the results are presented in **Table 3**.

Age, gender, SBP, heart rate, prior heart failure, prior stroke, and ECG changes were found to be significantly associated with the hazard (risk) of death in the long-term follow-up period. For example, the risk of death for a patient with prior heart failure was 2.41 times that for a patient without a history of heart failure; the 95% CI for this relative risk was 1.60, 3.63. Males had a risk of 1.78 (95% CI 1.22, 2.59; $P = 0.003$) compared with females.

Age was treated as a categorical variable in the analysis with three categories: <60, 60–70, and >70 years. For a categorical variable, one category must be chosen as the reference, while the other categories are compared with this group in the multivariate analysis. The choice of reference category in a study is usually based on the main hypothesis being tested. For example, in the PRAIS-UK analysis, it was expected that the youngest age group would have the lowest risk of death, so that was chosen as the reference group.

The interpretation of results for a categorical variable is similar to that for a binary variable. Taking the age effect as an example, the results in **Table 3** suggest that, compared with patients aged <60 years, the relative risk of death for patients aged 60–70 years and >70 years is 2.29 (95% CI 1.18, 4.44; $P < 0.014$) and 4.88 (95% CI 2.62, 9.06; $P < 0.001$), respectively. SBP is a continuous variable measured in units of 10 mm Hg, so the hazard ratio of 0.94 means that for every 10 mm Hg increase, the risk of death is multiplied by 0.94. In other words, the risk is decreased by 6% ($[1 - 0.94] \times 100$).

Five most common uses of regression models in clinical research

Multiple regression models have a variety of uses in clinical research. The five most common uses are to:

- adjust for differences in baseline characteristics
- identify the predictors of an outcome variable
- identify prognostic factors while controlling for potential confounders
- determine prognosis (prognostic models)
- determine diagnosis (diagnostic models)

These five uses are related, and many studies will use multiple regression for several or all of these purposes. We discuss them separately below.

1. Adjusting for differences in baseline characteristics

In a randomized clinical trial, if the randomization has created perfectly identical groups then the treatment groups will be equal in terms of both known and unknown factors. If this is the case then any association between baseline characteristics and the treatment will be balanced, and thus no confounding effect will need be adjusted for. A simple unadjusted test to estimate the treatment effect can then be used. However, despite randomization, treatment groups can sometimes be different with respect to some variables that are associated with the outcome variable and treatment. Under such circumstances, adjusted analysis for the baseline differences in these variables may become necessary (see **Chapter 25** for more about covariate adjustment analysis).

2. Identifying the predictors of an outcome variable

This is the most popular use of regression analysis in clinical research. Using multiple regression analysis, we can describe the extent, direction, and strength of the relationship between several independent variables and a dependent variable. The two examples used in the previous sections fall largely into this category [2, 3]. The sign of b_k indicates the direction of the effect of predictor x_k on the outcome statistic being modeled (the mean value of the outcome variable if the outcome is a continuous variable; the log of the odds of the outcome if the outcome is a binary variable; the log of the hazard of the outcome if the outcome is a time to event), whereas the value of b_k (or e^{b_k}) measures the magnitude of its effect.

The CI for b_k (or e^{b_k}) gives a range for the true population value, and the *P*-value is a measure of the strength of evidence for the effect. In the case of a linear regression analysis, a positive b_k implies a positive (or increasing) relationship between x_k and the continuous outcome variable, while negative values would suggest a protective effect of the baseline and outcome variable. For logistic and hazards regression, $e^{b_k} < 1$ ($e^{b_k} > 1$) suggests that increasing x_k is associated with decreasing (increasing) the odds or hazard of having an outcome.

3. Identifying prognostic factors while controlling for potential confounders

With advances in medical research, we have learned more about the multifactorial nature of many diseases. In the case of, eg, coronary artery disease (CAD), many risk factors have been identified through epidemiological studies and clinical trials, such as smoking, high blood pressure, and high cholesterol. If we want to assess the effect of a new study variable on the occurrence of CAD, we need to adjust the analysis for risk factors that are already established as predictors of the disease.

Wei et al. conducted prospective cohort studies among 40,069 men and women to investigate the association between fasting plasma glucose levels, cardiovascular disease, and all-cause mortality using a Cox proportional hazards model [4]. After multivariate adjustment for age, gender, study population, ethnicity, current smoking status, high blood pressure, total cholesterol, BMI, triglycerides, history of cardiovascular disease and cancer, and a family history of premature cardiovascular disease, patients with fasting plasma glucose <70 mg/dL (<3.89 mmol/L) and those with fasting plasma glucose 70–79 mg/dL (3.89–4.43 mmol/L) had a 3.3-fold and 2.4-fold increased risk of cardiovascular disease mortality, respectively, compared with the risk in patients with fasting plasma glucose 80–109 mg/dL (4.44–6.05 mmol/L). Participants with low fasting plasma glucose levels also had an increased risk of all-cause mortality. They concluded that participants with low fasting plasma glucose levels had a high risk of cardiovascular disease and all-cause mortality.

4. Establishing prognostic models

A multiple regression model can be used to establish a prognostic model, providing information on the prognosis of a patient with a particular set of known prognostic factors.

For example, Pocock et al. developed a prognostic model for estimating the 5-year risk of death from cardiovascular disease based on data from eight randomized trials [5]. Baseline factors were related to the risk of death from cardiovascular disease using a multivariate Cox model, adjusting for trial and treatment group (active treatment versus control). A risk score was developed from 11 factors: age, gender, SBP, serum total cholesterol concentration, height, serum creatinine concentration, cigarette smoking, diabetes, left-ventricular hypertrophy, history of stroke, and history of a previous heart attack. Their risk score was an integer, with points added for each factor according to its association with risk.

The 5-year risk of death from cardiovascular disease for scores of 10, 20, 30, 40, 50, and 60 was 0.1%, 0.3%, 0.8%, 2.3%, 6.1%, and 15.6%, respectively. For example, a score of 10 points (typical for a woman aged 35–39 years) had a 5-year risk of 0.1%; a score of 25 (typical for men aged 35–39 years), 0.5%. A score of 65 indicated a 25% risk, achieved in a few elderly men only. This prognostic model illustrates how different survival can be with the same disease but different patient characteristics.

5. Determining diagnostic models

Multiple regression models are sometimes used to determine diagnostic models, which identify the best combination of diagnostic information to determine whether a person has a particular disease. For example, Budoff et al. developed a model incorporating electron-beam tomography-derived calcium scores in a model for the prediction of angiographically significant CAD [6]. They examined 1,851 patients with suspected CAD who underwent coronary angiography for

Table 4. Assumptions and interpretations of multiple regression models.

Description	Linear regression	Logistic regression	Hazards regression
Outcome variable			
Type	Continuous	Binary	Time to event
Distribution	Normal	Bernoulli	Depends on the model
Censored	Not allowed	Not allowed	Allowed
Statistic being modeled	The mean value of the outcome variable	The log of the odds of the outcome	The log of the hazard of the outcome
Predictor variables			
Continuous (x_k)	b_k is the change in the mean value of the outcome associated with a one-unit change in x_k	b_k is the change in the log odds of the outcome associated with a one-unit change in x_k	b_k is the change in the log hazard of the outcome associated with a one-unit change in x_k
Binary (x_k)	b_k is the difference in the mean value of the outcome between two groups	b_k is the difference in the log odds of the outcome between two groups; $\exp(b_k)$ is the odds ratio for group 1 relative to group 0	b_k is the difference in the log hazard of the outcome between two groups; $\exp(b_k)$ is the hazard ratio for group 1 relative to group 0
Category (x_k)	b_k is the difference in the mean value of the outcome between a group and the reference group	b_k is the difference in the log odds of the outcome between a group and the reference group; $\exp(b_k)$ is the odds ratio comparing a group and the reference group	b_k is the difference in the log hazard of the outcome between a group and the reference group; $\exp(b_k)$ is the hazard ratio comparing a group and the reference group

clinical indications and performed an electron-beam tomographic scan in all patients. Total per-patient calcium scores and separate scores for the major coronary arteries were added to logistic regression models to calculate a probability of CAD, adjusting for age and gender. The ability of coronary calcium to predict obstructive disease on angiography had an overall sensitivity of 95% and specificity of 66%.

With calcium scores >20, >80, and >100, the sensitivity to predict stenosis decreased to 90%, 79%, and 76%, whereas the specificity increased to 58%, 72%, and 75%, respectively. The logistic regression model exhibited excellent discrimination (receiver operating characteristic curve area, 0.842 ± 0.023) and calibration. The study concluded that electron-beam tomographic calcium-scanning provides incremental and independent power in predicting the severity and extent of angiographically significant CAD in symptomatic patients.

Conclusion

This chapter provides an introduction to three statistical methods commonly used to assess the effects of intervention and risk factors on medical outcomes. Multivariate analysis is a very powerful tool in medical research that helps us to understand the multidimensional nature of risk factors of diseases and how these are interlinked.

The choice of analysis method depends on the form of the response variable: linear regression is used to analyze continuous responses, logistic regression for binary data, and hazards regression for survival times. **Table 4** briefly summarizes the basic assumptions and the interpretation of results from these three separate multiple regression methods. A common thread of these applications is to identify and control for possible confounding factors through multivariate analysis. This allows us to understand whether an association is independently important of other factors. More about the use of multiple regression methods can be found in Katz's book [7].

References

1. Llewellyn-Jones RH, Baikie KA, Smithers H, et al. Multifaceted shared care intervention for late life depression in residential care: randomised controlled trial. *BMJ* 1999;**319**:676–82.
2. Eagle KA, Goodman SG, Avezum A, et al. for the GRACE Investigators. Practice variation and missed opportunities for reperfusion in ST-segment-elevation myocardial infarction: findings from the Global Registry of Acute Coronary Events (GRACE). *Lancet* 2002;**359**:373–7.
3. Taneja AK, Collinson J, Flather MD, et al. Mortality following non-ST elevation acute coronary syndrome: 4 years follow up of the PRAIS UK Registry (Prospective Registry of Acute Ischaemic Syndromes in the UK). *Eur Heart J* 2004;**25**:2013–18.
4. Wei M, Gibbons LW, Mitchell TL, et al. Low fasting plasma glucose level as a predictor of cardiovascular disease and all-cause mortality. *Circulation* 2000;**101**:2047–52.
5. Pocock SJ, McCormack V, Gueyffier F, et al. A score for predicting risk of death from cardiovascular disease in adults with raised blood pressure, based on individual patient data from randomised controlled trials *BMJ* 2001;**323**:75–81.
6. Budoff MJ, Diamond GA, Raggi P, et al. Continuous probabilistic prediction of angiographically significant coronary artery disease using electron beam tomography. *Circulation* 2002;**105**:1791–6.
7. Katz MH. *Multivariable Analysis: A Practical Guide for Clinicians*. Cambridge, UK; New York: Cambridge University Press, 1999.

What are adjusted and unadjusted analyses?

To assess the treatment effect in randomized clinical trials, one may or may not take into account the baseline characteristics of the subjects (or *covariates*). It is this inclusion or exclusion of covariates in the analysis that distinguishes *adjusted* analyses from *unadjusted* analyses.

In the case of a clinical trial with a carefully conducted randomization, the unadjusted analysis will give an unbiased estimate of the effect of a treatment on an outcome of interest. However, there are situations where adjustment for baseline covariates will lead to improved estimates in terms of reduced bias and increased statistical efficiency [1].

Example: primary biliary cirrhosis trial

We can illustrate unadjusted and adjusted analyses using the following trial. Primary biliary cirrhosis (PBC) is a chronic but eventually fatal liver disease. A randomized double-blind clinical trial was designed to assess whether the use of azathioprine could increase the survival of patients compared to placebo [2,3]. A total of 248 patients were entered into the trial and followed for up to 12 years. The primary endpoint was the time to death from randomization. Clinical and histological information was recorded at entry to the trial.

We will use a subset of the PBC database, containing information on 191 patients who had entry values for all prognostic variables. Of particular interest to the investigators was the biochemical marker bilirubin. Some summary statistics of bilirubin by treatment group are presented in **Table 1**, and the overall trial results regarding the primary endpoint are summarized in **Table 2**.

Table 1 shows a baseline imbalance across the two treatment arms for bilirubin in terms of their average values and spread. Mean and median baseline bilirubin in the placebo group is 53.75 and 30.90 µmol/L, respectively, much lower than the 67.40 and 38.02 µmol/L for patients in the azathioprine group. The range was 431.39 µmol/L for the placebo group compared with 529.79 µmol/L for the azathioprine group. Bilirubin is known to be a strong predictor of survival time and it is expected that this imbalance will have some impact on the observed treatment effect on the primary endpoint. Due to the higher bilirubin levels in the active treatment group at baseline, a higher mortality rate may be expected in this group regardless of any treatment effect. In other words, the baseline bilirubin level could be a confounding factor in this study (see **Chapter 26**). We can assess

Table 1. Summary statistics for bilirubin level (μmol/L) at baseline by treatment group (primary biliary cirrhosis trial).

Statistics	Placebo	Azathioprine
No. of patients	94	97
Mean	53.75	67.40
Standard deviation	70.50	88.95
Median	30.90	38.02
Minimum	5.13	7.24
Maximum	436.52	537.03

Table 2. Summary statistics for survival outcome by treatment group (primary biliary cirrhosis trial).

Statistics	Placebo	Azathioprine
No. of patients	94	97
No. of deaths	49	47
Person-years	357	393.54
Incidence rate (/100)	13.73	11.94

the impact of the bilirubin level on the primary endpoint using the Cox proportional hazards model (see **Chapter 21** for more details).

To estimate the treatment effect without considering the baseline bilirubin imbalance in the analysis, we could use a Cox model with treatment only as an explanatory variable. This can be written as follows:

$$h_i(t) = h_0(t)\exp(b_1 Treatment_i)$$

where:

- $h_i(t)$ is the hazard of death for patient i
- $Treatment_i$ is the treatment the patient received (1 = azathioprine, 0 = placebo)
- e^{b_1} is the hazard ratio of death between azathioprine and placebo

Parameter estimates for the above model and the PBC trial are reported in **Table 3**. The estimated unadjusted treatment effect is 0.86 with 95% confidence interval (CI) (0.57, 1.28), $P = 0.455$, suggesting that the active treatment did not significantly improve survival.

Table 3. Comparison of unadjusted and adjusted hazard ratios of death from the Cox proportional hazards model (primary biliary cirrhosis trial).

Covariate	Hazard ratio	P-value	95% CI
Unadjusted analysis			
Treatment (A vs P)	0.86	0.455	0.57, 1.28
Adjusted analysis			
Treatment (A vs P)	0.65	0.044	0.43, 0.99
Log bilirubin	2.80	<0.001	2.25, 3.48

A = azathioprine; CI = confidence interval; P = placebo.

To control for the imbalance in bilirubin, the above Cox regression model can be expanded to include bilirubin as another explanatory variable:

$$h_i(t) = h_0(t)\exp(b_1 Treatment_i + b_2 \log[Bilirubin_i])$$

where:

- $\log(Bilirubin_i)$ stands for the logarithmically transformed bilirubin of patient i

This results in a new e^{b_1} or adjusted hazard ratio. The log transformation of bilirubin was introduced because it fitted the model better than other specifications of a bilirubin effect, such as a linear effect. The adjusted hazard ratio and its 95% CI are also displayed in **Table 3**. These suggest that, when the imbalance of bilirubin at baseline was taken into account, the active treatment was found to be significantly protective (hazard ratio = 0.65, 95% CI [0.43, 0.99], $P = 0.044$).

What is the rationale for adjusting for baseline covariates?

Randomization does not guarantee the removal of any imbalances in baseline characteristics among patients enrolled in a clinical trial. If such imbalances involve covariates that are strong predictors of an outcome variable, as in the PBC trial, it is possible that the estimates of treatment effect will be influenced by these baseline differences. The final effect on the outcome will depend on the magnitude of these differences and the strength of the correlation between the outcome and the covariate in question, with the latter being the most important contributing factor [4]. This has been demonstrated in the case of time-to-event data in the PBC trial, and particularly holds true in analysis of covariance (ANCOVA) models, where a continuous outcome is regressed on treatment group indicator and some continuous explanatory variables (covariates) [5].

A sensitivity analysis shows that, unless a baseline covariate is uncorrelated with the outcome, the unadjusted analysis might not yield the correct P-values under the null hypothesis of no treatment effect [5]. Therefore, adjustment for a baseline covariate is recommended if the covariate is correlated to the outcome (eg, a correlation coefficient >0.50 as suggested by Pocock et al) [5]. Interestingly, if the baseline covariate is strongly correlated with the outcome, there is still an advantage in adjusting for a baseline covariate even if this is perfectly balanced across the treatment arms [5].

A second reason for adjusting for prognostic covariates is the increase in precision of the estimated treatment effect [4,5]. This, however, only applies to linear regression models. Thus, from a study design perspective, there could be considerable gains (in terms of increased power and reduction in the sample size required) from collecting data on highly prognostic variables at baseline and then including them in any analysis. In particular, one could take baseline measurements of the outcome of interest, as these are likely to be strongly correlated with the values of the outcome at the endpoint.

Slightly different considerations apply to non-normal outcomes modeled using, for example, logistic or Cox regression models. In particular, adjustment for a baseline prognostic variable will not increase precision; rather, in general, an increase in standard errors will be observed [6,7]. However, in the PCB trial, the standard error for the treatment effect was reduced after adjusting for log bilirubin. A summary of the advantages and disadvantages of an adjusted analysis is displayed in **Table 4**.

What are the main methods of covariate adjustment analysis?

If imbalances are found for some baseline characteristics that are predictors of outcome variables, then covariate adjustment analysis can be performed to estimate adjusted treatment effects. As mentioned earlier, for highly prognostic covariates, the adjusted analysis might be preferable even in the absence of imbalance, especially for a continuous outcome. Adjustment is often performed through the application of multivariate regression methods, by including the relevant baseline variables as extra predictors.

Table 4. Advantages and disadvantages of an adjusted analysis.

Advantages	Disadvantages
Imbalances are accounted for in known prognostic factor(s) across treatment groups at baseline. Failure to control for such factors can lead to a biased estimate of the true treatment effect [2,3].	Choosing the covariates to be adjusted is inherently subjective since many plausible analyses are possible. Therefore, different results can be generated using different covariates.
Increased precision of the estimated treatment effect with normal outcomes modeled using regression models: adjustment for baseline imbalances will result in increased efficiency as explained variation is subtracted [4,5].	Covariates that are not collected at baseline but have a substantial impact on the primary endpoint cannot be accounted for in the adjusted analyses.
Reduction in bias with non-normal outcomes modeled using logistic or Cox regression models: in logistic regression, for example, the adjusted analysis yields a larger standard error of the odds ratio estimate for a treatment effect than the unadjusted analysis, but this could be more than offset by a more accurate estimate of the odds ratio [6,7].	The simplicity of interpreting the treatment difference obtained from unadjusted analyses is lost and results are harder to describe – eg, the estimated treatment effect from an unadjusted analysis of a two-way parallel trial can be interpreted as the difference in the primary endpoint between two patient populations receiving two different treatments. On the other hand, it is difficult to generalize the results obtained from an adjusted analysis since, eg, the estimated treatment effect takes into account peculiar characteristics of the data at hand.

There are a number of regression methods available and the choice of method depends on the type of outcome variable. For example, if the outcome variable is continuous, a *linear regression model* (such as ANCOVA) can be used to adjust for any imbalances, in particular baseline measurements of the outcome variable. Simulation studies have shown that this method has a higher statistical power for detecting a treatment effect compared to other approaches, such as the use of change (or percentage change) from baseline as a derived outcome in the analysis [8,9].

For binary outcome data, either a *stratified analysis* or a *logistic regression model* can be employed. In a stratified analysis, the treatment effect is estimated separately across the subgroups of a prognostic factor. The *Mantel–Haenzel* method permits the combining of subgroups, giving more weight to strata with more information and providing an adjusted overall estimate of the treatment effect. The advantage of such an analysis is the clarity of presentation, while the major limitation is that only a small number of covariates can be considered.

Finally, if the outcome is survival time, a *Cox regression model* should be used, as illustrated in the PBC trial. The adjusted hazard ratio is often compared with the unadjusted hazard ratio to assess the impact of any imbalances of baseline variables on the estimates of the treatment effect.

Avoiding imbalances and planning an adjusted analysis at the design stage

If a baseline variable has little or no impact on the primary outcome variable, then any imbalances between treatments are usually unimportant. On the other hand, if a baseline variable is strongly associated with the primary outcome, then even a modest level of imbalance can have an important influence on the treatment comparison. By identifying the possible baseline variables that might have a substantial effect on the primary endpoint, an 'adjustment' can be incorporated into the trial analysis, regardless of whether there are serious imbalances or not.

Two types of adjustment are often used at the design stage. The first strategy is to perform a stratified randomization, to ensure a reasonable balance across treatment groups in a limited number of baseline factors known to be strong predictors. This method of adjustment can be extremely useful when a single baseline predictor has a small number of groups (such as age groups) or a small number of prognostic factors. However, if there are several influential predictors, the number of strata needed will be large and this can lead to over-stratification (see **Chapter 7**).

The second strategy is to prespecify in the protocol which baseline covariates will be adjusted for and then present the results from the adjusted analysis. In many cases it will be possible to identify important prognostic variables before the start of the trial, by, for example, looking at previous studies. This strategy has the advantage of overcoming the problem of subjectively selecting predictors in an *ad hoc* manner in the analysis. The US Food and Drug Administration (FDA) and the International Conference on Harmonisation of Technical Requirements for Registration of Pharmaceuticals for Human Use (ICH) guidelines for clinical reports require that the selection of and adjustment for any covariates should be an integral part of the planned analysis, and hence should be set out in the protocol and explained in the reports [10].

Conclusion

In most clinical trials, estimates of treatment effects unadjusted for baseline covariates are produced and reported. The validity of an unadjusted analysis relies on the assumption that there are no important imbalances involving measured and unmeasured baseline covariates across treatment groups. When imbalances occur on measured predictors of outcome variables, adjusted analyses can be performed to account for this.

Adjustment can be carried out using various regression models by including the prognostic covariates alongside the treatment group indicator. The adjusted analyses can yield estimates that are more precise (in case of a normal regression model) and less biased (for non-normal outcomes). Ideally, a list of covariates to be adjusted for should be prespecified in the protocol. This will free the investigator from having to decide *post hoc* which covariates, if any, are to be included in the final analysis, a decision that is inherently subjective.

References

1. Gail MH, Wieand S, Piantadosi S. Biased estimates of treatment effect in randomized experiments with nonlinear regressions and omitted covariates. *Biometrika* 1984;**71**:431–44.
2. Christensen E, Neuberger J, Crowe J, et al. Beneficial effect of azathioprine and prediction of prognosis in primary biliary cirrhosis. Final results of an international trial. *Gastroenterology* 1985;**89**:1084–91.
3   Altman DG. Adjustment for covariate imbalance. *Biostatistics in Clinical Trials*. Chichester: John Wiley & Sons, 2001.
4. Senn SJ. Covariate imbalance and random allocation in clinical trials. *Stat Med* 1989;**8**:467–75.
5. Pocock SJ, Assmann SE, Enos LE, et al. Subgroup analysis, covariate adjustment and baseline comparisons in clinical trial reporting: current practice and problems. *Stat Med* 2002;**21**:2917–30.
6. Robinson LD, Jewell NP. Some surprising results about covariate adjustment in logistic regression models. *Int Statist Rev* 1991;**58**:227–40.
7. Chastang C, Byar D, Piantadosi S. A quantitative study of the bias in estimating the treatment effect caused by omitting a balanced covariate in survival models. *Stat Med* 1988;**7**:1243–55.
8. Vickers AJ. The use of percentage change from baseline as an outcome in a controlled trial is statistically inefficient: a simulation study. *BMC Med Res Methodol* 2001;**1**:6.
9. Senn S. *Statistical Issues in Drug Development.* Chichester: John Wiley & Sons, 1997.
10. FDA, Section 5.8 of the International Conference on Harmonization: Guidance on Statistical Principles for Clinical Trials. Available from: http://www.fda.gov/cber/gdlns/ichclinical.pdf. Accessed April 19, 2005.

Chapter 26

Confounding

Duolao Wang, Tim Clayton, and Ameet Bakhai

The aim of a clinical trial is to provide an accurate estimate of the effect of a therapy or procedure on an outcome such as death, compared with the effect of a control, such as a placebo. However, the estimate of this effect can be distorted by various sources of bias during the design, conduct, and analysis of a study. Confounding is one such bias that can distort the estimate of the treatment effect, due to an imbalance across treatment groups of a variable associated with the outcome. In this chapter, we describe what a confounding factor is and how it can impact a clinical trial, explain how confounding factors can be identified, and introduce some methods that can be used to control confounders during study design and analysis.

What is confounding?

A confounding factor is a variable that is related to both the treatment being investigated and the outcome [1,2]. Consider a hypothetical study in which drug X produces an overall reduction in the number of deaths of patients with hypertension compared with standard therapy. For screening purposes, a chest X-ray is performed before randomization and later it is found that half of the patients in the standard therapy arm have lung cancer compared with none in the drug X group. On closer inspection, the rate of death in the patients diagnosed with cancer was found to be four times higher than in the group of patients without cancer. From these later observations, we can state that the reason that drug X appeared to do better was because the patients in the standard therapy group suffered a higher rate of lung cancer deaths. Therefore, lung cancer is a *confounder* for the relationship between drug X and the likelihood of death in the study, since lung cancer (a cause of premature death) is unevenly distributed between the two treatment groups.

Confounders are more usually a problem in observational studies, where the exposure of a risk factor is not randomly distributed between groups [3]. An example from epidemiology would be a hypothetical observational study conducted to assess the effect of the type of work undertaken by mothers during pregnancy (office or manual) on the birth weight of the baby. Let us say that the results showed that babies born to women with manual jobs had a lower birth weight than those born to women working in offices. However, it is also established that the type of work done during pregnancy is associated with other maternal characteristics and the woman's age and nutritional status. Furthermore, these maternal characteristics are also known to be associated with the weight of the baby. Therefore, it is possible that our observed association between the type of work undertaken during pregnancy and the birth weight of the baby is due to these other characteristics. These characteristics are considered to be *confounding variables* if they falsely accentuate the relationship between a perceived risk factor and the outcome of pregnancy.

Sometimes confounders are inherent in the design of early-phase clinical trials. For example, dose-titration studies are used to assess the dose–response relationship in drug development [4]. In a dose-titration study, a subject will only receive the next higher dose if he/she fails to meet some objective response criterion at the current dose level, such as a reduction of systolic blood pressure by a prespecified amount. The major problem in this case is that the dose–response relationship is often confounded with time course – it can be argued that the relationship found in a dose-titration study is not due to the dose, but rather to some other factor related to the time course, such as the total length of time the patient is exposed to the drug irrespective of dose concentration.

Table 1. Hormone replacement therapy (HRT) trial example: overall study results.

Treatment	Improvement in mental function Yes	No	Total number of women	Proportion of women showing improvement
No HRT	64	336	400	16%
HRT	96	304	400	24%

Odds ratio = 1.66 (95% CI 1.16, 2.36; $P < 0.005$).

Table 2. HRT trial example: improvement in mental function by socioeconomic status and treatment.

Socioeconomic status	Treatment	Improvement in mental function Yes	No	Total number of women	Proportion of women showing improvement
High	No HRT	40	60	100	40%
	HRT	80	120	200	40%
Low	No HRT	24	276	300	8%
	HRT	16	184	200	8%

Odds ratio for women in the high socioeconomic status group = 1.00 (95% CI 0.61, 1.63; $P = 1.00$).
Odds ratio for women in the low socioeconomic status group = 1.00 (95% CI 0.52, 1.93; $P = 1.00$).
Mantel–Haenszel estimate of the odds ratio, controlling for the socioeconomic status = 1.00 (95% CI 0.67, 1.48; $P = 1.00$).
HRT = hormone replacement therapy.

What causes confounding?

We will use an extremely hypothetical example to explain how confounding can occur in a clinical study. It has been reported that hormone replacement therapy (HRT) improves mental function (such as reasoning and verbal skills) in postmenopausal women. Therefore, a study to evaluate the effect of HRT on mental function was conducted in 800 postmenopausal women. Half the women recruited were allocated to daily HRT, while the remainder were given placebo (the non-HRT group). The researchers evaluated the cognitive function of the women 5 years after recruitment, and the primary endpoint was whether mental function was improved or not above a predefined level. The overall results from the study are summarized in **Table 1**.

The overall results appear to suggest that while there were women in both groups whose mental function improved after 5 years, HRT treatment resulted in a significantly greater proportion of women showing improvement than placebo (24% vs 16%, odds ratio = 1.66 [95% CI 1.16, 2.36; $P < 0.005$]). However, when these data are analyzed by socioeconomic status (using the categories high or low socioeconomic status), as in **Table 2**, a different conclusion emerges.

Table 3. Hormone replacement therapy (HRT) trial example: association between socioeconomic status and treatment.

Treatment	Number in each socioeconomic status group (%)		Total
	Low	High	
No HRT	300 (75)	100 (25)	400
HRT	200 (50)	200 (50)	400

χ^2 = 53.27; P < 0.0001.

The results in **Table 2** show that there is no difference in the proportions of women with mental function improvement between the two treatment groups if they are considered separately by socioeconomic class. The proportion of women with improved mental function was 40% in the high socioeconomic status group and 8% in the low socioeconomic status group, regardless of treatment. Accordingly, the estimated odds ratio is 1.00 in each group for both levels of socioeconomic class. Therefore, socioeconomic status did indeed confound the association between HRT treatment and improvement in mental function, and so the apparent difference found by the original analysis in **Table 1** is spurious.

How can we confirm whether a variable is a confounder?

For a variable to be a confounder it must satisfy three conditions [1,2]:

- It must be associated with the treatment.
- It must be a predictor of the outcome being measured.
- It must not be a consequence of the treatment itself.

We can illustrate how to identify a confounder using the hypothetical HRT study as an example.

Step 1. Assess whether the potential confounder has an association with the treatment group

From the HRT example, it is clear that a variable can confound the relationship between treatment and outcome only if it is *unevenly* distributed between the treatment groups. In our example, 50% of the women taking HRT were of high socioeconomic status compared with only 25% of women in the non-HRT group, indicating that the distribution of socioeconomic status among the two treatment groups was imbalanced. The chi-square test shown in **Table 3** confirms that this imbalance was highly statistically significant (χ^2 = 53.27; P < 0.0001).

Table 4. Hormone replacement therapy (HRT) trial example: comparison of proportion of mental function improvement in each socioeconomic group.

Socioeconomic status	Improvement in mental function Yes	No	Total number of women	Proportion of women showing improvement
High	120	180	300	40%
Low	40	460	500	8%

Odds ratio = 0.13 (95% CI 0.08, 0.20; $P < 0.0001$).

Step 2. Assess whether the potential confounder is a predictor of the outcome

The second condition for a variable to be a confounder requires that the potential confounder must also be related to the outcome being measured. The relationship between socioeconomic status and improvement in mental function is examined in **Table 4**. The results show that the odds of having improved mental function in the low socioeconomic status group are only about 13% of that in the high socioeconomic status group. The low P-value suggests that there is strong evidence of a difference in improvement in mental function between the two socioeconomic groups in favor of the high socioeconomic status group. Based on these results, socioeconomic status is an important predictor of an improvement in mental function among postmenopausal women.

Step 3. Assess that the potential confounder is not a consequence of treatment

In the HRT example, it is not possible for the treatment allocation to influence the socioeconomic class of a woman on admission, since this is determined before treatment randomization. Hence we can conclude that socioeconomic status would not lie on the causal path between HRT treatment and the primary endpoint (improvement in mental function).

Hence, the socioeconomic status variable satisfies all the criteria for being a confounding factor.

Evaluating the degree of confounding

If a prognostic factor satisfies the three conditions for being a confounder, the next step is to evaluate the degree of confounding. This should be done by comparing the unadjusted (also known as crude) estimates of treatment affect – ie, the estimates that are unadjusted for the potential confounding factor – with the adjusted estimates. There is no specific test to determine whether a factor is a confounder in respect of any given treatment effect, but, if we adjust for a potential confounder in the analysis and find that the adjusted and unadjusted estimates of the treatment effect differ, this suggests that the unadjusted estimate is confounded by the factor under consideration. In the HRT example, the unadjusted odds ratio was 1.66, but this became 1.00 after stratification by socioeconomic status, suggesting that socioeconomic status is a positive confounder.

Positive and negative confounding

Positive confounding is said to occur when the effect of a confounder is to make the observed treatment effect appear stronger (ie, to move the odds ratio further away from 1 when the confounder is unaccounted for) [1], as in the HRT example. Confounding can also work in the opposite direction – known as negative confounding – where it can result in the treatment effect appearing to be weaker than it really is after adjusting for the confounder [1].

Controlling confounding through study design

The effect of confounding can be prevented at different stages in a clinical trial, but the most effective method is to restrict it at the design stage. In general, randomization – a cornerstone of clinical trials – is the most effective way of preventing confounding. The purpose of randomization is to ensure that each subject has an equal chance of being assigned to each treatment group, and that the treatment assignment cannot be predicted in advance [4,5]. Ideally, randomization should result in the balanced distribution of all potential confounders, whether known or unknown, across all treatment groups at baseline. For a large trial, a simple randomization scheme should achieve this. However, in smaller trials it is possible for an imbalance in one or more baseline characteristics to occur, which could result in confounding, even if this imbalance might not be sufficient to reach statistical significance. Therefore, attention should be paid to identifying potential confounders – which can be adjusted for at the analysis stage if necessary – especially when the sample size of a clinical trial is small.

When designing clinical trials, if we know from previous studies that some characteristics are important prognostic factors, we can limit their potential for confounding by means of a *stratified randomization method* [4,5]. Stratified randomization is used to ensure a reasonable balance between treatment groups of one or more potential confounding factors, such as age, gender, presence of diabetes, severity of illness, geographical location, and socioeconomic status (see **Chapter 7**).

For example, a randomized placebo-controlled trial was conducted to test the feasibility and safety of the withdrawal of inhaled corticosteroids (ICS) from treatment for cystic fibrosis (CF) in 240 children and adults who were already taking ICS. Experience from earlier studies suggested that three factors – atopy (present or absent), forced expiratory volume in the first second (FEV$_1$ [40%–60%, 61%–80%, and 81%–100%]) and age (<17 years, ≥17 years) – were the most important determinants of time to first respiratory exacerbation (the primary outcome measure of the trial). The intention was to balance treatment within each of these 12 strata (the number of strata is equal to: number of strata for atopy × number of strata for FEV$_1$ × number of strata for age = 2 × 3 × 2). Stratified randomization is then performed by generating a randomization list for each of the 12 strata using randomized-permuted blocks (which ensure that there are equal treatment numbers within each stratum at various points during recruitment). The aim of this method is to produce groups that are balanced by each of the three factors throughout the duration of the study.

One problem that can easily occur is over-stratification. Suppose that in the above example 10 centers were recruiting patients, then 120 strata would be needed for 240 patients. The higher the ratio of strata to patients, the harder it is avoid imbalances as there can be many incomplete blocks. Therefore, the chosen stratification factors should be restricted to the variables that are known to be of particularly prognostic importance.

An alternative method used in clinical trials is called *minimization* [4–6]. The aim of minimization is to ensure a balance of a number of potential confounding factors between treatment groups. Minimization – also called an adaptive randomization procedure – assigns subjects to a given treatment group in order to minimize the differences between the treatment groups on a number of selected confounding factors. This is based on the idea that, at any stage of the trial, the probability of allocating the next patient to the treatment that will minimize the overall imbalance between the groups according to the selected factors will be greater than 0.5. This method is employed in situations that involve many prognostic factors, and, in this case, patient allocation aims to balance the subtotals for each level of each factor. Note that for such a sequential scheme it is not possible to prepare a randomization list in advance, and there are practical difficulties in implementation.

Methods for controlling confounding during analysis

Despite steps taken during the design of a trial, it is still possible for an imbalance to occur that might impact the association between the treatment group and the measured outcome. Once confounders are identified, the next stage is to control for these in statistical analysis so that unbiased results can be obtained. There are two methods for this: *stratification* and *regression modeling* [1,2].

Stratification

The simplest way to control for a confounding factor is to perform the analysis within each stratification of the confounder and then to calculate a summary measure from these strata-specific estimators using a suitable weighting scheme.

The most common way of performing such a stratification analysis is to use Mantel–Haenszel methods, which adjust for a categorical confounding factor on the relationship between treatment and some binary outcome [1]. Using Mantel–Haenszel methods on the data from our earlier HRT example (**Tables 1** and **2**), the Mantel–Haenszel estimate of the odds ratio adjusted for socioeconomic class is calculated as 1.00 (95% CI 0.67, 1.48; $P = 1.00$). The adjusted result suggests that, in this example, HRT does not result in improved mental function in postmenopausal women.

Regression modeling

As the number of potential confounders or number of possible sub-strata for a confounder increases, controlling confounding through stratification presents problems. This is because unless the overall sample size is large, each stratum will contain only a very small number of patients. In this case, a multivariable regression model approach is the preferred analysis method. There are a number of specific regression models, and the most appropriate technique will depend on the type of data to be analyzed. For example:

- A linear regression model is most suitable for a continuous outcome measure such as blood pressure.
- A logistic regression model is the preferred option for a binary outcome such as the occurrence of death.
- A Cox regression model should be used for a time-to-event outcome such as time to next seizure or pain episode.

The regression model is a very powerful technique that allows for the estimation of the effects of a treatment and a whole range of prognostic factors, each one adjusted for the potential confounding effect of the others. For the HRT example, using the logistic regression model to adjust for confounding produces identical results to the Mantel–Haenszel method.

What is the difference between interaction (or effect modification) and confounding?

Consider a study investigating the effect of vitamin A supplements on childhood growth. Among children who are vitamin A deficient, it is likely that vitamin A supplements will increase growth, while supplements may have no effect in children who are not deficient in vitamin A. This is an example of interaction (or effect modification). This can be defined as a situation where the treatment effect (ie, vitamin A supplements) on the primary outcome (ie, height) varies according to the levels of a third factor (ie, the level of vitamin A before supplementation).

In the evaluation of a clinical trial, confounding and interaction effects are two different things. Confounding is a nuisance effect that distorts the observed treatment effect on an outcome of interest because the confounder is associated with the outcome and is unequally distributed between the treatment groups. We aim to control confounding in the design and analysis stages of a clinical trial to enable the true treatment effect to be estimated.

Interaction is a real effect, independent of the study design, that causes the treatment effect to vary according to the level of a third factor, which we want to detect. Exploring the nature of interaction can be very helpful in understanding the biological processes underlying an association between a treatment and an outcome. Interaction is discussed further in the next chapter.

Conclusion

Confounding is the situation where the observed association between a prognostic factor (such as treatment) and an outcome measure is made stronger or weaker by the imbalance of another factor. In a clinical trial, confounding factors can falsely obscure or accentuate the treatment effect. Therefore, attention should be paid to controlling for potential confounders during the design and analysis stages of clinical trials.

When designing a clinical trial, the most effective way to reduce the possibility of confounding is to employ a suitable randomization method. When analyzing the data, unexpected confounders can be controlled for by compensating for their imbalance, so that the net impact of the treatment effect can be estimated, while controlling for the effect of these confounders.

References

1. Gail MH, Benichou J. *Encyclopedia of Epidemiologic Methods*. Chichester: John Wiley & Sons, 2000.
2. Gordis L. *Epidemiology*. 2nd edition. Philadelphia: WB Saunders Company, 2000.
3. Bakhai A. Practical issues in trial design. Part 1: The place of observational studies and randomized controlled trials. *Clinical Researcher* 2001;**1**(4):28–9.
4. Chow SC, Liu JP. *Design and Analysis of Clinical Trials: Concept and Methodologies*. New York: John Wiley & Sons, 1998.
5. Pocock SJ. *Clinical Trials: A Practical Approach*. Chichester: John Wiley & Sons, 1983.
6. Pocock SJ, Simon R. Sequential treatment assignment with balancing for prognostic factors in the controlled clinical trial. *Biometrics* 1975;**31**:103–15.

Chapter 27

Interaction

Duolao Wang, Tim Clayton, and Ameet Bakhai

Interaction effects in clinical trials occur when a subject's response to a treatment varies according to the level of another variable such as age or gender. Identifying and understanding the real interaction effects can help us target therapies to subgroups of patients who may benefit most. In this chapter, we review the basis of this most important concept and describe different types of interaction effects in clinical trials. We also describe how an interaction effect can be evaluated and interpreted within a framework of a regression model.

Table 1. Mean reduction in systolic blood pressure (in mm Hg) by hypertensive drug treatment and smoking status in a hypothetical trial on 800 hypertension patients (200 in each group).

Smoking status	Hypertensive drug treatment	
	Placebo	Drug
Smoker	−2.07	−2.60
Nonsmoker	−1.94	−4.65

What is an interaction effect?

In a clinical trial, an interaction effect occurs when a treatment effect is dependent on another factor (eg, gender). For example, suppose a clinical study is carried out to investigate the effect of vitamin A supplements on childhood growth in a developing country. Vitamin A supplements might have a greater effect on growth in children from more deprived areas compared with children from less deprived areas. In this example, the effect of the treatment (vitamin A supplementation) on the primary outcome (height during childhood) varies according to the levels of a third pre-existing factor (the prior nutritional status of the child). Therefore, the treatment effect is dependent on nutritional status at baseline. In epidemiology, this phenomenon is often referred to as *effect modification* because the third variable modifies the treatment effect on outcome.

Example 1

Table 1 presents the results of a hypothetical clinical trial assessing the effect of a new antihypertensive drug on systolic blood pressure (SBP) among 800 patients with hypertension. The results show that the antihypertensive drug reduces SBP, but the drug's benefit appears to be greater for nonsmokers (a reduction in SBP of −2.71 mm Hg) than for smokers (a reduction in SBP of −0.53 mm Hg).

When to look for an interaction effect

During the design or analysis of a clinical trial, investigators are often interested in knowing whether the treatment effect of a study drug or therapy varies according to patient characteristics. For example, a treatment effect might decrease with age, or be larger in subjects in a particular diagnostic category. To address this, statistical tests of interactions between treatments and relevant covariates are often planned and performed. If such interactions are anticipated, or are of particular prior interest, then the planned confirmatory analysis will include a subgroup analysis, or will use a statistical model including interactions. In most cases, subgroup or interaction analyses are exploratory in nature and carried out after data collection.

Classification of an interaction effect

Interaction effects can be classified as *quantitative* or *qualitative* [1]. A quantitative interaction effect occurs when the magnitude of the treatment effect varies according to different levels (values) of another factor, but the direction of the treatment effect remains the same for all levels of the factor. A qualitative interaction occurs when the direction of the treatment effect differs for at least one level of the factor.

To illustrate the two interaction effects described above, consider a hypothetical trial of an antihypertensive drug. Suppose that one of the objectives of the trial is to assess whether the reduction in SBP is the same for smokers and nonsmokers. Treatment and smoking status both have two levels (for the former, the levels are placebo and active drug treatment; for the latter, the levels are nonsmoker and smoker), generating four possible combinations. Suppose that the primary endpoint is the change in SBP from baseline. The effect of each combination on the outcome can be displayed graphically to allow for visual inspection of the various interactions (**Figure 1**).

In **Figure 1**, mean change in SBP from baseline is on the vertical axis, while the horizontal axis represents smoking status. The mean change from baseline SBP by treatment can then be plotted at each level of smoking status, and a line can be drawn between the points for each treatment level. The distance between the two lines represents the treatment effect (the difference in the mean change in SBP between the active drug and the placebo).

In **Figure 1**, panel A shows a pattern of no interaction effect; this is characterized by two parallel lines that are equidistant at the two levels of smoking status (ie, the effect of the study drug is to reduce SBP by the same amount in smokers and nonsmokers). Panels B and C show a possible *quantitative interaction* between treatment and smoking status; the two lines do not cross and so the treatment effect does not change its direction, although the distance between the lines is different at each level of smoking status. In panels B and C, the results indicate that the active treatment is more effective at reducing SBP than placebo. While panel B demonstrates that the treatment leads to a greater reduction in SBP among nonsmokers than smokers, the opposite effect is observed in panel C.

In panel D, the difference in the mean reduction in SBP between the active treatment and placebo group is positive (a larger reduction in SBP on placebo than on active treatment) among smokers, but negative (a larger reduction in SBP on active treatment than on placebo) among nonsmokers. Panel D shows a possible *qualitative interaction* between treatment and smoking status. Since the

Figure 1. Plots demonstrating quantitative and qualitative interaction.
(A = no interaction; B and C = quantitative interaction; D = qualitative interaction).

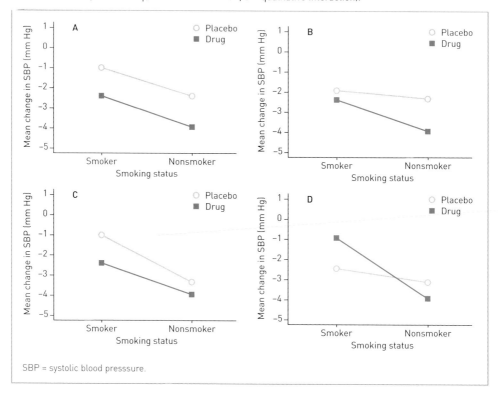

SBP = systolic blood presssure.

two lines cross each other, a qualitative interaction of this kind is also sometimes called a *crossover interaction*.

Evaluation of an interaction effect

To formally evaluate whether there is an interaction effect between two variables and the magnitude of that effect, statistical tests must be performed. There are a number of statistical methods for the evaluation of interaction effects [1–3]. The most commonly used method is to use a regression model. Which regression model to choose depends on the type of data to be analyzed. For example, linear regression is most suitable for a continuous outcome measure (eg, SBP), while a logistic regression is preferred for a binary outcome (eg, death) (see **Chapter 24**).

Using a linear regression model

Using data from the hypothetical trial in **Table 1**, a linear regression model can be applied to illustrate how to evaluate the interaction effect in a trial where the primary endpoint is a continuous variable. In this example, Y represents the change in SBP for each patient, X_1 represents the treatment variable ($X_1 = 0$ for placebo, and $X_1 = 1$ for active drug treatment) and X_2 represents the smoking status variable ($X_2 = 0$ for a nonsmoker, and $X_2 = 1$ for a smoker). A linear regression model that predicts Y based on X_1 and X_2 can then be expressed as:

$$Y = \alpha + \beta X_1 + \gamma X_2 + \varepsilon \qquad (1)$$

Where α is a constant, β and γ represent the effects of the treatment (X_1) and smoking status (X_2) on SBP (Y), respectively, and ε is a random error. The above model (1) assumes that the effects of X_1 and X_2 are additive and are independent of each other, and so it is often called the *main effect model*.

The interaction between treatment and smoking status can now be investigated by adding another term into the linear regression model (1):

$$Y = \alpha + \beta X_1 + \gamma X_2 + \delta(X_1 X_2) + \varepsilon \qquad (2)$$

This means that, in addition to the main effect of treatment (X_1) and smoking status (X_2), there is an interaction effect (δ) between treatment and smoking status ($X_1 X_2$). The value of $X_1 X_2$ is 1 for a patient who is a smoker on active treatment, and 0 otherwise. The model implies that the change in SBP differs according to different combinations of treatment and smoking status. In other words, the treatment effect differs by the smoking status. If δ is found to be statistically significantly different from 0 then there is evidence of an interaction between treatment and smoking status, suggesting that the effect of the treatment depends on the smoking status of patients.

Example 1 (continued)
Table 2 presents the results from fitting the two regression models described in equations (1) and (2), using the data in Example 1. The main effect model shows that the difference in mean SBP reduction is statistically significantly different, not only between the antihypertensive drug and placebo groups, but also between smokers and nonsmokers. However, whether the drug works differently for smokers and nonsmokers is uncertain. To address this uncertainty, the interaction term is introduced.

Table 2. Use of a linear regression model to evaluate an interaction effect between smoking status and treatment.

Regression analysis model	Variable	Regression coefficient	P-value	95% CI	
Main effect model	Constant	−2.49	<0.01	−2.75	−2.23
	Treatment (X₁)	−1.62	<0.01	−1.92	−1.32
	Smoking status (X₂)	0.96	<0.01	0.66	1.26
Main and interaction effect model	Constant	−1.94	<0.01	−2.23	−1.65
	Treatment (X₁)	−2.71	<0.01	−3.12	−2.30
	Smoking status (X₂)	−0.13	0.53	−0.54	0.28
	(Smoking status) (treatment) (X₁X₂)	2.18	<0.01	1.61	2.76

Table 3. Estimate of treatment effects on systolic blood pressure reduction by smoking status, using the results of the regression model in Table 2.

Regression analysis model	Variable	Regression coefficient	P-value	95% CI	
Main effect model	Smoker	−1.62	<0.01	−1.92	−1.32
	Nonsmoker	−1.62	<0.01	−1.92	−1.32
Main and interaction effect model	Smoker	−0.53	<0.01	−0.94	−0.12
	Nonsmoker	−2.71	<0.01	−3.12	−2.30

The null hypothesis for the interaction test is $H_0: \delta = 0$, ie, there is no interaction between smoking status and the treatment for reducing SBP. The linear model estimate for δ is 2.18 mm Hg (95% CI 1.61, 2.76) with the corresponding P-value for the test ($H_0: \delta = 0$) being <0.01. Therefore, there is statistically significant evidence of an interaction between smoking status and treatment.

Once a significant interaction effect is found, the modified effects for different combinations of treatment and smoking status should be calculated. **Table 3** presents the estimated treatment effect (difference in SBP reduction between drug group and placebo group) for smokers and nonsmokers. The main effect model indicates that the treatment difference is the same (−1.62 mm Hg) for smokers and nonsmokers. On the other hand, the interaction effect model suggests that the treatment effect is −2.71 mm Hg among nonsmokers compared with −0.53 mm Hg among smokers. As the direction of treatment effect is negative for both smokers and nonsmokers (−0.53 and −2.71, respectively), the interaction effect is a *quantitative interaction*.

Table 4. Number of patients allocated to each treatment in the GISSI-Prevenzione trial [4].

n-3 polyunsaturated fatty acids supplementation	Vitamin E supplementation		Total
	Placebo	Active	
Placebo	2,828	2,830	5,658
Active	2,836	2,830	5,666
Total	5,664	5,660	11,324

Other means of evaluating an interaction effect can also be used, such as the Mantel–Haenszel method [1–3]. An interaction test is sometimes called a homogeneity (or heterogeneity) test. For example, in a multicenter study, if there is no significant interaction between treatment and center, then the treatment effect is said to be *homogeneous* across different centers and an overall treatment effect can be obtained by pooling all centers together. On the other hand, if a significant interaction is found between the treatment and the center, then the treatment effect is *heterogeneous* across different centers. Under such circumstances, pooling the estimate of treatment effect together from different centers might produce a misleading overall result.

Examples of types of interaction effects seen in clinical trials

The objective of evaluating an interaction effect in a clinical trial is to assess whether the treatment effect is the same among different levels (values) of another factor or factors. The factor might be the other drugs under evaluation in a factorial design, or some stratification variable – such as severity of the underlying disease, gender, or other important prognostic factors. In the following discussion, different types of interactions will be described in different clinical trial settings.

Example 2: Treatment-by-treatment interaction in a factorial design

The GISSI-Prevenzione (Gruppo Italiano per lo Studio della Streptochinasi nell'Infarto Miocardico Prevenzione) trial investigated the effects of vitamin E (α-tocopherol) and n-3 polyunsaturated fatty acids (PUFA) supplementation in patients who had recently suffered a myocardial infarction [4]. In this trial, 11,324 patients surviving a recent myocardial infarction (≤3 months previously) were randomly assigned to receive supplements of *n*-3 PUFA (1 g daily, $n = 2,836$), vitamin E (300 mg daily, $n = 2,830$), both vitamin E and *n*-3 PUFA ($n = 2,830$), or neither (control, $n = 2,828$), using a 2×2 factorial design. The primary combined efficacy endpoint was a composite of death, nonfatal myocardial infarction, and stroke.

Table 5. Rate of primary endpoint (number of primary endpoint) by treatment in the GISSI-Prevenzione trial [4].

n-3 polyunsaturated fatty acids supplementation	Vitamin E supplementation		Total
	Placebo	Active	
Placebo	14.64% (414)	13.11% (371)	13.87% (785)
Active	12.55% (356)	12.69% (359)	12.62% (715)
Total	13.59% (770)	12.90% (730)	

Table 6. Use of a logistic regression model to evaluate the interaction effect between n-3 polyunsaturated fatty acids (PUFA) and vitamin E supplementation in the GISSI-Prevenzione trial [4].

Regression analysis model	Variable	Regression coefficient	P-value	95% CI	
Main effect model	n-3 PUFA	0.90	0.05	0.80	1.00
	Vitamin E	0.94	0.27	0.84	1.04
Main and interaction effect model	n-3 PUFA	0.84	0.02	0.72	0.97
	Vitamin E	0.88	0.10	0.76	1.02
	(n-3 PUFA) (vitamin E)	1.15	0.21	0.93	1.43

The number of patients randomized to each arm of the trial is summarized in **Table 4**. In **Table 5** the event rates for each of the four arms are given, as well as the total event rates for the n-3 PUFA and vitamin E arms. The difference in the event rate between subjects receiving placebo and active n-3 PUFA is 0.42% (= 13.11% – 12.69%) for subjects receiving active vitamin E, and 2.09% (= 14.64% – 12.55%) for subjects receiving placebo (instead of active vitamin E). Similarly, the difference in the event rate between those receiving placebo and active vitamin E is –0.14% (= 12.55% – 12.69%) for subjects receiving active n-3 PUFA, and 1.53% (= 14.64% – 13.11%) for subjects receiving placebo (instead of active n-3 PUFA).

These descriptive statistics suggest that the difference in the event rate for one treatment may depend on the level of the other treatment, or, in other words, that there is a possible interaction effect between two treatments. To explore this formally, two logistic regression models were fitted (a main effect model and an interaction effect model), where the outcome variable was the occurrence of the primary endpoint. The results are displayed in **Table 6**.

The results from the main and interaction effect logistic regression model in **Table 6** suggest that there is no evidence of an interaction effect between the two treatments (for the interaction term, $P = 0.21$). In other words, the observed treatment effects were the result of chance. Therefore, the reduction in the primary endpoint event rate attributed to n-3 PUFA is not affected by taking vitamin E,

Table 7. Reduction in mean systolic blood pressure (SBP) by center in a hypothetical multicenter study.

Center number	Number of patients	Mean SBP (mm Hg) Drug A	Drug B	Difference in SBP between drug B and drug A (mm Hg)	Rank by difference
1	100	−3.01	−1.42	1.59	3
2	100	−4.92	−5.78	−0.86	8
3	100	−3.39	1.36	4.75	1
4	100	−5.70	−6.75	−1.06	9
5	100	−4.88	−8.43	−3.55	10
6	100	−4.26	−4.19	0.07	7
7	100	−3.74	−3.16	0.58	5
8	100	−3.25	−0.25	3.01	2
9	100	−4.59	−4.31	0.29	6
10	100	−3.05	−2.31	0.74	4

so the results from the main effect model should be reported. In reporting a factorial design trial, it should be clear that the potential interaction effect between treatments has been considered.

Example 3: Treatment-by-center interaction in a multicenter trial

The above example demonstrates how to test for an interaction between two treatments. However, in clinical trials it is sometimes necessary to check for an interaction between the treatment and other important prognostic factors. Of special importance is treatment-by-center interaction in multicenter studies. A multicenter study is a single study involving several study centers (sites or investigators) [5], which should permit an overall estimation of the treatment difference for the targeted patient population across different centers (see **Chapter 16**). When analyzing a multicenter study, it may be appropriate to explore whether there is a treatment-by-center interaction.

Consider a hypothetical multicenter trial for assessing the efficacy of two drugs (A and B) in reducing SBP among hypertensive subjects. The study is a randomized, multicenter trial that involves 1,000 patients in 10 centers (each center has 100 patients). The mean changes in SBP from the baseline after 5 weeks of treatment are given in **Table 7**, and the mean change in SBP against study centers is plotted in **Figure 2**. In this figure, the centers are ranked according to the magnitude of the difference in mean change in SBP between drugs A and B.

As can be seen from **Table 7**, seven centers show a difference in the positive direction, while three centers show a change in a negative direction. Regression analysis indicates that a significant *qualitative interaction* between treatment

Figure 2. Mean change in systolic blood pressure (SBP) from baseline by center for a hypothetical multicenter study.

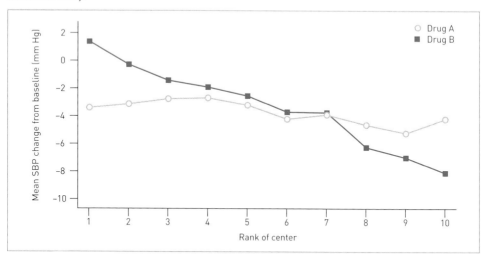

and center occurred ($P < 0.001$). If the interaction is ignored and a main effect regression analysis is performed, the overall treatment effect is estimated to be 0.56 mm Hg (95% CI 0.20, 0.91; $P < 0.01$). However, this positive significant result is somewhat misleading because it is not reproducible in the three centers showing a negative change. In other words, if we randomly select a center from the pool of centers and repeat the study with the same protocol, there is a relatively high chance that a totally opposite result will be observed. The three centers with a negative change have 300 patients who show different results. As a consequence, the reproducibility and generalizability of the targeted patient population and the treatment setting are questionable.

In other words, if there is no evidence of treatment-by-center interaction, the data can be pooled for analysis across centers. By carrying out an analysis with combined data, an overall estimate of the treatment effect across centers is provided. On the other hand, if an interaction effect between treatment and center is found, the overall (or average) summary statistic can be misleading and, hence, considered to be inadequate [5,6]. In this case, it is preferable to describe the nature of the interaction and to indicate which centers contribute towards the interaction [5].

Treatment-by-period interaction in a crossover trial

In the earlier stages of drug development, crossover trials are frequently used to investigate the pharmacokinetics of a study drug. In any crossover trial a so-called *treatment-by-period interaction* can be present. This means that the effect of the treatment is influenced by the period of the trial that the patient is in. Even after an adequate washout interval (where the subject is free of drugs), the effect of either treatment can be influenced by whether it is administered first or second, particularly if patients can sense any real therapeutic effects. For example, in a crossover trial testing two antihypertensive drugs, both drugs are more effective in the second period than in the first.

If this period effect is large, it can be minimized by randomly allocating equal numbers of subjects to different sequences and applying some form of statistical adjustment. In a bioequivalence trial, such an interaction might be present even in the absence of any carry-over (long term residual) effect. The problem is that we cannot tell whether the interaction is due to carry-over or a period-by-treatment interaction, as these two effects are confounded and can never be separated. Therefore, the problem of carry-over is best avoided by ensuring that a crossover trial is properly designed (see **Chapter 10**).

Conclusion

An interaction effect in a clinical trial is where there is a change in the magnitude or direction of the association between a treatment and an outcome according to the level of a third variable. Unlike a confounding effect which can be controlled during a clinical trial, an interaction effect is an unexpected inherent modification of the treatment effect, and can only be explored and assessed once the data have been collected.

The identification of interaction effects can assist in targeting specific therapies at subgroup populations who are more likely to benefit from the therapy. Interaction effects can also help treatment mechanisms to be understood, furthering research in the early stages of drug development. In the later phases of drug research, interaction effects might affect the labeling and prescribing of the product.

In summary, it is important to identify and understand interaction effects, and specific statistical methods might be required to elucidate and quantify these effects. Finally, it is important to note that interaction tests should be used cautiously in data analysis, as most trials are not powered to detect such interaction effects, and the results of such tests are always exploratory in nature [7].

References

1.   Gail M, Simon R. Testing for qualitative interactions between treatment effects and patient subsets. *Biometrics* 1985;**41**:361–72.

2. Gail MH, Benichou J, editors. *Encyclopedia of Epidemiologic Methods*. Chichester: John Wiley & Sons, 2000.

3. Gordis L. *Epidemiology*, 2nd edition. London: WB Saunders Company, 2000.

4. GISSI-Prevenzione Investigators. Dietary supplementation with n-3 polyunsaturated fatty acids and vitamin E after myocardial infarction: results of the GISSI-Prevenzione trial. *Lancet* 1999;**354**:447–55.

5. Chow SC, Liu JP. *Design and Analysis of Clinical Trials: Concepts and Methodologies*. New York: John Wiley & Sons, 1998.

6. Pocock SJ. *Clinical Trials: A Practical Approach*. New York: John Wiley & Sons, 1983.

7. Pocock SJ, Assmann SE, Enos LE, et al. Subgroup analysis, covariate adjustment and baseline comparisons in clinical trial reporting: current practice and problems. *Stat Med* 2002;**21**:2917–30.

Chapter 28

Repeated Measurements

Duolao Wang and Zoe Fox

In many clinical trials, particularly pharmacokinetic and pharmacodynamic studies, an outcome or marker measurement is recorded at different time points for each subject, generating repeated measurement data, which are often correlated. Failure to take account of such correlation in the analysis could produce biased estimates of true treatment effects. There are various strategies that can be used to analyze such data, depending on the questions you wish to answer and the type of data you will be collecting. In this chapter, we present an overview of the various strategies for dealing with repeated measurements of a continuous outcome, and explore in more detail the use of summary measures, which convert mutiple data points into a singular measure (eg, mean or area under the curve).

Figure 1. Repeated measurements of systolic blood pressure (SBP) for 10 patients in a clinical trial.

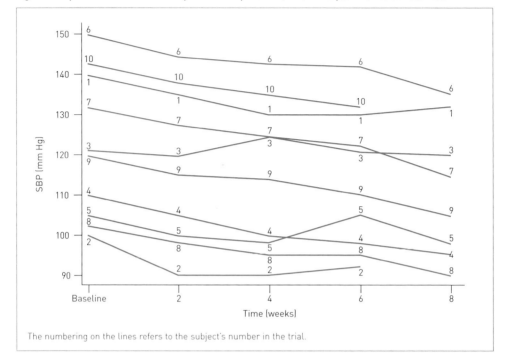

The numbering on the lines refers to the subject's number in the trial.

What are repeated measurements?

A repeated measurement in a clinical trial is an outcome variable that is measured two or more times for each subject, usually over a period of time, eg, before, during, and/or after an intervention or treatment. **Figure 1** illustrates repeated measurements of systolic blood pressure (SBP) at baseline, 2, 4, 6, and 8 weeks for 10 patients in a clinical trial.

Repeated measurements are commonly encountered in pharmacokinetic and pharmacodynamic studies, eg, collection of blood samples at preselected time points in order to measure the blood plasma concentration of a drug. Many factors (eg, gender, race, and weight) can influence the absorption and elimination of a study drug. As a result, some people might exhibit consistently higher blood plasma concentrations of a drug than others during the study period. This phenomenon is generally referred to as *tracking*. In **Figure 1**, the patients who have a higher SBP (such as subjects 1, 6, and 10) or a lower SBP (such as subjects 2, 4, 5, and 8) tend to have consistently higher or lower SBP throughout follow-up.

Key considerations when dealing with repeated measurement data

There are two key considerations when dealing with repeated measurement data. The first consideration is how to deal with the correlation between the repeated measurements for an individual (known as the correlation structure). This is the principal distinction between the different methods of analysis [1–3]. To draw valid scientific inferences, the correlation structure must be taken into account. Failure to control for such correlation effects can lead to biased results: the statistical significance of the observed treatment effects may be over estimated and spuriously significant conclusions could be drawn [1,2].

Secondly, not all repeated measurement data are complete – individuals might be lost to follow-up, withdraw consent, or die during the study – consequently, some measurements might be missing [4]. In **Figure 1**, data on SBP are missing for subjects 2 and 10 at 8 weeks.

What strategies are used to analyze repeated measurement data?

Four main strategies for handling repeated measurement data have been used in clinical research [3,5,6]. They are:

- analysis at a predefined time point
- time-by-time analysis
- use of statistical models
- use of summary measures

Analysis at a predefined time point

The first strategy is to analyze the response outcome at a predefined time point [5]. This approach is most suitable when the response to the treatment at a particular time point is of clinical interest. The change in response from baseline can also be measured to control for individual variations in baseline values. However, the strategy does not utilize information from other time points, thus wasting potentially valuable information. To address this problem, a time-by-time analysis is sometimes performed [5].

Time-by-time analysis

An alternative to analysis at a predefined time point is time-by-time analysis. A group mean (the mean of all the patients' data) can be calculated at each separate time point and a statistical analysis carried out – a time-by-time analysis.

For example, in a study comparing coronary-artery bypass surgery with and without cardio-pulmonary bypass and cardiac arrest (on- and off-pump surgery), Khan et al. compared mean troponin T levels for off-pump and on-pump patients at 0, 6, 12, 24, 48, and 72 hours after randomization [7]. It was found that at 6 and 12 hours postoperatively, troponin T levels were significantly higher in the on-pump group than the off-pump group ($P < 0.001$ for both comparisons), but this difference disappeared by 24 hours.

It should be noted that although analysis at each time point is often requested by clinicians, this method of analysis should not be encouraged because false-positive results may be generated due to multiple testing (ie, a significant result may be found due to chance). In addition, this method ignores within-subject correlation. If a significant difference is found between treatment arms at one time point, differences are likely to be significant at subsequent time points. Hence, time-by-time analysis is best used when there are a small number of time points and the intervals between them are large [5].

Use of statistical models

The use of statistical models in the analysis of repeated measurement data is becoming increasingly popular [1–3,5,6]. These models can be particularly useful when the object of the study is to assess the average treatment effect over the duration of the trial. During the last 20 years, statisticians have considerably enriched the methodology available for the analysis of such data [1,5].

These models offer a variety of approaches for handling both correlation between repeated measurements and missing values. Of these, the mixed model has been widely used in the analysis of repeated measurement data in clinical trials, for two reasons [2,5]:

- it can accommodate a wide variety of ways in which the successive observations are correlated with one another
- it does not require complete data from all subjects

Use of summary measures

The most straightforward method of analyzing repeated measurement data is to use a summary measure. This method is sometimes known as response profile analysis [5,6]. There are two steps to a summary measure approach. The first step is to calculate a summary statistic from the repeated measurements for each subject, eg, the mean, maximum, area under the curve (AUC). The second step is to compare the difference in the summary statistic by treatment groups, by using a standard statistical technique such as a t-test, a nonparametric test, or an analysis of variance.

The summary measure needs to be chosen prior to the analysis of the data and it should be representative of some relevant aspect of the subject's response profile. In some situations, more than one summary measure is needed. This is the main statistical method that is used in the analysis of pharmacokinetic and pharmacodynamic data. As the most straightforward method of analysis, the use of a summary statistic is the focus of this article and will be discussed in greater detail below.

The summary measure approach

The use of the summary measurement approach has two main advantages. Firstly, the analysis is easily interpreted because it is based on summary statistics that have been chosen because of their clinical relevance to the study objective [6].

Secondly, the analysis avoids the problem of correlation structure [5,6]. Once a summary measure is constructed, the number of repeated measurements is reduced to a single quantity for each subject. Therefore, values for different subjects can be thought of as independent – a key requirement of most standard statistical methods.

Most importantly, the trial designer needs to think carefully about the questions to be addressed to determine the best summary measure to use. Making the right decision before data are collected can lead to improvements in the design of the trial.

Commonly used summary statistics

Some commonly used summary measures are summarized in **Table 1**. Their applications and limitations are explained in the following sections.

Mean

The simplest and most commonly used summary measure is the mean of the response over time, since many clinical trials are most concerned with differences in the overall treatment effect rather than more subtle effects. The mean is particularly useful if the individual profiles show no clear pattern or trend with time (see **Figure 2** for a SBP profile). For the data in **Figure 1**, the mean SBP over five visits for subject 6 is 143.2 mm Hg, whereas the mean SBP over four visits for subject 10 is 137.0 mm Hg.

Obviously, this method has a serious drawback: it does not take into account the variability in response variable with time. For example, in **Figure 1**, there is a clear downward trend in SBP for subjects 6 and 10 after drug administration, but the

Table 1. Summary measures for repeated measurements, their applications and limitations.

Summary measure	Data type	Application	Limitations
Mean	No clear pattern or trend	Use to describe the central level of an outcome variable when assessing drug efficacy	Sensitive to missing information Ignores within-subject variation
Maximum	Single peak	Use to describe the maximum drug concentration in a pharmacokinetic study	Sensitive to missing information Sensitive to sampling time points
Time to maximum	Single peak	Use to describe the speed of drug absorption in a pharmacokinetic study	Sensitive to missing information Sensitive to sampling time points
Area under the curve	Peaked or no clear pattern	Assess an overall extent of drug concentration	Ignores within-subject variation
Percentage of time the outcome variable is above or below a certain value	Multiple peaks or troughs	Use when assessing the fraction of time that the drug is effective for during the study period, especially for pharmacodynamic studies	To get a stable estimate, many time points are needed
Number of occasions on which the outcome variable is above or below a certain value	Multiple peaks or troughs	Use to assess the frequency of fluctuations of pharmacodynamic parameters such as pH, blood pressure, and heart rate	To get a stable estimate, many time points are needed
Rate of change	Linear or non-linear trend	Evaluate a rate of change in an outcome variable by fitting a linear or non-linear model	Coefficients are measured with varying levels of precision depending on missing values

overall mean only describes the middle data point. In this case, the overall mean is not an ideal statistic to use to represent the SBP over the course of the study.

This method is also susceptible to outliers in the data (ie, a measurement might be unusually high/low at one visit and consequently influence the overall mean). For example, if the measurement at week 4 for subject 10 had been 168.0 mm Hg, then the overall mean would have increased to 148.2 mm Hg. This would be higher than the mean for subject 6, but would obviously not be representative of the entire profile for subject 10.

Maximum

Another easily interpreted summary statistic is the maximum value of the response variable during the observation period. This can be used to assess the maximum effect of a study drug in a trial or the maximum drug concentration in a pharmacokinetic study.

For example, in a study examining the immunological response to highly active anti-retroviral therapy (HAART) in different age groups, the maximum CD4 T-cell count over 31 months of follow-up was calculated for each subject individually, and then summarized and compared between age groups [8]. The

Figure 2. Repeated measures with no clear pattern or trend for a subject that could be better summarized by a mean.

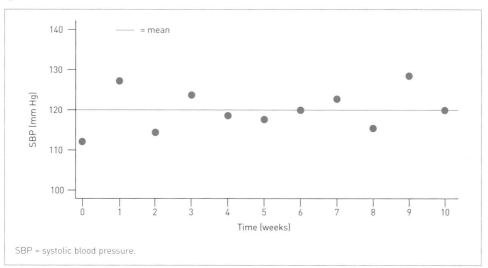

SBP = systolic blood pressure.

maximum CD4 T-cell count was determined for four age quartiles. The median maximum CD4 T-cell count by increasing age quartile was 500×10^6 cells/L, 448×10^6 cells/L, 430×10^6 cells/L, and 419×10^6 cells/L ($P < 0.0001$), illustrating that older patients had a lower maximum CD4 count and indicating a poorer response to HAART. This result was consistent with the other results of the study such as the maximum CD4 T-cell gain (251×10^6 cells/L, 246×10^6 cells/L, 212×10^6 cells/L, and 213×10^6 cells/L, for increasing age quartiles [$P = 0.0003$]) and was still significant after adjustments for other variables influencing CD4 T-cell response.

Time to reach the maximum

A statistic related to the maximum value is the time to reach the maximum. This is a measure of how quickly a subject responds to the drug. Although the previous two statistics avoid the problem of correlation structure seen with repeated measurement data, by reducing multiple measurements to a single index correlation they are susceptible to missing observations. The missing values could be higher than the actual measurements that were recorded and could come at earlier time points. If the time point at which the unknown theoretical maximum value would be achieved is not selected in the design stage, inaccurate estimates will be obtained for both the maximum value and the time to reach it (see **Chapter 13**).

Figure 3. Calculation of C_{max}, T_{max}, and *AUC* for a subject's plasma concentration profile.

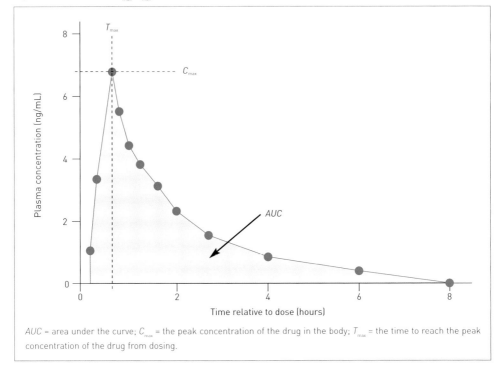

AUC = area under the curve; C_{max} = the peak concentration of the drug in the body; T_{max} = the time to reach the peak concentration of the drug from dosing.

In pharmacokinetic studies, the peak plasma concentration (C_{max}) and the time to achieve it (T_{max}) are used to assess the speed or rate of absorption of a study drug. C_{max} and T_{max} can be derived from a subject's plasma concentration profile, as shown in **Figure 3**. The data in **Figure 3** suggest that in this subject the study drug has a very rapid absorption, reaching a peak of about 6.67 ng/mL in less than an hour after administration.

Area under the curve

A method that makes use of all available response values, as well as the lengths of the time intervals, is an *AUC* approach (see **Figure 3**). Mathematically, *AUC* can be calculated for any time serial data in which an outcome variable is observed at different time points (with equal or unequal intervals) by using the trapezoidal rule, but it is particularly useful in situations where the total uptake of a drug concentration is of interest. The unit for *AUC* is the unit of drug concentration multiplied by the unit of time, eg, for the *AUC* calculated from the pharmacokinetic profile in **Figure 3**, the unit is hour.ng/mL.

In bioequivalence studies, C_{max} and AUC are often used as primary endpoints to assess bioequivalence between test and standard drug formulations, with respect to the rate of, and extent of, absorption of a study drug. Like the mean, the AUC does not take variability in response for a particular subject into consideration.

When calculating an AUC by the trapezoidal rule, missing values are conventionally treated in the following ways. If missing values occur before the first or after the last observed response value, they do not contribute to the AUC calculation – in **Figure 3**, the plasma concentration is non-quantifiable before 0.25 hours and after 8 hours. If the missing value occurs between two observed data points, it is assumed that the outcome variable lies on a straight line between these points. For example, in **Figure 3** the drug concentration between 4 and 6 hours is assumed to be linearly distributed. Various other methods can be used to extrapolate missing values for different types of data, such as last observation carried forward. Each method has its advantages in different settings: for detailed information see Reference [9].

Percentage of time/number of occasions that a response variable is above/below a certain value

The use of percentage or number of follow-up measurements that are larger or smaller (depending on the clinical relevance) than a prespecified value specifically takes into account fluctuations in the response variable during the course of a study. The former gives the fraction of time that an outcome variable is above or below a clinically meaningful value, whereas the latter reflects the frequency of fluctuation around this selected value during the observation period. These summary measures are useful when there are many peaks and troughs in a response profile with a very large number of time points. They are frequently used in pharmacodynamic studies in which pH values or vital signs (eg, blood pressure, heart rate, respiration rate) are recorded at small time intervals.

For example, a blinded trial was conducted in healthy volunteers to determine whether drug A was comparable to drug B in the suppression of gastroesophageal reflux provoked by a standard meal, by using ambulatory esophageal pH monitoring. The primary efficacy parameter was the percentage of time for which the esophageal pH fell below 4, and the second efficacy parameter was the number of occasions on which esophageal pH fell below 4. **Figure 4** shows a pH profile for a subject, in which the pH was recorded every 6 seconds over 4 hours. For this subject, the percentage of time and number of occasions for which the pH falls below 4 are 0.75% and 5, respectively.

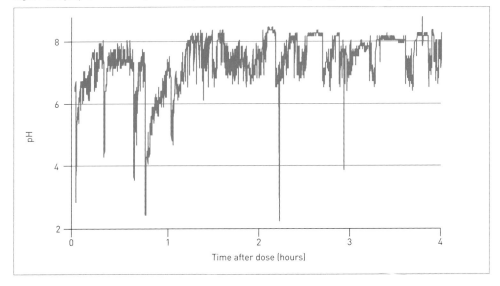

Figure 4. A pH profile for a subject taking part in a trial of a new drug for gastroesophageal reflux.

Rate or gradient of change in a response variable

The statistical approaches discussed so far mainly relate to data where the value of the outcome variable under consideration fluctuates in the absence of a unified monotonic trend for all subjects during the study period. Conversely, in situations where the response variable increases or decreases steadily with time, eg, in the case of growth data, it is possible to ask more detailed questions about how the outcome variable changes with time. This can be done by calculating the slope (or regression coefficient) of the decline/increase for each individual and comparing these slopes using standard techniques.

For the SBP data in **Figure 1**, most subjects show a trend towards decreasing SBP. Therefore, a linear regression line can be fitted for each of the 10 subjects – the fitted lines are displayed in **Figure 5**. The estimated slopes in the figure range from –3.9 for subject 7 to –0.1 for subject 3, illustrating the different rates of change in SBP for the subjects after drug administration. The change in SBP during the study period was large for subject 7, dropping by 3.9 mm Hg on average at each visit, whereas the change in SBP for subject 3 was much smaller. We can assess which drug reduces SBP fastest by comparing the mean rates of the two treatment groups.

If the data are non-linear then a non-linear model should be fitted for each subject's data. For example, in a pharmacokinetic study to describe the rate of elimination, a log-linear model is always fitted; the coefficient of the log-linear model is used to describe the rate of drug elimination.

Figure 5. A linear regression line for the systolic blood pressure (SBP) data for the 10 subjects receiving a drug for hypertension.

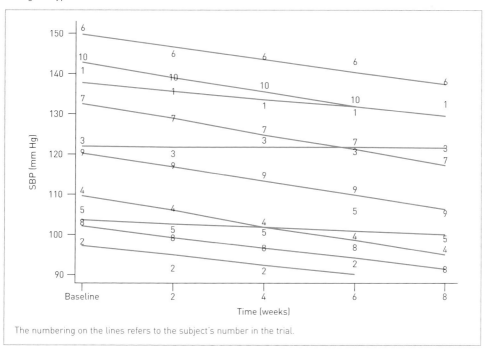

The numbering on the lines refers to the subject's number in the trial.

Conclusion

The key issues when choosing which method of summary measure analysis to use are the questions you wish to answer and the type of data collected. The summary measures chosen need to have a clear clinical relevance and should be deduced at the design stage. In most trials, more than one summary measure may be used to analyze repeated measurement data, to address different aspects of the study question.

References

1. Diggle PJ, Liang KY, Zeger SL. *Analysis of Longitudinal Data*. Oxford: Clarendon Press, 1994.
2. Brown H, Prescott R. *Applied Mixed Models in Medicine*. Chichester: John Wiley & Sons, 1999.
3. Everitt BS. The analysis of repeated measures: a practical review with examples. *Statistician* 1995:**44**:113–35.
4. Touloumi G, Pocock SJ, Babiker A, et al. Impact of missing data due to selective dropouts in cohort studies and clinical trials. *Epidemiology* 2002:**13**:347–55.
5. Dunn G, Pickles A. Longitudinal data analysis. Overview. In: Armitage P, Colton T, editors. *Encyclopedia of Biostatistics*. New York: John Wiley & Sons, 1998:2352–63.

6.   Matthews JN, Altman DG, Campbell MJ, et al. Analysis of serial measurements in medical research. *BMJ* 1990;**300**:230–5.

7.   Khan NE, De Souza A, Mister R, et al. A randomized comparison of off-pump and on-pump multivessel coronary-artery bypass surgery. *N Engl J Med* 2004;**350**:21–8.

8.   Viard JP, Mocroft A, Chiesi A, et al. Influence of age on CD4 cell recovery in human immunodeficiency virus-infected patients receiving highly active antiretroviral therapy: evidence from the EuroSIDA study. *J Infect Dis* 2001;**183**:1290–4.

9.   Cozzi Lepri A, Smith GD, Mocroft A, et al. A practical approach to adjusting for attrition bias in HIV clinical trials with serial marker responses. *AIDS* 1998;**12**:1155–61.

Chapter 29

Multiplicity

Dorothea Nitsch, Duolao Wang,
Tim Clayton, and Ameet Bakhai

In a clinical trial, information is often collected with multiple
endpoints and baseline variables. In addition, outcomes are
often measured at several different time points. It is tempting
to analyze this information by performing many statistical tests
such as comparisons of multiple endpoints, or undertaking
many separate subgroup analyses or comparisons of outcome
measures at several time points during the course of the study.
Consequently, the problem of 'multiple testing' or multiplicity
can occur where many statistical tests are performed, increasing
the probability of false-positive results (ie, the probability that
at least one result is significant at $P < 0.05$ by chance). In this
chapter, we discuss the issue of multiplicity in the context of
clinical research, and highlight some strategies for dealing
with it.

Introduction

The most simple randomized clinical trial involves the comparison of two treatments with respect to just one outcome measure. In this case, the observed data can be evaluated with a statistical significance test where a traditional threshold for significance (such as $P < 0.05$) is chosen as evidence of a true difference between the two treatments. The problem of multiplicity arises when a clinical trial is used to test several hypotheses simultaneously, rather than just a single test for a single hypothesis based on a single event outcome [1].

The key to understanding the problem of multiplicity is that we may consider a treatment effect to be statistically significantly superior to the control treatment when indeed the difference arose by chance. This is called a Type I error (see **Chapter 18**). To elaborate, consider a randomized double-blinded placebo-controlled clinical trial evaluating drug A for reducing systolic blood pressure (SBP) among hypertensive patients. The null hypothesis is that there is no difference in mean SBP between patients receiving drug A (μ_1) and placebo (μ_2) ($H_0 : \mu_1 = \mu_2$). The alternative hypothesis states there is a significant difference between treatments ($H_a : \mu_1 \neq \mu_2$).

If the null hypothesis is rejected due to a chance significant (false-positive) finding, we say that a Type I error has occurred. For example, a Type I error has occurred if we claim that drug A reduces SBP when in fact there is no difference between drug A and placebo in the reduction of SBP. The probability of committing a Type I error is known as the level of significance, denoted by α. This is traditionally set at $\alpha = 0.05 = 5\%$, suggesting that this scenario will occur in one out of every 20 studies.

If a statistical model is constructed for detecting the difference in a parameter such as the mean between two identical populations (ie, no true differences), with a certain pre-set statistical limit α, then the probability of a Type I error will be increased as further tests are conducted using different samples from the two same populations and the same limit α. In other words, the chance of finding at least one significant result (overall Type I error) increases with the number of tests, even though there are no true differences between the comparison groups. For instance, assuming that all tests are independent, the probability of one of them being spuriously significant is $[1 - (1 - \alpha)^n]$, where n is the number of tests (see **Figure 1**).

From this graph, we can see that if five such tests are performed, the Type I error is increased to over 0.20. In other words, if five independent tests are used to test null hypotheses that are in fact true using the significance limit of 0.05 for each

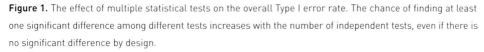

Figure 1. The effect of multiple statistical tests on the overall Type I error rate. The chance of finding at least one significant difference among different tests increases with the number of independent tests, even if there is no significant difference by design.

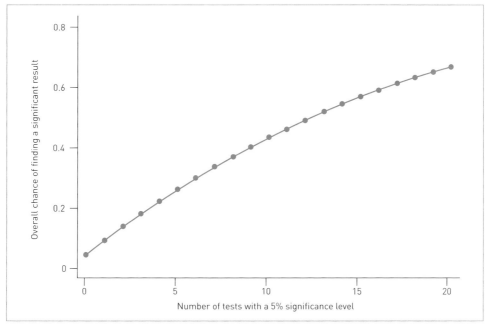

single test, there is more than a 20% chance that at least one of these tests will produce a *P*-value ≤0.05. If 10 such tests are performed, the Type I error is increased to about 0.40; and with 14 tests, the likelihood is higher than 0.50.

The above results suggest that the use of multiple testing with a critical significance level based on a single test ("Do any of the statistical tests reach the significance level of 0.05?") is an inappropriate way of testing more than the original null hypotheses. This suggests that results from the use of multiple testing with a critical significance level based on a single test should be interpreted with caution; approaches to this problem are discussed later in the chapter. **Figure 1** also highlights that using a statistical tool developed for a single defined question needs careful consideration when answers to more than one question are sought. In general, however, tests will tend to be correlated and the probabilities of making at least one Type 1 error may be expected to be less than those shown in **Figure 1** (see **Figure 1** in **Chapter 31** for simulation results).

How does multiplicity occur in the setting of clinical trials?

Multiple endpoints

In contemporary practice, trials compare two treatments in terms of several outcomes. This might be because we are keen to appreciate the impact of a new treatment on several outcomes (such as mortality, disease incidence, and quality of life) or because for some diseases there might not be a single dominant measure of outcome. This is common in trials addressing chronic disease conditions such as arthritis or neuropathy in which pain or joint mobility are the outcomes of interest.

An example of this problem can be found in a recently published trial in children with osteogenesis imperfecta [2]. This disease is characterized by fragile bones, which break easily. The trial evaluated olpadronate (a bisphosphonate) with respect to its skeletal effects in children. There were three primary outcomes:

- incidence of fractures of long bones
- changes in bone mineral density and content
- functionality

It is clinically sensible to address this series of outcomes together, as no single endpoint is sufficient to address the primary objective of the study. However, caution is needed in the interpretation of the results since many separate statistical tests may be needed.

Multiple endpoints also arise in studies of diseases that have major morbidity outcome measures, such as the occurrence of a stroke, heart attack, or death; outcomes commonly used in cardiovascular trials.

Multiple treatments

The decision to evaluate multiple treatments, combinations of treatments, or different doses of the same treatment within a trial with several parallel arms almost always implies some form of multiple comparison study. An example might be the simultaneous investigation of two treatments, both individually and in combination, on the disease-free survival of postmenopausal women with early breast cancer [3]. The number of possible treatment combinations increases rapidly with the number of treatments, and so do the number of statistical tests performed.

Repeated measurements

In many clinical trials, an outcome or marker measurement is recorded at different time points for each subject, generating repeated measurement data. To analyze such data, a time-by-time analysis is sometimes used: group means are calculated at each separate time point, and separate statistical analyses are carried out at each of the time points (see **Chapter 28**). This also leads to the problem of multiple comparisons and therefore increases the possibility of a false-positive result.

Subgroup analyses

A clinical trial is usually concerned with the overall impact of a treatment on the trial population. However, individuals within a trial population vary in their characteristics. Common secondary analyses involve the investigation of whether differences between treatments vary between different subgroups of the study population. For example, we might test whether males or females benefit more from a certain treatment, or specifically diabetic patients, or patients above a certain age. Such analyses are called subgroup analyses. The statistical issues related to these are complex and prone to confusion and often involve multiple testing, in addition to the problem that trials are often not powered to detect treatment differences amongst subgroups (see **Chapter 23**) [4].

Interim analyses

Interim analyses are usually undertaken during the conduct of a trial for ethical and economical reasons, with the possibility that the trial might be terminated early if significant treatment differences in efficacy or safety outcomes are found. It is worth noting that successive analyses conducted on the growing body of trial data will also lead to an increase in the overall Type I error rate at the final analysis of the trial, unless adjustments are made (as discussed in the next section) (see also **Chapter 31**).

Strategies for dealing with multiplicity

Multiplicity needs to be considered at the design stage of the trial and when writing a statistical analysis plan – *before* any analysis is undertaken. We discuss three possible strategies for handling multiplicity in trials.

Change limits to *P*-values of single test

The first strategy is to plan a predefined correction for the inflated Type I error. If the significance level for each individual test is reduced, then the overall level of significance can be kept at 0.05 for the entire series of tests. There are different types of statistical corrections that are based on this approach.

A commonly used approach is the *Bonferroni correction* to the nominal significance level [5]. The significance level of each subtest is set to be the overall significance level divided by the total number of tests performed – eg, with five tests, the critical level of significance for each of the five subtests is set at 0.01 (= 0.05 / 5) instead of 0.05. By performing such a correction, the probability that one or more of the tests will produce a statistically significant result if the null hypothesis is true is approximately 0.05, maintaining the traditional significance level.

An example of this is seen in a multicenter trial of hormonal emergency contraception for healthy women [6]. One part of the outcome assessment included testing for differences in the occurrence of one or more side-effects (nausea, changes in menstrual bleeding, headache, etc). In total there were 10 side-effects that were potentially due to emergency contraception, giving an adjusted significance level of 0.005. After Bonferroni correction, mifepristone was still significantly associated with less and delayed menstrual bleeding compared to levonorgestrel because the P-value obtained for this test was <0.0001, smaller than the threshold for significance of 0.005.

The Bonferroni correction is very conservative, ie, this correction assumes that each of the outcomes tested is independent. The situation can arise where several of the results are all less than $P = 0.05$ but, according to the Bonferroni correction, the result would be nonsignificant. Under such circumstances, the Bonferroni procedure will be an over-correction for multiple testing.

There are several other correction methods available for reducing the likelihood of a Type I error, discussed in detail by Hsu [7]. There are also various statistical amendments that can be made to the P-values in interim analysis. Three of the most popular methods are the O'Brien–Fleming, Pocock, and Peto–Haybittle rules (see **Chapter 31**) [8]. For example, the previously mentioned trial that evaluated several treatments in postmenopausal women with breast cancer planned one single interim analysis with an adjusted nominal P-value for interim analysis of efficacy using a Peto–Haybittle stopping rule [9]. The Peto–Haybittle stopping rule is similar to the Bonferroni rule in that it is very conservative – the results of one or more repeated interim analyses with respect to efficacy are interpreted as significant only if $P < 0.001$ [10].

Define the relative meaning of several outcomes

A second strategy is to specify in the protocol the pattern of statistically significant findings in the individual response variables that will be taken as conclusive for the study as a whole. For example, a trial might have many endpoints (say six) measuring different aspects of disease outcome. In such a case, it may be stated that statistical significance (at the 5% level) must be achieved on the first two primary outcomes and on one of the remaining four primary endpoints in order to allow the conclusion of a positive outcome to the trial. Such an approach makes no formal correction for inflated overall Type I error, but it avoids the possibility that an overall positive result will be interpreted from positive results on only one of several variables, thereby reducing the overall Type I error quite substantially.

Just wait for the results and then decide

The last strategy is to do nothing to correct for inflated Type I error, to test each comparison at the 5% level of significance, and, whenever appropriate, to add cautions to the trial report warning of the potential effects of multiple testing [11]. The problem with this strategy is that it puts the burden on the reader to assess whether any positive results generated from the trial are valid, or are likely to be due to the spurious output of multiple testing. This approach can be attractive when the outcome variables are expected to be highly associated, and can be used as an alternative or as a supplement to the second strategy described above. The current practice of medical journals is not to demand any correction for multiple testing. A balanced caution in the interpretation of the usually large number of statistical tests performed is preferred to undue flexibility in suppressing unexpected findings.

Specific strategies for dealing with several endpoints

Multiple endpoints exist in almost every trial. We will now discuss some specific methods based on the strategies mentioned above, which are used to deal with several endpoints. They all demonstrate that a possible loss of detailed information has to be weighed against a gain in terms of reducing false-positive findings.

Specify the priorities of the endpoints in advance

This approach is most commonly applied in clinical trials practice. One example is the previously mentioned World Health Organization trial of emergency contraception [6]. The trial protocol prespecified the sequence of planned analyses and defined primary and secondary endpoints. The primary endpoint in this trial was unintended pregnancy, and the secondary endpoints were side-effects due to the various treatments. The main conclusion of the trial with respect to the primary endpoint was that there was no evidence for a difference between the various hormonal methods of emergency contraception with respect to unintended pregnancies. As mentioned above, treatments differed in their side-effect profiles, with less menstrual bleeding under mifepristone. The main conclusion was that all studied regimes seem to be efficacious for emergency contraception.

Combine outcomes into a single summary statistic

A quality of life questionnaire is a classic example of a summary endpoint that synthesizes a large amount of information into a single measure (score) of outcome. Patients answer a whole list of questions, and a summary measure indicating their quality of life is then generated. This strategy is also useful in the analysis of data with repeated measurements when a summary measure is derived from those multiple measures. This summary measure is then used to evaluate a possible treatment difference in a single statistical test. For example, the area under the curve and peak value (C_{max}) are often used as a primary endpoint in bioequivalence studies (see **Chapters 13** and **28**).

Define a combined composite endpoint

Another strategy is to define a composite endpoint as the first occurrence of any of a list of several major events of interest. An example of this is the RITA (Randomized Intervention Trial of Angina) 3 trial, which assessed an initial conservative strategy (medical therapy) versus an initial interventional strategy (angiography and subsequent revascularization, if indicated) in patients with unstable angina or non-ST-segment elevation myocardial infarction (MI) [12].

The co-primary trial endpoints were the occurrence of the first of either death, nonfatal MI, or refractory angina at 4 months, and death or nonfatal MI at 1 year. The co-primary endpoints reflect major complications of unstable angina that the treatment strategies aim to reduce. The interventional treatment prevented about a third of these complications at 4 months compared to the conservative strategy. However, caution is needed in interpreting the results as this difference was entirely driven by a reduction in refractory angina, and there were few differences between the groups in terms of deaths or nonfatal MIs.

Use a multivariate approach/overall hypothesis accounting for all the endpoints

A further problem that must be considered when dealing with multiple outcome measures is that there can be a greater tendency for patients to have several outcomes together than just one: so a patient avoiding a heart attack is also likely to avoid a reduction in his quality of life. There are specific statistical methods that adjust for such correlations between endpoints, while the capacity for clinical interpretation of each component is maintained.

One of these methods, the *Wei–Lachin procedure* [13], was used in a trial investigating the effects of mitoxantrone in patients with multiple sclerosis [14]. In this trial, five clinical measures indicating the severity of multiple sclerosis (changes of two different severity scores reflecting the disability of patients, number of relapses requiring steroid treatment, time to first treated relapse, and changes in the standardized score of neurological status) were tested in one overall hypothesis that the treatment affects all of those measures.

Table 1. Different types of multiplicity and possible strategies for adjusting for multiplicity.

Type of multiplicity	Possible strategies
Multiple endpoints	Specify primary and secondary endpoints in advance
	Define a summary statistic as an endpoint
	Predefine meaningful composite endpoints
	Choose a multivariate global test statistic
	Use Bonferroni correction
Multiple treatments	Predefine priorities or use a global test statistic to test for any difference
Subgroup analyses	Predefine a limited number of subgroups in the protocol to be analyzed with interaction tests
	Use Bonferroni correction if uncritical testing of many subgroups
Interim analysis	Predefine P-values for efficacy that statistically account for the frequency of interim analysis, with more stringent P-values for early analyses

There were visible merits in using a multivariate approach in this trial, because all five primary outcomes by themselves and as a whole gave a credible and consistent answer in terms of an overall direction, indicating a benefit of treatment. However, in situations where trials have uninformative or inconsistent results, such a multivariate statistical approach with a possible borderline global result might give controversial answers that have to be interpreted with caution, thereby taking account of the clinical setting of the trial. In certain situations such paradoxes may be natural, eg, if death is prevented then nonfatal events may increase in frequency, such as disease flair-ups during the extended survival period [15].

Conclusion

The basic principles of statistical testing apply to a single test of a single null hypothesis. However, the problem of multiplicity or multiple statistical comparisons is a common one in clinical research, arising when several comparisons are undertaken from which to draw conclusions. Repeated or multiple testing of different outcome variables or many different treatments within the same trial will tend to increase the likelihood of finding a statistically significant difference by chance alone, inflating the overall Type I error, which can undermine the validity of the statistical analyses unless accounted for.

There are several strategies with which to deal with the problem of multiple testing – either at the design or at the analysis stage. A table of summary points is provided (see **Table 1**). The simplest advice would be to design the trial by specifying the priorities of analysis in terms of primary and secondary importance, and reducing the significance threshold if needed.

References

1. Bland JM, Altman DG. Multiple significance tests: the Bonferroni method. *BMJ* 1995;**310**:170.
2. Sakkers R, Kok D, Engelbert R, et al. Skeletal effects and functional outcome with olpadronate in children with osteogenesis imperfecta: a 2-year randomised placebo-controlled study. *Lancet* 2004;**363**:1427–31.
3. Baum M, Budzar AU, Cuzick J, et al. Anastrozole alone or in combination with tamoxifen versus tamoxifen alone for adjuvant treatment of postmenopausal women with early breast cancer: first results of the ATAC randomised trial. *Lancet* 2002;**359**:2131–9.
4. Assmann SF, Pocock SJ, Enos LE, et al. Subgroup analysis and other (mis)uses of baseline data in clinical trials. *Lancet* 2000;**355**:1064–9.
5. Bonferroni CE. Teoria statistica delle classi e calcolo delle probabilita. *Publicazioni del R Instituto Superiore die Scienze Economiche e Commerciali di Firenze* 1936;**8**:3–62 (in Italian).
6. von Hertzen H, Piaggio G, Ding J, et al. Low dose mifepristone and two regimens of levonorgestrel for emergency contraception: a WHO multicentre randomised trial. *Lancet* 2002;**360**:1803–10.
7. Hsu JC. *Multiple Comparisons – Theory and Methods*. London: Chapman & Hall, 1996.
8. Jennison C, Turnbull BW. *Group Sequential Methods with Applications to Clinical Trials*. London: Chapman & Hall, 2000.
9. Chow SC, Liu P. *Design and Analysis of Clinical trials: Concepts and Methodologies*. New York: John Wiley & Sons, 1998.
10. Comelli M. Multiple Endpoints. In: *Encyclopaedia of Biopharmaceutical Statistics*. Chow SC, editor. New York: Marcel Dekker Inc, 2003:333–43.
11. Vardy A. Statistics. In: *Handbook of Clinical Research*, 2nd edition. Lloyd J, Raven A, editors. London: Churchill Medical Communications, 1994:334–63.
12. Fox KA, Poole-Wilson PA, Henderson RA, et al. Interventional versus conservative treatment for patients with unstable angina or non-ST-elevation myocardial infarction: the British Heart Foundation RITA 3 randomised trial. Randomized Intervention Trial of unstable Angina. *Lancet* 2002;**360**:743–51.
13. Wei LJ, Lachin JM. Two-sample asymptotically distribution free tests for incomplete multivariate observations. *J Am Stat Assoc* 1984;**79**:653–61.
14. Hartung HP, Gonsette R, Konig N, et al. Mitoxantrone in progressive multiple sclerosis: a placebo-controlled, double-blind, randomised, multicentre trial. *Lancet* 2002;**360**:2018–25.
15. Senn S. Multiplicity. Section 10. In: *Statistical Issues in Drug Development*. Chichester: John Wiley & Sons, 1997:141–52.

Chapter 30

Missing Data

Maurille Feudjo-Tepie, Christopher Frost,
Duolao Wang, and Ameet Bakhai

Missing information is unfortunately common in randomized controlled trials given that patients may miss visits, withdraw from a trial, or data may be lost. Since it is impossible to avoid missing some data, the challenges are: (1) to design a clinical trial so as to limit the occurrence of missing data; (2) to control or assess its potential impact on the trial conclusions. Targeting the latter, in this chapter we discuss some of the problems associated with missing data values, for simplicity focusing on situations where the response variable is continuous. Based on data from a hypothetical trial, we illustrate some useful ways of coping with missing data in longitudinal studies.

What are missing data?

In clinical trials, after treatment group assignment, each participant is scheduled for follow-up, during which time the primary outcome and other variables will be measured on at least one occasion. It is common for participants to miss some of their scheduled visits. It is also common for information to be misplaced or not entered, despite being collected successfully [1,2]. In both of these situations, we say we are faced with a *missing data problem*.

Missing responses can be easily identified when the number of measurements per participant is fixed (balanced study). However, in studies with varying numbers of measurement visits per participant (unbalanced studies), it might not be possible to identify some of the nonresponses (missing data) unless all scheduled measurement occasions are strictly recorded.

In some of the literature, unobserved latent variables and/or random effects are also treated as missing data [3,4]. This is not the type of missing data considered here. We are concerned with missing outcome variables, ie, measurements that could potentially have been obtained. This is in contrast to latent or random variables that could never have been observed.

What are the common types of missing data?

There are numerous reasons why data may be missing at the analysis stage. These reasons can include the trial design (eg, if some participants miss some visits by design, such as trial closure), loss of successfully collected information, and participant refusal or withdrawal. While knowledge of these reasons is important, the analyst is most interested in their potential impact on the results of the analysis. This impact depends on the relationship between the process giving rise to the missing data and other variables included in the analysis.

Rubin gives a useful taxonomy and terminology, widely accepted, for the different mechanisms that can generate missing data, based on their potential influence on the results of an analysis [5]. He classifies three different types of missing data:

- missing completely at random (MCAR)
- missing at random (MAR)
- missing not at random (MNAR), also termed non-ignorable missing data

In MCAR, the probability that a response is missing is completely unrelated to both the observed information and the hypothetical response value that would have been observed were it not missing. In MAR, the probability that a response is missing depends on some or all of the observed variables and responses. However conditional on the observed data, this probability is unrelated to the hypothetical value that would have been observed were the data not missing. A process that is neither MCAR nor MAR is termed MNAR.

In practice, it might not be possible to state with confidence whether a particular missing data mechanism is MCAR, MAR, or MNAR. However, this classification is useful and if we can decide which assumption is most plausible then it provides a good guide to the type of analysis that should be adopted to account for the missing data.

What are the potential effects of missing data?

Three types of concern typically arise in the analysis of missing data [6]:

- loss of efficiency
- complications in data handling and analysis
- introduction of bias

The importance of each of these is determined by the missing data mechanism (MCAR, MAR, or MNAR) and the way in which the data are analyzed. For example, if the missing data mechanism is MCAR then an analysis that excludes participants with incomplete data will not introduce bias, but will not necessarily be efficient. An analysis in which missing values are replaced with 'plausible' values (eg, by carrying forward the last observed measurement) might increase precision, but might also introduce bias if the method for choosing the plausible values is inappropriate.

When the missingness is not MCAR, however, a simple analysis restricted to participants with no missing values (completers), or even to all available data, can introduce serious bias – eg, if data were missing due to the side-effects of a drug causing participants to drop out. Indeed, with MAR and MNAR processes, it is necessary to consider an analysis strategy that takes account of the influence of missingness process.

What are the commonly used strategies for dealing with missing data?

When the response is continuous, there are several commonly used strategies available for handling missing data. We will consider these in four categories:

- analysis of complete cases only
- analysis of all available data without data replacement
- last observation carried forward (LOCF) and other *ad hoc* methods for replacing missing values
- multiple imputations for replacement

Analysis of complete cases only

A complete case analysis involves analysis of only those participants who have no missing values. When dealing with a process that is MCAR, such an analysis will be unbiased. However, discarding data on participants with some missing values can lead to a loss of efficiency. Molenberghs et al. point out that this loss of efficiency can be particularly severe when there are a large number of measurement occasions [7]. If data are not MCAR then an analysis of complete cases will, in general, be biased [7].

Analysis of all available data

Analysis of all available data is generally preferable to analysis of complete cases. Indeed, if the data are MAR (rather than MCAR) then a valid analysis can be obtained through a likelihood-based analysis of all available data, ignoring the missingness mechanism (provided that parameters describing the measurement process are functionally independent of parameters describing the missingness process [8,9]).

Since an analysis of all available data can still generate unbiased parameter estimates, researchers have coined MAR data as 'ignorable missingness'. It should, however, be borne in mind that the missing data can only be ignored if an appropriate analysis is carried out. We describe such an analysis in a later section.

Last observation carried forward

LOCF is another popular strategy, particularly when participants drop out, or the trial terminates, on a set date (in contrast to intermittent missing values). Here, the last observed value for a participant who drops out is carried forward to each of the subsequent missed measurement occasions. The analysis that follows does not distinguish between the observed and 'carried forward' data.

This approach is simple and easy to implement, but it is based on the assumption that had the participant remained in the trial until completion, the participant's measurements would have remained exactly the same as at the time of dropping out. A number of problems have been documented with this approach [7]. Time trends in the data, when combined with differential dropout rates between groups, can introduce severe bias. This method also ignores the fact that, even if a participant's disease state remains constant, measurements of this state are unlikely to stay exactly the same, introducing a spurious lack of random variability into the analysis.

Other alternatives to LOCF are occasionally adopted: carrying forward the worst case, carrying forward the best case, or carrying forward the baseline value [10,11]. These methods have drawbacks similar to those of LOCF and we therefore recommend that these strategies be used predominantly to conduct a sensitivity analysis.

Multiple imputation

LOCF and other strategies where previously observed values (last, worst, or best observed) are carried forward to fill in the missing values belong to a class of methods termed *imputation* methods [12]. They can be labeled *nonparametric* or *data-based* imputation methods, as opposed to *parametric* or *model-based* imputation [13].

Parametric imputation involves replacing missing values with predictions from a statistical model; in nonparametric imputation, the missing value is replaced with an observed value. Provided that an appropriate statistical model is used (one that takes account of the observed predictors and responses that are related to the missingness mechanism) then parametric imputation can give rise to unbiased parameter estimates under MAR. However, the fact that only a single imputation of each missing value is made, and that there is no allowance for imprecision in such imputations in the analysis, introduces spurious precision into the estimates.

Multiple imputation can be used to take appropriate account of uncertainty in the imputed values [8]. Provided that an appropriate model is used for imputation, this approach can result in valid unbiased estimates under MAR. Horton and Lipsitz present the multiple imputation method as a three-stage process [14].

- Firstly, sets of 'plausible' values for missing observations are created. Each of these sets is used to fill in the missing value and create a 'completed' dataset.
- Secondly, each of these datasets is analyzed.
- Finally, the results are combined, taking account of imprecision in parameter estimates from each 'completed' dataset and variation between datasets.

Multiple imputation is now readily available in public domain software such as SOLAS version 3.0 and above, SAS 8.2 and above, S-Plus, and MICE [15–18]. In the analysis of clinical trials, multiple imputation is most useful for dealing with missing covariates. When it is only the outcome variable that is missing, a correctly specified model for all of the available data will give similar results for less computational effort. Multiple imputation is therefore rarely used for imputing outcome variables in clinical trials.

Methods for MNAR data

Of the methods we have described, only a likelihood-based analysis of all the data and multiple imputation are capable of producing valid, unbiased estimates if the missing data are MAR. However, in practice, it is difficult to be certain that the data are indeed MAR, and to exclude the possibility that the missingness mechanism is MNAR. Unfortunately, when the data are MNAR we cannot ignore the missing data process as with MAR, and none of the approaches we have described will result in unbiased estimates.

There have been suggestions for MNAR models – eg, Diggle and Kenward provide such a modeling procedure for a continuous response [8]. However, such models require strong and untestable distributional assumptions [8]. A pragmatic approach is to make such models a component of a sensitivity analysis carried out to investigate the robustness of results obtained using a plausible MAR-based analysis [7,9].

Comparison of different strategies for dealing with different types of missing data

In this section, we will use simulated data to illustrate patterns of missing data and the consequences of using different analytical strategies.

The simulation model for the full dataset

Consider a randomized controlled trial with 2,000 participants in each of two treatment groups (A and B) and four follow-up visits, with the primary outcome being the response at the final visit. For simplicity, let us say that the outcome variable is not measured at baseline. Let us suppose that in group A, at the first visit, the true mean level of the variable of interest is 150 units, and that this increases by 10 units at each follow-up visit.

Furthermore, suppose that in group B the true mean level is 10 units higher than in group A at each follow-up visit, and that the correlation structure of the

Figure 1. Response profiles for 20 participants from Dataset I.

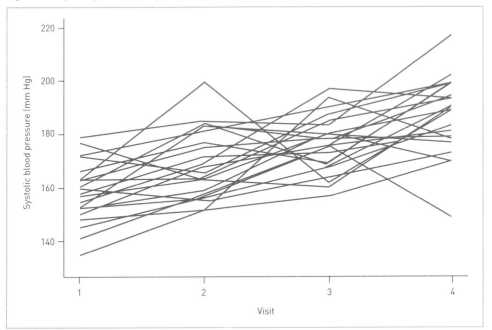

repeated measures is exchangeable with between- and within-subject standard deviations both equal to 10 units. Formally, this model can be written:

$$R_{ij} = 150 + 10V_{2j} + 20V_{3j} + 30V_{4j} + 10T_i + u_i + \varepsilon_{ij}$$

$$\text{with } u_i \sim N(0,100) \text{ and } \varepsilon_{ij} \sim N(0,100)$$

where:

- R_{ij} = the response for the ith participant at the jth visit
- V_{kj} = 1 if $j = k$ and 0 otherwise
- T_i = 1 if the ith participant is in group B and 0 if the ith participant is in group A

Using this equation, we simulated 4,000 participants to give a dataset (Dataset I). **Figure 1** shows the response profile of 20 randomly selected participants. **Figure 2** presents the mean responses over visit by treatment, reflecting the patterns described in the equation.

Figure 2. Mean response over visit (full dataset: Dataset I).

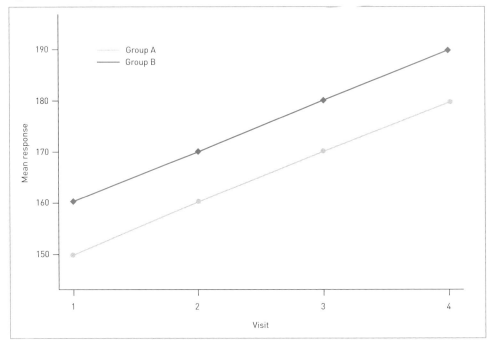

Datasets with missing values

We derived a second dataset (Dataset II) from observations that were MCAR by giving each participant a 20% chance of dropping out of the study before the second visit (irrespective of response and treatment group). Participants attending for the second visit were given a 20% chance of dropping out before the third visit, and participants attending for the third visit were given a 20% chance of dropping out before the final visit.

Dataset III is an MAR scenario. All participants with an observed value >150 units at the first visit were continued to the second visit, whilst all participants with an observed value <150 units at the first visit were given a 60% chance of dropping out by the second visit. Missing values were generated in a similar way at the third and fourth visits: the cut-offs for determining participants at risk of dropping out were 160 and 170 units at the preceding visit, respectively. These data are MAR because the probability of a missing observation is totally driven by the observed data.

In contrast, Dataset IV is an MNAR scenario. All participants who would have had an observed value <160 units at the second visit were deemed to be missing at that and all subsequent visits. Similarly, all participants who would have had an

Table 1. Four simulated datasets with different types of missing data.

	Visit 1 Group		Visit 2 Group		Visit 3 Group		Visit 4 Group	
	A	B	A	B	A	B	A	B
Dataset I: no missing data								
N	2000	2000	2000	2000	2000	2000	2000	2000
Missing	0	0	0	0	0	0	0	0
Mean	149.6	160.2	159.8	170.1	169.8	180.0	179.5	190.0
SD	14.2	14.4	14.2	14.2	14.0	14.1	14.3	14.1
Dataset II: missing completely at random (MCAR)								
N	2000	2000	1624	1559	1320	1242	1037	971
Missing	0	0	376	441	680	758	963	1029
Mean	149.6	160.2	159.9	170.3	169.8	180.2	179.7	190.4
SD	14.2	14.4	14.2	14.3	13.9	14.2	14.0	13.9
Dataset III: missing at random (MAR)								
N	2000	2000	1385	1701	1025	1494	795	1395
Missing	0	0	615	299	975	506	1205	605
Mean	149.6	160.1	162.2	171.7	174.3	182.9	186.1	193.5
SD	14.2	14.4	14.0	13.7	13.3	13.3	13.8	13.2
Dataset IV: missing not at random (MNAR)								
N	2000	2000	992	1520	662	1262	473	1110
Missing	0	0	1008	480	1338	738	1527	890
Mean	149.6	160.1	171.3	175.9	182.1	186.8	193.8	197.5
SD	14.2	14.4	18.5	10.4	9.0	10.5	9.6	10.4

observed value <170 units at the third visit were deemed to be missing at that and the final visit, and participants who would have had an observed value <180 units at the final visit were deemed to be missing at that visit.

Table 1 presents the observed mean (standard deviation) response at each visit and for each group, as well as the numbers of missing and non-missing observations for each of the datasets. **Figure 3** plots the proportion of missing data at each visit. Different patterns can be observed for the different scenarios. For the MCAR scenario in Dataset II, the proportion of the data that is missing at each visit is similar in the two groups. However, in Datasets III and IV, where the chance of data being missing is related to the value of the responses (observed responses in III, unobserved in IV) and where responses differ between the two groups, clear differences are seen in the proportions that are missing in the two

Figure 3. Proportion of missing information by visit for different missing data scenarios.

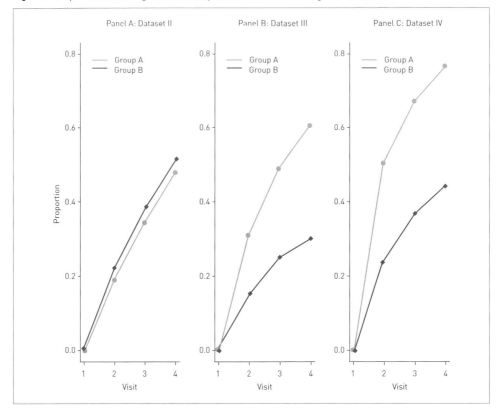

groups. These patterns of missing data can help us to understand the underlying mechanisms of missing data in the analysis of real clinical trials

Statistical analysis
Each of the four datasets was analyzed using three different methods:

- analysis of all available data
- analysis of complete cases only
- LOCF

The model used in all the analyses was the same as that used in the generation of the full dataset, with the addition of interaction terms between visit and treatment group so as to investigate potential interaction effects between visit and treatment caused by different missing schemes. **Figure 4** presents the fitted mean responses by treatment group and visit, whilst **Table 2** presents the estimated treatment effects (standard errors) at the final visit.

Figure 4. Fitted visit-specific mean responses for four missing data scenarios and three analysis strategies.

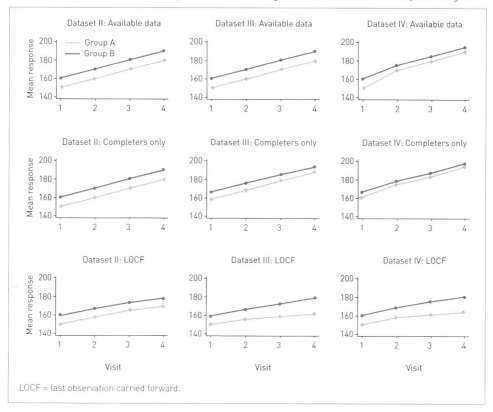

LOCF = last observation carried forward.

There are a number of observations from these results. Firstly, for MCAR (Dataset II), the estimated treatment effects at the final visit are close to the true value for all three approaches, as expected. The standard error for the analysis of all available data is smaller than that from the analysis of complete cases only, reflecting the fact that the complete case analysis discards informative data. Despite the LOCF analysis leading to an underestimation of the mean levels in each group at all visits other than the first, the LOCF analysis does give an unbiased estimate of the treatment effect in this case.

Turning to Dataset III (MAR), **Figure 4** shows that only the analysis of all available data gives rise to fitted response curves that are similar to those for the full dataset (**Figure 2**). **Table 2** confirms that this is the only method that results in an unbiased estimate of the treatment effect at the final visit. It is important to emphasize that such unbiased estimates at a particular visit are only obtained when the linear mixed model is used to simultaneously model the outcomes at each follow-up visit.

Table 2. Comparison of estimates of treatment effect for different missing data scenarios with three different analysis strategies.[a]

Missing schemes	Datasets	Strategy for dealing with missing data		
		All available data	Completers only	LOCF
No missing data	I	10.4 (0.45)	10.4 (0.45)	10.4 (0.45)
MCAR	II	10.4 (0.58)	10.7 (0.63)	8.9 (0.51)
MAR	III	10.0 (0.58)	7.4 (0.56)	17.3 (0.60)
MNAR	IV	5.6 (0.61)	3.6 (0.59)	18.3 (0.59)

[a]The treatment effect is defined as the difference in mean response between groups A and B at the fourth visit as estimated from the mixed model analysis. The figures in brackets stand for the standard error of the treatment effect. LOCF = last observation carried forward; MAR = missing at random; MCAR = missing completely at random; MNAR = missing not at random.

Analysis of all available data at the final visit in isolation would not yield unbiased estimates. Analysis of completers only, whether through the repeated measurements model or through simple comparison of means at the final visit (**Table 1**), underestimates the treatment effect. The reason for this is that participants with 'low' levels tend to be lost to follow-up, and there are more such losses in group A. In contrast, LOCF overestimates the treatment effect because LOCF takes no account of the general increase in levels with time, with this effect having greater impact in group A, where there are more losses to follow-up, than in group B.

Not surprisingly, when there is a large amount of MNAR data (Dataset IV), none of the methods provides a reliable estimate of the treatment effect.

Conclusion

When some values are missing in a randomized clinical trial there are implications for both efficiency and bias. The extent of the bias in the analysis depends very much on the cause of missing data in the trial in question. In the absence of specific knowledge about the reasons why data are missing, a graphical exploration of the pattern of missing data is likely to give the analyst some hints.

There is a large amount of statistical literature on the analysis of studies with missing data. There is a growing consensus that *ad hoc* imputation methods such as LOCF should be avoided. When data can reasonably be assumed to be MCAR or MAR, unbiased methods of analysis do exist. In the latter case, it is usually necessary to carry out an appropriate analysis of all the available data at all follow-up visits in order to estimate unbiased treatment effects at a particular single visit. Multiple imputation provides an alternative approach when data can be assumed to be MAR. The situation is more complex when dealing with data that are MNAR. The best that can be done in such situations is to investigate the robustness of the results obtained using an MAR-based analysis with a sensitivity analysis.

References

1. Murray GD. Missing data in clinical trials. In: *Encyclopedia of Biostatistics*. Armitage P, Colton T, editors. New York: John Wiley & Sons, 2000:2637–41.
2. Bailey I, Bell A, Gray J, et al. A trial of the effect of nimodipine on outcome after head injury. *Acta Neurochir* 1991;**110**:97–105.
3. Marcoulides GA, Moustaki I. *Latent Variable and Latent Structure Models*. Mahwah, NJ: Lawrence Erlbaum Associates, 2002.
4. Liu Z, Almhana J, Choulakian V, et al. Recursive EM algorithm for finite mixture models with application to internet traffic modeling. *Second Annual Conference on Communication Networks and Services Research*, 2004, May 19–21. Fredericton, Canada: IEEE/Computer Society Press: 198–207.
5. Rubin DB. Inference and missing data. *Biometrika* 1976;**63**:581–92.
6. Barnard J, Meng XL. Applications of multiple imputation in medical studies: from AIDS to NHANES. *Stat Methods Med Res* 1999;**8**:17–36.
7. Molenberghs G, Thijs H, Jansen I, et al. Analyzing incomplete longitudinal clinical trial data. *Biostatistics* 2004;**5**:445–64.
8. Rubin DB. *Multiple Imputation for Nonresponse in Surveys*. New York: Wiley-Interscience, 2004.
9. Little RJ, Rubin DB. *Statistical Analysis with Missing Data*, 2nd edition. New York: Wiley-Interscience, 2002.
10. Frison L, Pocock SJ. Repeated measures in clinical trials: analysis using mean summary statistics and its implications for design. *Stat Med* 1992;**11**:1685–704.
11. Ting N. Carry-Forward Analysis. In *Encyclopedia of Biopharmaceutical Statistics*. Chow SC, editor. New York: Marcel Dekker, 2000:103–9.
12. Rubin DB. Multiple imputation after 18+ years. *J Am Stat Assoc* 1996;**91**:473–89.
13. Hox JJ. A review of current software for handling missing data. *Kwantitatieve Methoden* 1999;**62**:123–38.
14. Horton NJ, Lipsitz SR. Multiple imputation in practice: comparison of software packages for regression models with missing variable. *Am Stat* 2001;**55**:244–54.
15. Van Buuren S, Oudshoorn CGM. Multivariate imputation by chained equations. MICE V1.0 User's manual, 2000.
16. SAS\STAT Software: Changes and Enhancement, Release 8.1. SAS Institute, Inc.
17. SOLAS™ for missing data analysis and imputation. Statistical Solutions.
18. Schafer JL. *Analysis of Incomplete Multivariate Data*. London: Chapman & Hall, 1997.

Chapter 31

Interim Monitoring and Stopping Rules

James F Lymp, Stephen L Kopecky,

Ameet Bakhai, and Duolao Wang

Interim monitoring has, for a variety of reasons, become increasingly important and common in clinical trials. Ethical considerations require that patient safety be monitored and that decisions regarding treatment benefit, or lack thereof, be made as quickly as possible. However, care must be taken not to jump to early conclusions based on limited evidence. As a consequence, many statistical methods have been developed for the design of clinical trials, and these methods account for the interim monitoring process. In this chapter, we discuss the motivations for interim monitoring, show how inappropriate statistical methods can lead to erroneous conclusions, and present an outline of some statistical methods that can be used for appropriate interim monitoring in clinical trials.

What is interim monitoring?

The interim monitoring of clinical trials has become increasingly important and common for a variety of reasons. The reasons for monitoring might be ethical, scientific, economic, or a combination of these.

Interim monitoring is the process of collecting and reviewing trial information over the course of a clinical trial. This information includes patient safety data, treatment efficacy data, logistics (such as patient accrual rates), and quality-assurance information (such as the number of data-entry errors).

What are the main reasons for interim monitoring?

Potentially, the two main products of interim monitoring in clinical trials are a decision to stop the trial early or a decision to change the study protocol. The primary ethical reason for interim monitoring is to ensure patient safety. Monitoring can help to:

- ensure that adverse event frequency and toxicity levels are acceptable
- ensure that patients are not recruited into a trial that is going to be unable to reach a definitive result
- ensure that randomization of patients is stopped as soon as there is sufficiently clear evidence either for or against the treatment being evaluated
- address unexpected problems with the study protocol such as exclusion criteria delaying recruitment

The scientific reasons for interim monitoring are to improve the integrity of the trial and, in situations where intervention has a stronger effect than expected (either positively or negatively), reach conclusions early in the study.

Interim monitoring is also beneficial economically because it can help trials to be more efficient and prevent the use of resources on trials that either already have reached, or are unlikely to reach, an answer.

Which trials should have interim monitoring?

In the US, according to federal regulations (21 CFR 312.32 (c) [1]), all clinical trials need to be monitored for safety. However, there is no fixed rule for determining which trials should be monitored for efficacy endpoints or quality-assurance purposes. It depends on the degree of severity of the condition being treated, the toxicity level of the investigational intervention, and the duration of the enrollment and follow-up periods. If the enrollment and follow-up periods are too short, then interim monitoring for efficacy endpoints will not be useful because the study will be completed before any decisions are made on the basis of this monitoring.

For every trial, the amount of interim monitoring should be determined as a result of discussions between the investigators, the sponsors, and the regulatory bodies. Monitoring may occur at regular time periods during the recruitment and follow-up stages, or during enrollment on reaching certain proportions of target recruitment (eg, 25% of target, 50% of target). These discussions should also focus on whether an independent data and safety monitoring board (DSMB) needs to be formed. The US Food and Drug Administration is currently drafting DSMB guidelines, and these have been discussed previously.

What procedures are used for interim monitoring?

The first step is to determine the level of monitoring – that is, in addition to monitoring for safety, deciding whether to monitor for efficacy, futility, or secondary endpoints. The second step is to decide whether the monitoring will be done by the trial investigators or by an independent DSMB. The monitoring group then decides how frequently to meet and what data should be collected for discussion.

The DSMB can be treatment-blinded or be made aware of treatment allocation, but always has to maintain complete confidentiality. Usually, only the statistician working with the DSMB has access to the treatment codes.

As an example, consider a pivotal trial that is designed to compare a new drug therapy with placebo and that has an accrual period of 3 years, a follow-up period of 5 years, and survival as the primary endpoint. Due to the length and pivotal nature of the trial, an independent DSMB would be involved. The DSMB might decide to monitor laboratory measurements and adverse event reports to gauge safety, and monitor survival rates in order to gauge efficacy and futility. The DSMB might then decide to meet every 6 months from the start of accrual to monitor for safety, and once every year to monitor for efficacy and futility.

Figure 1. The effect of repeated statistical tests (on the same data) on the Type I error rate. The results are based on 200,000 simulations of two groups of binomial data with a 50% chance of success in both groups and a final sample size of 100 per group. Equally spaced chi-squared tests were used. The graph shows that the greater the number of interim analyses carried out, the greater the chance of Type I errors.

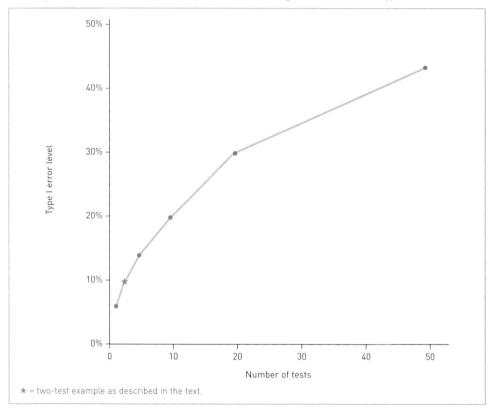

★ = two-test example as described in the text.

What statistical methods can be used for interim monitoring?

One issue that arises when monitoring a trial is choosing statistical analysis methods for assessing the safety, efficacy, and futility endpoints. The primary problem occurs when carrying out multiple hypothesis tests during the course of a clinical trial. In the usual hypothesis-testing situation, the Type I error (or false-positive) – the rejection of the null hypothesis when it is actually true – is controlled at some level of significance, typically 5%. The overall Type I error level increases with the number of tests, as shown in **Figure 1**. For example, if the 5% level is used on two tests – one at the midpoint of the trial and one at the end of the trial – the overall Type I error level is actually 9%. This means that in 9% of trials with no treatment effect, the null hypothesis that there is no effect would be falsely rejected.

Figure 2. Variation of the test statistic with respect to time in a simulated clinical trial with no treatment effect. The standardized normal test statistic is computed and plotted after each pair of patients in the trial. Horizontal dashed lines are drawn at zero and at ±1.96, the two-sided 5% boundary for the test statistic.

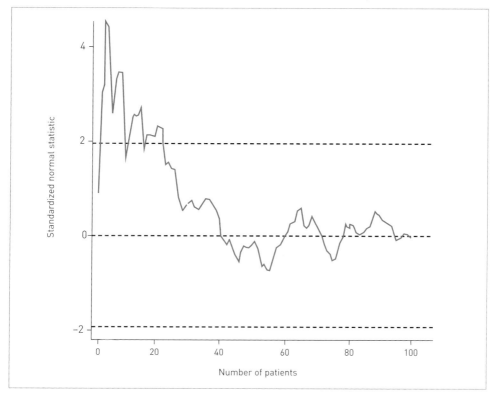

Figure 2 shows a plot of the test statistic over the course of a simulated study in which there is no treatment effect. The test statistic could be many things, eg, the standardized difference in means, the log odds ratio, or the log hazard ratio. Note that, in this simulation, the test statistic is above the two-sided 5% boundary early in the trial. This trial might have been stopped prematurely if hypothesis testing were done after each pair of patients.

The examples in **Figures 1** and **2** highlight the need to exercise caution when repeating statistical tests during the course of a clinical trial. Interim monitoring therefore involves the problem of multiplicity risking a Type 1 error occurring (see **Chapter 29**). There are many possible solutions to this problem. The most commonly used solutions, and those that we focus on here, are group sequential methods. A thorough review can be found in *Group Sequential Methods with Applications to Clinical Trials* by Jennison and Turnbull [2]. Other less common methods are based on Bayesian statistics, decision theory, or conditional power analysis.

Figure 3. Standardized normal statistic two-sided 5% boundaries for two different group sequential methods in a trial with five tests. The graph shows that the Pocock method more easily results in the early termination of trials, while the O'Brien–Fleming method results in easier rejection of the null hypothesis at the end of the trial.

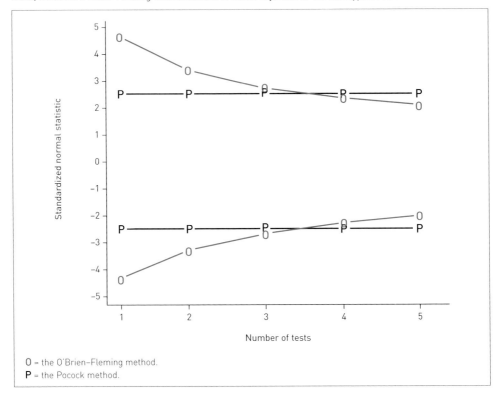

O = the O'Brien–Fleming method.
P = the Pocock method.

The most common group sequential methods currently in use are attributed to Pocock [3], O'Brien and Fleming [4], and Lan and DeMets [5]. For ease of presentation, we will describe these methods for situations in which the test statistic has a standard normal distribution. However, the methods are generalizable to other settings.

Recall from **Chapter 17**, that for a significance threshold of $P \leq 0.05$ the test statistic value is 1.96. The Pocock method adjusts this critical value from the usual value of 1.96 to some higher number that depends on the number of tests being performed. The number is chosen so that the overall Type I error remains 5% despite mutiple tests.

The Pocock method, although controlling the overall Type I error, creates a situation in which the power to detect the true treatment difference at the end of a trial is reduced, and this reduction is greater with higher numbers of interim

Figure 4. Sample *P*-values for two different group sequential methods in a trial with five tests. The graph shows that the Pocock method makes it easier to stop a trial early and the O'Brien–Fleming method makes it easier to reject the null hypothesis at the end.

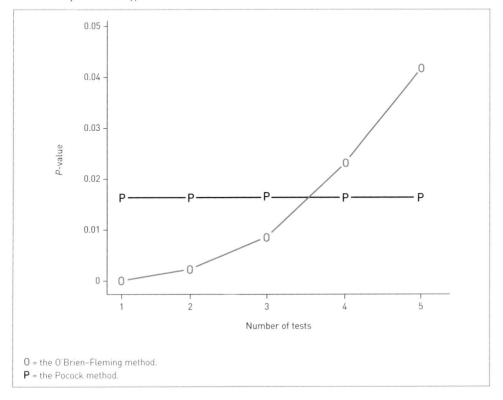

0 = the O'Brien–Fleming method.
P = the Pocock method.

tests. The O'Brien–Fleming method uses a conservative early approach that addresses the issue of power at the end of the trial. In other words, some of the Type I error is removed from the earlier tests and moved to the later tests. The O'Brien–Fleming method also makes it more difficult to reject the null hypothesis of no treatment effect early in the trial. **Figures 3** and **4** illustrate these two group sequential methods in a trial with four interim analyses plus a final analysis.

The Lan–DeMets method generalizes the Pocock and the O'Brien–Fleming methods in two important ways. The Pocock and O'Brien–Fleming methods rely on equally spaced intervals, in terms of number of patients, between tests. The Lan–DeMets method, also referred to as an alpha spending approach, allows for unequally spaced intervals. As a consequence, the Lan–DeMets method allows for differences between the planned and actual sample sizes during the course of the study, and even unplanned analyses as well. While the Pocock method spreads the Type I error equally throughout the study, the O'Brien–Fleming method places almost all of the Type I error on the final analysis. The Lan–DeMets method is flexible enough to incorporate either of these approaches and also allow for compromise between the two, depending on recruitment rates.

It is possible to use group sequential methods not only for treatment-difference trials but also for equivalence trials, one-sided tests, and asymmetric boundaries. An example of an asymmetric boundary might be to use an O'Brien–Fleming method to monitor the benefit of the new intervention and a Pocock method for monitoring detrimental effects of the new intervention. Different methods could be used in the same trial to monitor different endpoints. For example, an O'Brien–Fleming method might be used to monitor efficacy at the same time as using the Pocock method to monitor safety.

What situations can drive early trial termination?

There are four main outcomes from interim monitoring:

- trial continues as planned
- trial continues with protocol amendments (more patients or centers, or requests about details of adverse events for closer scrutiny or amendment to inclusion/exclusion criteria due to unexpected observations)
- trial is halted temporarily for further safety data or for protocol amendment and further training in the new protocol
- trial is stopped prematurely and permanently due to early divergence of treatment effects (either in favor of or against the new treatment)

Interim monitoring allows the DSMB to evaluate whether a divergence of event rates between groups is occurring. This divergence usually has to be present for two consecutive interim analyses. It will then result in early trial termination to avoid further disadvantage to patients in the higher event rate group. If the DSMB is blinded then the higher event rate may or may not be in favor of the new treatment. If the DSMB is unblinded then they will know if the new treatment has greater benefit or not. For example, the BHAT (Beta-blocker Heart Attack Trial) was terminated 9 months early, mainly because the observed treatment benefit with beta blockers was judged significant and likely to remain so during the 9 months remaining in the trial [6].

Similarly, if a new treatment is unlikely to be superior, ie, there is no curve divergence some way through the trial, the trial may be stopped under futility rules since it is unlikely to have future benefit if the drug effect is supposed to be demonstrated in the first few months. CARET (Beta-Carotene and Retinol

Efficacy Trial) was such an example [7], where at the second interim analysis the cumulative incidence of lung cancer was higher in the active treatment arm than in the placebo group. This led to the DSMB and steering committee recognizing the extremely limited prospect of a favorable overall effect.

In addition, if serious adverse event rates are unacceptably higher in the new treatment group than in the control group, the trial may be terminated or suspended until protocol modifications can be instituted. A trial by the Medical Research Council Lung Cancer Working Party (MRC LU16) was stopped because the interim analysis showed that although the palliative effects of treatment were similar in the treatment groups, there was increased hematological toxicity and significantly worse survival in the study treatment (oral etoposide) group [8].

Furthermore, the DSMB can also recommend extending (longer follow-up) or expanding (increasing numbers of patients recruited) the trial if the projections suggest a more definitive result will only arise with this amendment. This may occur if the assumed event rates in the control group are not met; either due to recruitment of a low risk group, or because medical advances in such a patient group have improved morbidity beyond the expectations of such patients when the power calculations for the trial were originally performed, or if dropouts are higher than expected. Finally, if similar large trials report conclusively then it might be unnecessary and unethical to continue the current trial. The DSMB is, therefore, very critical to the success of a trial.

Conclusion

Interim monitoring is a critical part of clinical trials research. The benefits of interim monitoring and appropriate statistical analysis methods are to increase the ethical, scientific, and economic value of clinical trials for patients, investigators, and sponsors alike. For this reason it is of key importance that members of the DSMB be chosen wisely and have sufficient expertise, knowledge, and independence to be able to make tough decisions about trial progress. Further information on data monitoring and interim analysis can be found in references [9] and [10].

References

1. Title 21, Code of Federal Regulations, Part 312.32 (c).
2. Jennison C, Turnbull BW. *Group Sequential Methods with Applications to Clinical Trials.* London: Chapman and Hall, 1999.

3. Pocock SJ. Group sequential methods in the design and analysis of clinical trials. *Biometrika* 1977;**64**:191–9.

4. O'Brien PC, Fleming TR. A multiple testing procedure for clinical trials. *Biometrics* 1979;**35**:549–56.

5. Lan KKG, DeMets DL. Discrete sequential boundaries for clinical trials. *Biometrika* 1983;**70**:659–63.

6. DeMets DL, Hardy R, Friedman LM, et al. Statistical aspects of early termination in the beta-blocker heart attack trial. *Control Clin Trials* 1984;**5**:362–72.

7. Omenn GS, Goodman GE, Thornquist MD, et al. Effects of a combination of beta carotene and vitamin A on lung cancer and cardiovascular disease. *N Engl J Med* 1996;**334**:1150–5.

8. Girling DJ. Comparison of oral etoposide and standard intravenous multidrug chemotherapy for small-cell lung cancer: a stopped multicentre randomised trial. Medical Research Council Lung Cancer Working Party. *Lancet* 1996;**348**:563–6.

9. Grant AM, Altman DG, Babiker AB, et al; DAMOCLES study group. Issues in data monitoring and interim analysis of trials. *Health Technol Assess* 2005;**9**:1–238.

10. DeMets DL, Furberg CD, Friedman L. *Data Monitoring in Clinical Trials: A Case Studies Approach.* New York: Springer Verlag, 2005.

Part V

Reporting of Trials

Chapter 32

Overview of Reporting

Dorothea Nitsch, Felicity Clemens,
Duolao Wang, and Ameet Bakhai

In order to interpret the findings of a clinical trial, the reader
has to understand the rationale for and the conduct of a clinical
trial, and whether and how the findings relate to further clinical
practice. The phrase 'clinical trial' encompasses a whole
range of defined processes that are not necessarily familiar
to a reader of a clinical trials report. Therefore, a report of
a clinical trial should include information about exactly how
the trial was conducted and how this might affect the results.
The CONSORT (Consolidated Standards of Reporting Trials)
statement is the standard guide for clinical trials reports
in medical publications. In this chapter, we explain the
key features of the CONSORT statement.

Different types of reports

A well-written clinical trial report is the sound basis of passing on research findings. The most cited forms of research reports in academic life are those in medical journals and conference presentations. However, equally important in the medical field are regulatory submissions for new therapies or press releases for the lay public. As with any written description of past work, the focus and style of a report should be tailored to the audience in such a way that its results are correctly understood. Perhaps the most difficult form of reporting is a press release, which targets the general lay audience. While aiming to be simple it should not promote over-interpretation of the findings, which the media commonly encourages for news value.

Structure and quality of a clinical report

The purpose of any report of a clinical trial is to clearly convey a very few key points or 'headline findings' based on the main aims of the study; these should be borne in mind throughout the write-up as the main thrust of the report should focus on these key points. Before starting to write a report the author should think about the reasons for writing that particular report and its audience/readership.

At the stage of writing a clinical research report, the aim of the study and the research hypothesis have usually been sufficiently clarified. The style of the report must be tailored to the audience for which it is intended while still ensuring that the 'headline findings' of the trial are conveyed in a clear and accurate way. For example, is it a press release aimed at enhancing public knowledge of the results? Is it a regulatory submission aiming to get a new treatment licensed? In the latter case there are usually clear guidelines about the requirements and format of the reporting laid out by the regulatory authorities, which can be accessed via their websites. Reports for interim analyses with the data and safety monitoring board should also meet regulatory standards.

In this chapter, we focus on writing a clinical trial report for a medical journal. The audience of a report depends on the journal that is chosen for publication. Hence, the language should be adapted in such a way that the journal's readership should be able to grasp the methodology of the study and its results.

The commonly accepted format of a trial report is an introduction and literature review, followed by methods, results, discussion, and a conclusions section. An abstract should precede the introduction and a comprehensive list of references should follow the conclusions. Acknowledgment of all trial personnel and investigation at each center may either be at the end of the paper or available on the journal or trial website.

The format follows the key questions:

- Why did you perform the trial? (Introduction)
- How did you conduct the trial? (Methods)
- What did you find? (Results)
- What does it mean? (Discussion)

In its *introduction* a trial report should give sufficient background knowledge for the reader to understand the study aim and the hypothesis of interest; it might include an overview of relevant literature and how the proposed study will improve the situation.

The *methods* section of a trial report should contain sufficient information on the study design, data collection, and statistical analysis to allow critical interpretation of the results. An important criterion of a good quality report is that its methods should be laid out in such a way that the intended reader is able to critically appraise the value of the results.

The *results* section should contain baseline tables to describe the features of the study population at entry to the study, further information on completeness of follow-up, and results with respect to treatment efficacy and side-effects. The *discussion* should aim to put the findings into the context of current research, and highlight potential questions for further research. Any intended reader with sufficient background knowledge should be able to infer the conclusions on the basis of the results presented.

In other words, the methods and results should be presented in such a way that a reader is enabled to critically draw conclusions; for nonspecialist readers there is a danger of accepting the results of studies without sufficient criticism on the potential limitations of the study findings. For this reason, in the setting of clinical trials, the CONSORT (Consolidated Standards of Reporting Trials) statement has been elaborated, and has been adopted by many leading clinical journals as a common standard for reporting.

The *abstract* and the *conclusions* section of a trial report can be seen as the interface between two groups of people: the trialist, with his/her specialist knowledge of the clinical area and the mechanics, processes, and results of the trial itself; and the audience, which might comprise specialist medical readers or the general lay public. As such, these sections must carefully guard against misinterpretation of the results whilst being tailored to the needs of the target audience – a task that requires great care.

Interpreting a trial report

There are two distinct forms of validity of a study: *internal* and *external* validity. Internal validity is defined as the ability of a trial to study the hypothesis of interest. External validity is the generalizability of the study findings, ie, the extent to which the results can be applied to clinical practice.

Internal validity

Internal validity is concerned with study design and conduct. The study design is chosen in such a way that biases and errors are minimized. These include systematic errors, confounding, and random errors; in clinical trials, the randomization and selection procedures aim to ensure a lack of confounding and selection bias.

Key factors are a randomization scheme with masking so that neither doctors nor patients are aware of the participants' intended allocation, as well as blinding to the treatment allocation during follow-up. False-negative and false-positive findings due to random error can be avoided by choosing a sufficiently large study population (see **Chapter 9**). Study size and statistical analyses should be chosen with reference to the hypothesis of interest.

External validity

External validity is a function of the selection of the study population, treatment regimens, and outcome measures. The study population should represent the population that is intended to receive the treatment in the population at large, should there be a positive result. Treatment regimens should be practicable and relevant to clinical practice. Outcome measures should reflect measures of clinical interest (ideally these should be hard outcomes, such as mortality or morbidity) or at least routine measurements that apply to clinical practice. Since diagnostic criteria and treatment guidelines change over time, it is essential that the reader understands the context of the study with respect to current and past clinical guidelines, and clinical practice.

Sufficient information

All of the above points should have been clarified during the planning of the trial. Large clinical studies often publish a study design paper early in the process, where the rationale, assumptions, and study design are laid out in detail. However, the interpretation of a trial report relies on the reader's ability to identify potential limitations in the design and conduct of a trial. Therefore, any clinical report incorporating results should still contain sufficient information for the reader to judge key points of internal and external validity. The CONSORT statement provides a checklist to help authors cover all the relevant points (**Table 1**).

CONSORT Statement

The CONSORT statement has been very influential in providing a standard for the quality of a clinical trial report in medical publications. A full explanation can be found on the CONSORT website, which is freely accessible [1]. In this section, we highlight key points of the CONSORT statement.

In order to enable the reader to evaluate the flow of patients through a study, a flow chart (as shown in Figure 1 of **Chapter 33** of this book) is a helpful graphical summary. A checklist provided by CONSORT (**Table 1**) describes several items that should be included when reporting a clinical trial. Items 1–14 and 16–18 relate to the internal validity of the study, while items 2–4, 6 and 15 are particularly important to address the generalizability of the findings; these should be highlighted by the authors themselves, as mentioned in item 21.

Randomization
Randomization is essential to ensure that there is no confounding. Hence, it should be mentioned in the title and abstract of the study (item 1), and further explained in detail in the methods (items 8–10). Different randomization schemes can be used depending on the numbers of patients allocated to a particular treatment in different study centers. Reporting the method of allocation concealment and its implementation helps the reader to identify potential problems in masking and blinding (item 11).

Sample size
A trial needs to include sufficient numbers of patients in order to detect the effect of interest (item 7). The sample size calculations depend on the form of the planned statistical analysis and on making reasonable assumptions about the expected treatment effect, summary statistics of the primary endpoint in the control group, etc (see **Chapter 9**).

Defined outcome
Statistical analyses are tailored to a defined hypothesis of interest (item 5 and 12). If statistical analyses are used for hypotheses other than those originally planned then there is a danger of false-positive chance findings. Therefore, the primary outcome has to be defined in advance (item 6).

Table 1. Checklist of items to include when reporting a randomized trial.

PAPER SECTION and topic	Item	Description
TITLE & ABSTRACT	1	How participants were allocated to interventions (eg, 'random allocation', 'randomized', or 'randomly assigned').
INTRODUCTION		
Background	2	Scientific background and explanation of rationale.
METHODS		
Participants	3	Eligibility criteria for participants and the settings and locations where the data were collected.
Interventions	4	Precise details of the interventions intended for each group and how and when they were actually administered.
Objectives	5	Specific objectives and hypotheses.
Outcomes	6	Clearly defined primary and secondary outcome measures and, when applicable, any methods used to enhance the quality of measurements (eg, multiple observations, training of assessors).
Sample size	7	How sample size was determined and, when applicable, explanation of any interim analyses and stopping rules.
Randomization – sequence generation	8	Method used to generate the random allocation sequence, including details of any restrictions (eg, blocking, stratification).
Randomization – allocation concealment	9	Method used to implement the random allocation sequence (eg, numbered containers or central telephone), clarifying whether the sequence was concealed until interventions were assigned.
Randomization – implementation	10	Who generated the allocation sequence, who enrolled participants, and who assigned participants to their groups.
Blinding (masking)	11	Whether or not participants, those administering the interventions, and those assessing the outcomes were blinded to group assignment. When relevant, how the success of blinding was evaluated.
Statistical methods	12	Statistical methods used to compare groups for primary outcome(s); methods for additional analyses, such as subgroup analyses and adjusted analyses.
RESULTS		
Participant flow	13	Flow of participants through each stage (a diagram is strongly recommended). Specifically, for each group report the numbers of participants randomly assigned, receiving intended treatment, completing the study protocol, and analyzed for the primary outcome. Describe protocol deviations from study as planned, together with reasons.
Recruitment	14	Dates defining the periods of recruitment and follow-up.
Baseline data	15	Baseline demographic and clinical characteristics of each group.
Numbers analyzed	16	Number of participants (denominator) in each group included in each analysis and whether the analysis was by 'intention-to-treat'. State the results in absolute numbers when feasible (eg, 10/20, not 50%).
Outcomes and estimation	17	For each primary and secondary outcome, a summary of results for each group, and the estimated effect size and its precision (eg, 95% confidence interval).
Ancillary analyses	18	Address multiplicity by reporting any other analyses performed, including subgroup analyses and adjusted analyses, indicating those prespecified and those exploratory.

Continued.

Table 1 contd. Checklist of items to include when reporting a randomized trial.

PAPER SECTION and topic	Item	Description
Adverse events	19	All important adverse events or side-effects in each intervention group.
DISCUSSION Interpretation	20	Interpretation of the results, taking into account study hypotheses, sources of potential bias or imprecision, and the dangers associated with multiplicity of analyses and outcomes.
Generalizability	21	Generalizability (external validity) of the trial findings.
Overall evidence	22	General interpretation of the results in the context of current evidence.

Reproduced from the CONSORT Statement (www.consort-statement.org).

Allocated treatment

In order to avoid bias and preserve the purpose of randomization, analyses should be carried out by allocated treatment and not by received treatment (item 16). In pharmaceutical trials, statistical methods are usually predefined in protocols before the onset of the trial. This ensures that analyses are chosen prior to obtaining data, and not on the basis of significant *post-hoc* findings after receiving the data (item 12 and 18).

Coherence and clarity

Results should correspond to the methods section. Comparison of the flow chart and the methods section will inform the reader of the success of the study design with respect to enrollment, allocation, and completion. Baseline data are informative with respect to the success of randomization (item 15), and a table showing adverse reactions might explain reasons for dropout (item 19). Results of analyses should be displayed clearly, as outlined in the methods section (items 16–18).

If a trial report follows the guidelines outlined in the CONSORT statement then a critical reader should arrive at an interpretation of results similar to that of the authors (item 20). External validity is more difficult to judge for a reader who is not familiar with clinical implications and recent research in the field; however, even an informed reader will need information on eligibility criteria and interventions (items 3 and 4), the features of randomized patients (item 13 and 15), and timing of recruitment and follow-up (item 14) to judge the applicability of the results to practice. Authors themselves should discuss generalizability and interpret the results in light of the overall evidence (items 21 and 22).

Problem areas in trial reporting: examples

Randomization

The idea of correct randomization to ensure an unbiased comparison is very old. However, its importance was not acknowledged in early trial reports. According to a review in 1990, a third of published trials provided no clear evidence that groups were randomized [2]. Indeed, there were indications of *post-hoc* assemblies of groups, with some trials using simple randomization schemes, often with too similar sample sizes in both groups than would be expected by chance. Furthermore, in about 40% of published trials from this time the baseline comparisons were inadequately handled [2].

Intention-to-treat analysis

A survey in 1999 showed that only 50% of trial reports mentioned 'intention-to-treat' analysis [3]. This can have serious implications on the interpretation of the results. For example, in a trial comparing medical and surgical treatment for stable angina pectoris, some patients allocated to surgical intervention died before being operated on [4]. If these deaths are not attributed to surgical intervention using an intention-to-treat analysis then surgery will appear to have falsely low mortality.

Publication bias

Until recently, medical literature was dominated by a bias towards reporting very significant positive effects or very large point estimates, but avoiding trials with neutral or negative results. This led to distorted views – an effect known as *publication bias* [5]. The scientific community is changing and now encourages the publication of all trials. This is of particular relevance in meta-analyses, which seek to support external validity against other studies.

Effect sizes

Care should be taken in examining effect sizes. Effect sizes are sometimes reported in such a way that the treatment effect seems massive. For example, a trial of cholestyramine (a lipid-lowering drug) in men with high cholesterol reported a 17% relative reduction in risk for both fatal and nonfatal coronary events, whereas the absolute risk difference was only 1.7%. Because this study incorrectly used only one-sided tests, there remains uncertainty about the real effect of cholestyramine [6].

Changes to regulatory definitions/guidelines

As mentioned earlier, regulatory definitions or guidelines might change during the course of a trial. For example, the RITA (Randomized Intervention Trial of Angina) 3 trial used a different definition of myocardial infarction from that published some years later by the European and US cardiology societies [7].

The RITA 3 trial was set up to investigate the policy of early intervention versus conservative medical management in unstable angina. During the follow-up of the trial, the definition of myocardial infarction changed. Therefore, the investigators carried out two analyses: one using the original trial definition of the endpoint myocardial infarction, and another using the new definition. This approach explained some discrepancies in estimated effects of previous and contemporary trials in the field [7].

Incorrect reporting

We discuss examples related to testing more than one outcome or testing for multiple subgroup effects in more detail in other chapters of this book (see **Chapters 23** and **29**). Particular examples related to incorrect reporting can be found in Pocock et al [8]. The description and discussion of inclusion criteria and trial procedures are particularly important to judge external validity. This field in particular has sparked many discussions and is probably a factor for the relatively low adherence to guidelines found in clinical practice [9]. The tension between treating a single patient who might or might not correspond to the inclusion criteria of a particular published trial is difficult to solve.

Prerandomization run-in

Additionally, prerandomization run-in periods can lead to a distorted picture. Active run-in periods in which patients are excluded if they have adverse outcomes are likely to invalidate the applicability of the trial to the clinical situation. For example, trials examining carvedilol in the setting of heart failure excluded up to 9% of patients in the run-in period because of adverse events (some of which were fatal), with subsequent much lower complication rates postrandomization than in the run-in phase [10,11].

Press releases

The requirements of a press release are different from those of a publication in a medical journal. The key findings and overall structure of the report must be the same – however, the style in which they are conveyed is different. The audience consists of the general public, so press releases should avoid technical jargon or extensive explanation of the processes of the study. The report must also be very careful not to over-emphasize the clinical significance of the findings and to make sure that the study population is explicitly stated. Short sentences should be used, and graphs should be avoided altogether. Percentages may be quoted, but their denominators should also be explicitly given; other measures of effect, such as odds ratios, should be explained in words. Some statement should be made about the power of the study, again avoiding technical jargon. It is useful to give some estimate of the overall prevalence or incidence of the condition of the study, and the possible public health impact of the trial's results, but this should avoid extrapolation from the study population to the population at large. Finally, the title of a press release must always reflect the key findings of the trial.

The danger of over-simplified information cannot be over-estimated. An example highlighting the problem of imprecise global information uptake by health care providers and patients can be found in RALES (Randomized Aldactone Evaluation Study) [12,13]. This study published beneficial findings of spironolactone in heart failure. Spironolactone was used prior to this trial, mainly in dosages of 100–300 mg/day in patients with liver cirrhosis. In contrast to patients with heart failure, patients with liver cirrhosis are unlikely to receive angiotensin-converting enzyme (ACE) inhibitors concomitant with spironolactone, and are therefore at a much lower risk of developing hyperkalemia with large doses of spironolactone.

When the results of RALES became available, large doses of spironolactone were prescribed to heart failure patients in conjunction with ACE inhibitors without adequate monitoring of potassium, despite the fact that the spironolactone dosage in the trial ranged from 25 to 50 mg/day with close potassium monitoring according to the trial protocol. Hospitalizations of patients due to life-threatening hyperkalemias rose massively and, in contrast to the predicted effects of the RALES trial, the rates of readmission for heart failure or death from all causes did not decrease after publication of the trial results.

Conclusion

Clinical trial reports should be concise and understandable. They are usually targeted at a medically trained reader, which implies that the reader may not be an expert on statistical issues that are implicit in trial design and analysis, however the report should clarify the assumptions and methods behind these issues. The CONSORT statement is helpful in outlining the main points of a report that have to be covered in order to ensure a correct and critical interpretation and presentation of the results.

By following such international guidance on publications, reports provide sufficient information in a concise manner, allowing the presented results to be scrutinized fully, and helping clinicians to decide how best to translate the findings into practice.

References

1. Moher D, Schulz KF, Altman DG; for the CONSORT group. The Consort Statement: Revised recommendations for improving the quality of reports of parallel-group randomized trials. Available from: www.consort-statement.org. Accessed April 1, 2005.

2. Altman DG, Dore CJ. Randomisation and baseline comparisons in clinical trials. *Lancet* 1990;**335**:149–53.

3. Hollis S, Campbell F. What is meant by intention to treat analysis? Survey of published randomised controlled trials. *BMJ* 1999;**319**:670–4.

4. European Coronary Surgery Study Group. Coronary-artery bypass surgery in stable angina pectoris: survival at two years. *Lancet* 1979;**1**:889–93.

5. Horton R. Medical editors trial amnesty. *Lancet* 1997;**350**:756.

6. The Lipid Research Clinics Coronary Primary Prevention Trial results. I. Reduction in incidence of coronary heart disease. *JAMA* 1984;**251**:351–64.

7. Fox KA, Poole-Wilson PA, Henderson RA, et al. for the Randomized Intervention Trial of unstable Angina (RITA) investigators. Interventional versus conservative treatment for patients with unstable angina or non-ST-elevation myocardial infarction: the British Heart Foundation RITA 3 randomised trial. *Lancet* 2002;**360**:743–51.

8. Pocock SJ, Hughes MD, Lee RJ. Statistical problems in the reporting of clinical trials. A survey of three medical journals. *N Engl J Med* 1987;**317**:426–32.

9. Rothwell PM. External validity of randomised controlled trials: "to whom do the results of this trial apply?" *Lancet* 2005;**365**:82–93.

10. Australia–New Zealand Heart Failure Research Collaborative Group. Effects of carvedilol, a vasodilator-beta-blocker, in patients with congestive heart failure due to ischemic heart disease. *Circulation* 1995;**92**:212–18.

11. Packer M, Bristow MR, Cohn JN, et al. The effect of carvedilol on morbidity and mortality in patients with chronic heart failure. U.S. Carvedilol Heart Failure Study Group. *N Engl J Med* 1996;**334**:1349–55.

12. Pitt B, Zannad F, Remme WJ, et al. The effect of spironolactone on morbidity and mortality in patients with severe heart failure. Randomized Aldactone Evaluation Study Investigators. *N Engl J Med* 1999;**341**:709–17.

13. Juurlink DN, Mamdani MM, Lee DS, et al. Rates of hyperkalemia after publication of the Randomized Aldactone Evaluation Study. *N Engl J Med* 2004;**351**:543–51.

Chapter 33

Trial Profile

Duolao Wang, Belinda Lees, and Ameet Bakhai

The use of a trial profile or flow chart is now considered to
be essential for the reporting of randomized controlled trials.
It allows the reader to determine the number of participants
randomly allocated, receiving the intended treatment,
completing the study protocol, and analyzed for the primary
outcome. In this chapter, we describe the content of a trial
profile, illustrate its use in the reporting of randomized
controlled trials with different designs, and look at the current
practice of major medical journals on the use of trial profiles.

What is a trial profile?

A trial profile diagrammatically summarizes the flow of participants through each stage of a randomized controlled trial. A flow chart is recommended to display this information clearly. The CONSORT (Consolidated Standards of Reporting Trials) guidelines for reporting parallel-group randomized controlled trials state that researchers should use a trial profile "specifically for each study population and report the numbers of participants randomly assigned, receiving intended treatment, completing the study protocol, and analyzed for the primary outcome." Deviations from the planned study protocol should also be described, and reasons given [1].

What should be included in a trial profile?

Figure 1 shows the template recommended by CONSORT for the reporting of the flow of participants through each stage of a randomized trial. Essentially, a trial profile consists of five components:

1. Enrollment. Ideally, this should include the number of patients screened for inclusion into the trial; this will allow the reader to determine whether the participants are representative of all patients seen with the disease.

2. Randomization. The number of participants fulfilling the inclusion and exclusion criteria, and the number randomly allocated to a treatment arm should be given. This allows the overall size of the trial to be determined and enables the reader to see whether the study uses an intention-to-treat analysis.

3. Treatment allocation. This is the number of participants allocated to each group who actually receive the treatment. The reasons for not receiving treatment after randomization as allocated should be given, such as withdrawal of consent by the subject.

4. Follow-up. This is the number of participants who completed follow-up as allocated by treatment arm. Reasons for not completing follow-up or treatment should be given.

5. Analysis. The number of participants included in the analysis should be given by study group, with reasons for excluding patients.

Since a trial profile gives only a brief summary of the flow of participants, a text description is sometimes also given in a report to provide further information on

Figure 1. The CONSORT flow chart. Template for reporting the flow of participants through each stage of a randomized controlled trial [1].

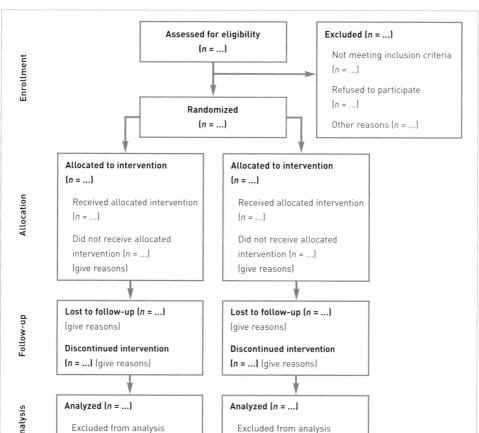

the conduct of the trial. For instance, the date the trial started and stopped, and the duration of follow-up are often described in the text. Also, since the numbers of participants included in the efficacy and safety analyses are often different, the report should give descriptions of the efficacy and safety populations.

What is the purpose of a trial profile?

A trial profile is a clear way of showing whether or not the participants received the treatment as allocated (and if not, why not), and also whether they were lost to follow-up or excluded from the analysis. This is important because patients who

Figure 2. Trial profile for a parallel design study investigating the use of *Mycobacterium vaccae* in the treatment of pulmonary tuberculosis (TB) [2].

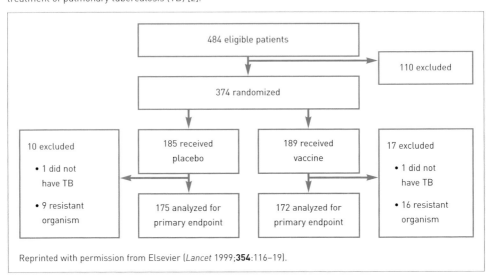

Reprinted with permission from Elsevier (*Lancet* 1999;**354**:116–19).

are excluded after allocation and are not available for follow-up (eg, because of a side-effect of treatment, or worsening of the disease process) might not be typical of the other participants in the study and this can bias the results. The trial profile will allow the reader to determine whether an analysis is intention-to-treat – ie, whether the analysis has been performed on all those patients who were randomized to the group they were originally allocated to (regardless of their subsequent treatment) or only on those who completed the entire study (per protocol analysis).

It might be necessary to adapt the flow chart to suit the needs of a particular trial. For example, there may be a large number of patients who do not receive the allocated treatment as planned, so that the box describing treatment allocation would need to be expanded to describe the reasons for this and the number of patients for each reason (categorized into broad divisions if needed).

Examples of trial profiles

In this section, three trial profiles from published studies with different trial designs will be described: a two-way parallel design, a *2 × 2* factorial design, and a two-way crossover design. Although the CONSORT guidelines on trial profiles were designed for reporting parallel-group randomized controlled trials, the profile can be adapted to describe the flow of participants in factorial and crossover design trials.

Figure 3. Trial profile for a factorial-design study investigating the use of vitamin E and n-3 polyunsaturated fatty acid (PUFA) supplementation in patients suffering a recent myocardial infarction [3].

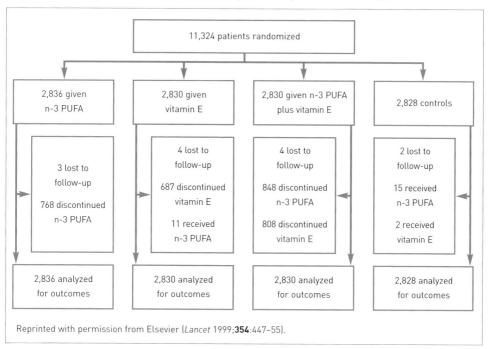

Reprinted with permission from Elsevier (*Lancet* 1999;**354**:447–55).

Two-way parallel design

Figure 2 shows a trial profile from a two-arm parallel design study. The study investigated whether the time to achieve a negative sputum culture among patients with newly diagnosed tuberculosis would be decreased by adding *Mycobacterium vaccae* to standard short-course anti-tuberculosis chemotherapy. Patients were randomized to an injection of either saline (placebo) or *Mycobacterium vaccae* [2]. This is an example of a trial profile in which the information on all five of the components of trial execution is clearly provided. The profile indicates that 175 patients from the placebo group and 172 patients from the vaccine group were used for the primary endpoint analysis. However, safety analysis was based on 185 placebo patients and 189 vaccine patients. The reasons for this discrepancy are described in the report [2].

2 × 2 factorial design

Figure 3 illustrates a *2 × 2* factorial study, which can be reported as a four-arm parallel trial. This study investigated the effects of vitamin E or n-3 polyunsaturated fatty acid (PUFA) supplementation in patients who had suffered a recent myocardial infarction [3]. The primary combined efficacy endpoint was death, non-fatal myocardial infarction, and stroke. From October 1993 to September

Figure 4. Trial profile for a crossover-design study of the use of azithromycin as a treatment for children with cystic fibrosis [4].

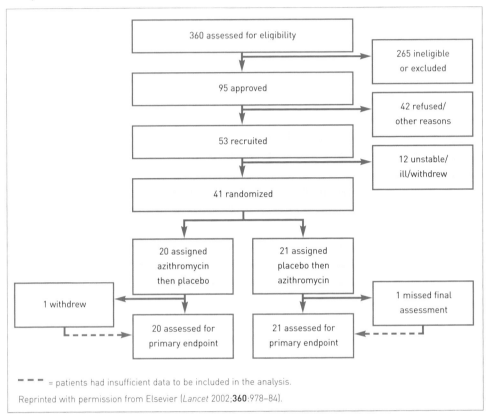

= patients had insufficient data to be included in the analysis.

Reprinted with permission from Elsevier (*Lancet* 2002;**360**:978–84).

1995, 11,324 patients were randomly assigned supplements of *n*-3 PUFA (1 g daily, *n* = 2,836), vitamin E (300 mg daily, *n* = 2,830), both n-3 PUFA and vitamin E (*n* = 2,830), or none (control, *n* = 2,828). The trial profile shows the flow of patients through the various stages of the study in each of the four treatment arms: no further descriptive text is needed [3].

Two-way crossover design

In a crossover trial, participants switch treatments at different time periods or stages of the study. Usually the treatment sequences are treated as parallel groups in a trial profile, rather than the treatment arms. **Figure 4** shows the trial profile of a crossover trial of azithromycin in children with cystic fibrosis [4]. In this study, 41 children with cystic fibrosis participated in a randomized, placebo-controlled crossover trial. Initially, they received either azithromycin or placebo for 6 months. Then, after a 2-month washout period (free of either treatment), they were

Table 1. Results of a survey on the use of trial profiles in clinical trials published in four general medical journals between July and October 1999.

		The Lancet	New England Journal of Medicine	BMJ	JAMA
Number of clinical trials		38	24	18	14
Number of trials with a profile		36 (95%)	3 (13%)	5 (28%)	12 (86%)
Components of trial profile	Enrollment	36	3	5	12
	Randomization	36	3	5	12
	Treatment allocation	36	3	5	12
	Follow-up	35	3	4	12
	Analysis	11	0	0	1
Text description of flow of participants only		2 (5%)	21 (86%)	12 (67%)	2 (14%)
Trial profile and text description of flow of participants		29 (76%)	2 (8%)	4 (22%)	7 (50%)

assigned to the treatment they had not already received (crossed over). The primary outcome was median relative difference in forced expiratory volume in 1 second between azithromycin and placebo treatment periods.

The trial profile indicates that one patient withdrew and one patient missed their final assessment, but it is not clear in which periods these events occurred. Therefore, the authors explained in the text that one patient in the azithromycin/placebo group withdrew after 4 months of the second treatment period, and one patient in the placebo/azithromycin group missed the 6-month assessment in the first treatment period.

Current practice of medical journals on the use of trial profiles

To investigate the practice of medical journals regarding the use of trial profiles when reporting studies, 94 clinical trial reports were identified that were published in four general medical journals during July to October 1999 before the release of the revised CONSORT statement (38 in *The Lancet*, 24 in the *New England Journal of Medicine*, 18 in the *BMJ*, and 14 in *JAMA*).

In **Table 1**, a summary of the number of studies giving trial profiles and the number giving a text description of flow of participants are provided for these published clinical trials. The use of a trial profile was more frequent in *The Lancet* and *JAMA* (95% and 86% respectively) compared with the *New England Journal of Medicine* (13%) and the *BMJ* (28%). However, it is important to note that a simple trial without any follow-up or exclusions might not require the flow of participants to be described by a trial profile; simple text explanations may suffice.

In the survey described above, the percentage of the reports using only a text description to describe the flow of participants was 5% for *The Lancet*, 86% for the *New England Journal of Medicine*, 67% for the *BMJ*, and 14% for *JAMA*, and the percentage using a text description together with a trial profile was 76%, 8%, 22%, and 50%, respectively.

Table 1 also shows whether the five suggested components of trial profiles were included in the trial profiles included in the survey. All of those studies that published a trial profile included information on enrollment, randomization, follow-up, and treatment allocation, but very few gave the analysis population in the trial profile – instead, this was often provided in the text.

Conclusion

The use of a trial profile is helpful for reporting the design and results of a randomized clinical trial. Trial profiles diagrammatically and transparently summarize a great deal of data that can be interpreted rapidly, holding to the axiom that a picture is worth a thousand words. We support the CONSORT guidelines and recommend that the template should be used wherever possible and that, at the very least, the trial profile should include the number of patients randomly assigned, receiving treatment, completing the study protocol, and included in the final analysis for the primary outcome.

References

1. Moher D, Schulz KF, Altman DG; for the CONSORT Group. The CONSORT Statement: Revised recommendations for improving the quality of reports of parallel-group randomized trials. Available from: www.consort-statement.org. Accessed March 23, 2005.

2. Durban Immunotherapy Trial Group. Immunotherapy with *Mycobacterium vaccae* in patients with newly diagnosed pulmonary tuberculosis: a randomized controlled trial. *Lancet* 1999;**354**:116–9.

3. GISSI-Prevenzione Investigators. Dietary supplementation with n-3 polyunsaturated fatty acids and vitamin E after myocardial infarction: results of the GISSI-Prevenzione trial. *Lancet* 1999;**354**:447–55.

4. Equi A, Balfour-Lynn IM, Bush A, et al. Long term azithromycin in children with cystic fibrosis: a randomized, placebo-controlled crossover trial. *Lancet* 2002;**360**:978–84.

Chapter 34

Presenting Baseline Data

Belinda Lees, Duolao Wang, and Ameet Bakhai

The presentation of baseline data is essential for the proper reporting of a randomized clinical trial. Baseline data describe the characteristics of the population participating in the trial. They are usually recorded at randomization and include patients' demographic characteristics, disease-related risk factors, medical histories, and concurrent medical treatments. In this chapter, we discuss some of the uses of baseline data in clinical trials, data that should be included as baseline data in publications, and issues relating to the significance testing of baseline data.

Why should baseline data be described?

Baseline data describe the characteristics of the population participating in the trial. This should allow you to assess the generalizability of the trial by comparing the characteristics of the trial's patient population with the overall patient population with that disease, thus confirming the external validity of the trial.

In large studies where randomization has been performed correctly, the baseline variables should be well balanced between treatment groups, confirming that randomization has been successful. If the treatment groups are imbalanced with respect to their baseline variables then the results obtained might be biased – particularly when such variables might affect the outcome (eg, disease severity).

Reporting baseline data also allows for the identification of imbalances between treatment groups that might subsequently become confounders. Such potential confounders can create an apparent difference in outcome between groups where none really exists, or they can even mask an effect that truly exists.

If the investigator is aware in advance of which baseline characteristics might act as potential confounders then, when designing the study, procedures such as stratification or minimization can be incorporated into the randomization algorithm to balance these characteristics. This will help to ensure that any important variables that might affect the outcome are balanced across groups. For example, in a trial of a treatment for lung disease in cystic fibrosis it might be important to ensure that the groups are balanced for baseline lung function measurements. This is particularly important in smaller studies, where there is an increased risk of imbalance in baseline variables due to chance.

What should be included in baseline data?

It is essential to provide baseline data when you report randomized controlled trials. Most major medical journals now require you to follow the CONSORT (Consolidated Standards of Reporting Trials) guidelines [1], which are a set of recommendations aimed at improving reporting through the use of a checklist and a flow chart. The checklist pertains to the content of the title, abstract, introduction, methods, results, and discussion. Item 15 of the CONSORT guidelines states that baseline demographics and clinical characteristics should be described for each group.

Baseline data should always be measured prior to randomization, as close to the time of randomization as possible. This is particularly important when the variable being measured (eg, disease severity) could affect the outcome of the study.

Table 1. Typical baseline data for a randomized trial comparing the effects of percutaneous coronary intervention (PCI) with coronary artery bypass graft (CABG) surgery in the management of multivessel coronary disease [2].

	PCI (*n* = 488)	CABG (*n* = 500)
Demographic characteristics		
Men	390 (80%)	392 (78%)
Mean age ± standard deviation (years)	61 ± 9.2	62 ± 9.5
Disease risk factors		
Smoking status		
Current smoker	77 (16%)	72 (14%)
Ex-smoker	259 (53%)	286 (57%)
Canadian Cardiovascular Society classification		
Class IV	94 (19%)	108 (22%)
Class III	116 (24%)	133 (27%
Mean left-ventricular ejection fraction	57%	57%
Medical history		
Previous myocardial infarction	214 (44%)	234 (47%)
Previous cerebrovascular accident	5 (1%)	14 (3%)
Previous transient ischemic attack	7 (1%)	11 (2%)
Previous peripheral vascular disease	31 (6%)	35 (7%)
Family history of cardiovascular disease	235/487 (48%)	240/499 (48%)
Type 1 diabetes	19 (4%)	9 (2%)
Type 2 non-insulin-dependent diabetes	49 (10%)	65 (13%)
Hypertension	212 (43%)	235 (47%)
Hyperlipidemia	258 (53%)	251 (50%)
Disease status		
Number of segments with significant stenosis	3.2	3.2
Number of vessels		
Two-vessel disease	303 (62%)	262 (52%)
Three-vessel disease	183 (38%)	236 (47%)
Diseased vessel territory		
Left main stem	4 (1%)	3 (1%)
Left anterior descending (proximal)	235 (48%)	222 (44%)
Left anterior descending (other)	214 (44%)	241 (48%)
Circumflex	342 (70%)	374 (75%)
Right coronary artery	361 (74%)	395 (79%)
One occluded vessel	77 (16%)	70 (14%)
Two occluded vessels	4 (1%)	12 (2%)

Reprinted with permission from Elsevier (*The Lancet* 2002;**360**:965–70).

Table 1 shows typical baseline data for a randomized controlled trial comparing the effects of percutaneous coronary intervention (PCI) with coronary artery bypass graft (CABG) surgery in the management of multivessel coronary disease [2]. The primary endpoint for this study was the rate of repeat revascularization after each treatment. The baseline data included demographic variables (eg, age, gender) and factors that were likely to affect outcome (eg, left ventricular ejection fraction, number of diseased vessels, presence of comorbidities such as history of stroke, smoking, and diabetes mellitus). Factors that could modify any benefit of the treatment (eg, current medication) should also be reported.

If a large study includes subgroup analyses then the characteristics of these subgroups should be included. For example, in a surgical study of aortic valve replacement, patients receiving CABG might have a poorer outcome than those not receiving concomitant CABG, since a longer, more complex operation is required. From the baseline data provided, the reader can determine whether the characteristics of the subgroup receiving CABG with valve replacement are similar to those of the patients receiving valve replacement only.

The measurement of the baseline characteristics should also be clear. For example, in a trial on hypercholesterolemia, when reporting baseline lipid measurements it should be specified if the patients are fasting. Similarly, in a trial on hypertension it should be stated whether average blood pressure was assessed by a 24-hour ambulatory blood pressure monitor, or as measured in a clinic.

Continuous variables, such as age or height, should be reported as a mean value and the standard deviation should be given. If the data are not normally distributed (ie, skewed) then the median and range should be reported. Categorical variables, such as gender or ethnic group, should be reported as frequencies and percentages.

It is very important not to include too many variables in the table of baseline data as this makes interpretation of the data confusing for the reader. It is recommended that giving all patient data as well as individual group data should be avoided and also that significance tests are not included in the table.

Should significance tests be carried out?

The use of significance tests when comparing treatment groups for imbalances in baseline characteristics is a controversial issue [3]. Many statisticians argue that if randomization has been performed correctly then it is not necessary to carry out a statistical analysis of differences in baseline measurements between groups [4]. This is because the more variables are tested, the more likely it is that one variable will be found to be significantly imbalanced between treatment groups by chance alone (see **Chapter 29**). In this sense, the comparison of baseline data is a misuse of significance testing since it is not being used to test a useful scientific hypothesis [4,5].

In addition, there might be differences between groups in one or more baseline variables that are not statistically significant, but that are clinically important – particularly if they affect the outcome. Therefore, statistical testing leading to a nonsignificant difference might give false assurance about the differences between groups. The contents of the table of baseline measurements and any relevant differences should be discussed in the results section of a manuscript.

What can be done if imbalances occur?

It is important to perform significance testing if it is suspected that the randomization or blinding procedure is flawed in some way [6]. For baseline characteristics that are predictors of outcome variables, if important imbalances are found then covariate adjustment analysis should be performed to estimate adjusted treatment effects [5,7]. This is often done with multivariate regression methods during analysis, which take into account confounding factors and imbalances in relevant variables at baseline.

There are a number of regression methods available and the choice of method depends on the type of outcome variable. For example, if the outcome variable is continuous, a linear regression model (including analysis of covariance) can be used during the analysis to adjust for any imbalances and potential confounders that occur despite randomization [5]. If the outcome is binary then a logistic regression model should be employed. When the outcome is survival time, a Cox regression model is usually used.

Conclusion

Baseline data are crucial for describing the study population and establishing the external validity of a trial. It is particularly important to include demographic variables and any measurements taken at randomization that might have an impact on the treatment effect. By comparing the distributions of several baseline variables according to treatment group, we can provide a clear picture of the patients included and identify imbalances that have arisen by chance. The occurrence of severe imbalances in a trial might suggest failure of the randomization or blinding procedures. In this case, covariate adjustment analyses must be made to calculate the unbiased treatment effect. This topic is discussed further in **Chapter 25.**

References

1. Moher D, Schulz K, Altman D; for the CONSORT Group. The CONSORT statement: Revised recommendations for improving the quality of reports of parallel-group randomised trials. Available from: www.consort-statement.org. Accessed March 23, 2005.
2. SoS Investigators. Coronary artery bypass surgery versus percutaneous coronary intervention with stent implantation in patients with multivessel coronary artery disease (the Stent or Surgery trial): A randomised controlled trial. *Lancet* 2002;**360**:965–70.
3. Altman DG, Dore CJ. Randomisation and baseline comparisons in clinical trials. *Lancet* 1990;**335**:149–53.
4. Altman DG. Comparability of randomised groups. *Statistician* 1985;**34**:125–36.
5. Senn S. Testing for baseline balance in clinical trials. *Stat Med* 1994;**13**:1715–26.
6. Kennedy A, Grant A. Subversion of allocation in a randomised controlled trial. *Control Clin Trials* 1997;**18**(Suppl. 1):S77–8.
7. Pocock SJ, Assmann SE, Enos LE, et al. Subgroup analysis, covariate adjustment and baseline comparisons in clinical trial reporting: current practice and problems. *Stat Med* 2002;**21**:2917–30.

Chapter 35

Use of Tables

Hilary C Watt, Ameet Bakhai, and Duolao Wang

Clinical trial data are almost invariably displayed in statistical tables. Familiarity with the structure of these tables, therefore, allows a quick and logical appreciation of results. Use of a standardized column and row format, as well as informative headings, enables tables to stand alone and convey information in a concise manner. Such tables also allow a rapid comparison between treatment effects. In this chapter, we discuss different types of tables used in clinical trial reports, providing standard examples of the most common formats.

Introduction

The main results of clinical trials research are often reported in tables and figures within a research report or in a peer-reviewed manuscript. Very few research or study reports contain text alone. The benefits of collating results into tables are that they are concise and usually follow a logical order. Tables reduce the need for text, and allow an easy comparison of treatment effects. Furthermore, most statistical software can be programmed to generate tables; therefore, it is easy to produce revised tables if patients are added (or removed) from the dataset. Incorporating such revisions into text is more time consuming.

Ideally, the reader should be able to interpret tables and figures with little or no reference to the text. Once recruitment statistics have been reported (usually in a trial profile or a flow chart) then a baseline table should follow, with demographic and clinical characteristics of the patients, for each arm of the trial [1]. Constructing an appropriate baseline table is described in more detail in **Chapter 34**. Results tables usually follow, presenting clinical outcomes for each trial arm in adjacent columns, usually with additional column(s) to directly compare the arms. Finally, adverse events, prespecified secondary outcomes, outcomes at additional time points, and subgroup analyses results are tabled.

Whilst tables are essential for reporting results, detailed information on the methods used for the study are best provided in text format. These might elaborate on the specific method of randomization used, use of nonparametric or unusual statistical tests, construction of subgroups, and handling of missing data, as required. It is also unnecessary to use a table when very little information needs to be presented, particularly considering that tables require relatively more effort to produce and handle (certainly for journal editors), and that the inclusion of too many tables and figures duplicating information makes a report more difficult to produce, read, and appreciate [2].

Indeed, endless tables make it almost impossible to memorize the results and to find the more important information without guidance in the accompanying text. When large reports are necessary/standard practice, such as reports for data monitoring boards, it is a time-consuming and skilful task to extract the pertinent information. A single results line might contain the reason for delaying or terminating an entire study. Therefore it is important to be sensible about the construction of tables, bearing in mind the intended audience.

Table 1. Cause of death in a trial of magnesium supplementation for acute stroke [3]. Data are number of patients (%).

Cause of death	Placebo (n = 1198)	Magnesium (n = 1188)	P-value
Stroke	109 (9)	116 (10)	0.62
Coronary heart disease	15 (1)	18 (2)	0.60
Cardiac (noncoronary)	2 (0.2)	2 (0.2)	1.00
Vascular (noncardiac)	16 (1)	20 (2)	0.51
Cancer	0	2 (0.2)	0.25
Pneumonia	47 (4)	56 (5)	0.37
Other	7 (0.6)	13 (1)	0.16
Total	196 (16)	227 (19)	0.086

Reproduced with permission from Elsevier (*Lancet* 2004;**363**:439–45).

The standard table

Table 1 gives an example of a standard outcomes table showing deaths in each treatment arm. Glancing at it initially, we are presented with numbers and percentages by cause of death in a study comparing placebo and the active treatment of magnesium. It is a trial testing the effect of magnesium supplements on patients who have had an acute stroke within the preceding 12 hours (some of this information is summarized in the table heading, which has been expanded for the purpose of this chapter). The final column gives the *P*-value. Since there is one *P*-value per line, these clearly represent comparisons within each row, between the two treatments in each column, ie, between the placebo and the magnesium groups.

The authors follow the standard practice of giving both the percentages (useful for comparing directly between the two groups) and the numbers (useful for giving the informed reader some idea of the precision of the percentages quoted). The numbers of patients recruited are shown at the top, while in each row the numbers of patients experiencing the event are also shown. The reader can therefore calculate percentages for each outcome in each group for him/herself; the calculated percentages agree with those shown.

We must assume that there are no missing data since the percentages have been calculated using the same denominators for each column for each cause of death; if there were missing data, then it would be desirable to add the appropriate denominator in each column beside the absolute number of outcomes (eg, "109/1198 [9%]" for strokes in the placebo group). In this example, there is

Figure 1. Primary and secondary trial endpoints [3].

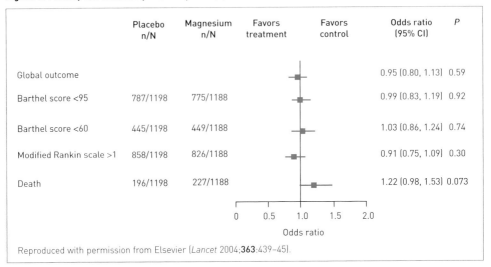

	Placebo n/N	Magnesium n/N	Favors treatment	Favors control	Odds ratio (95% CI)	P
Global outcome					0.95 (0.80, 1.13)	0.59
Barthel score <95	787/1198	775/1188			0.99 (0.83, 1.19)	0.92
Barthel score <60	445/1198	449/1188			1.03 (0.86, 1.24)	0.74
Modified Rankin scale >1	858/1198	826/1188			0.91 (0.75, 1.09)	0.30
Death	196/1198	227/1188			1.22 (0.98, 1.53)	0.073

Odds ratio: 0   0.5   1.0   1.5   2.0

Reproduced with permission from Elsevier (*Lancet* 2004;**363**:439–45).

no specified follow-up time for this specific table, which implies that the table lists any deaths that occurred during the course of the trial. In other cases, it might be helpful to specify the duration of follow-up; for instance, the first column could then be given a title such as "Main outcome at 12 months". This table could also be improved by presenting the risk difference/ratio and its 95% confidence interval (CI) for each outcome (see **Chapter 20**).

Complex tables: tables and figure combinations and two-dimensional comparisons

In some instances, a table might incorporate a figure within it. This is common practice in meta-analysis reports, as well as for reporting subgroup analyses in single clinical trials. **Figure 1** gives an example showing different outcome measures in a randomized trial, incorporating a table and figure combination. It also lists several forms of outcomes (global outcome, mobility, functionality, and death) on the left-hand side, followed along the row by absolute ratios of events within treatment groups, followed by a graphical comparison between the two treatment arms, and lastly supported by an odds ratio and a *P*-value of the treatment difference.

The ratios provided allow the reader to calculate crude or unadjusted odds ratios – eg, for Barthel score <95, the odds ratio can be calculated as $775 / (1188 – 775) / (787 / [119 8 – 787]) = 0.98$ – which are similar but not identical to the quoted odds ratios (0.99 for our row). Detailed reading of the statistical methods section states that the authors have adjusted their odds ratios for the stratification variables, namely age group, the side of the body affected by the stroke, time to randomization, and type of stroke – hence the reason for the discrepancy between the two ratios. Ideally, this adjustment should have been noted in a footnote to the table.

The text also explains the reason for the missing numbers against the "global outcome" (because it is a composite odds ratio for death or disability), which might again have been included in a table footnote. The figure within the table gives no additional information to the text of the table (representing merely the odds ratios and CIs graphically), but presents it in a more user-friendly way, allowing the reader to quickly appreciate which outcomes are improved by the active treatment.

In this example, there is a slight suggestion that the death rate is increased, since the estimated odds ratio is above 1, as well as most of the CI. However, the fact that the CI does encompass the odds ratio of 1 (ie, from 0.98 to 1.53) and the P-value = 0.07 (ie, >0.05) suggests that this is also compatible with no difference in death rates between the treated and control arms. Most other outcomes, including the global outcome, show very little difference between the two arms, with CIs including the odds ratio of 1, and nothing approaching statistical significance. For key outcome results, it is becoming traditional to present this very useful combination of both a figure and table.

On occasions it is necessary to incorporate subheadings within a table. **Table 2** shows an example of such a table, based on cost data from a randomized trial for the evaluation of a new model of routine antenatal care. The costs are appropriately reported separately for each country and also separately, using subheadings, for the provider's costs and the costs borne by the women. As well as giving descriptive statistics for the costs according to treatment (ie, means and standard deviations), the table also directly reports a comparison between the two models, ie, the authors quote a mean difference with 95% CIs. The use of this summary measure means that the reader can deduce the mean cost saving that would accrue by using the new method on, say, 100 women (by multiplying the mean difference in costs by 100), and the level of precision of this estimate, based on differing costs for different women (ie, attributable to sampling variation, as reported in the 95% CI).

The cost units are given in the footnotes (since they do not apply to all the data in any one column), as well as detailed information needed to interpret this information fully, namely on how local currencies were converted into US$. Such

Table 2. Costs to providers and women in Cuba and Thailand [4].

| Type of cost | New model | | Standard model | | Mean difference |
	Number of women	Mean (SD)	Number of women	Mean (SD)	(95% CI)
Providers' costs[a]					
Cuba	2870	885.4 (1632.0)	2734	956.8 (1294.2)	−71.4 (−148.8, 2.5)
Thailand	3278	167.2 (144.7)	3091	206.1 (172.9)	−38.9 (−46.3, −30.9)
Women's out-of-pocket costs[a]					
Cuba	170	174.4 (470.2)	170	242.4 (174.4)	−68.0 (−144.0, 7.7)
Thailand	205	11.9 (16.7)	226	18.4 (27.1)	−6.5 (−10.8, −2.19)
Women's time in access to care[b]					
Cuba	170	15.9 (17.3)	170	25.0 (23.5)	−9.1 (−13.5, −4.7)
Thailand	205	14.8 (12.1)	226	29.7 (19.2)	−14.9 (−18.0, −11.8)

[a]Average cost per pregnancy 1998, US$ purchasing power conversion. The official exchange rates on January 1, 1998, were: $US1 = 1.00 Cuban Peso = 52.3 Thai Baht. The purchasing power parity rate on January 1, 1998 was US$1 = 0.42 Cuban Peso = 26.9 Thai Baht. These were calculated on the basis of costs of a basket of selected food items in each country. This allowed a common purchasing power parity conversion method to be used.
[b]Average time per pregnancy in hours.

Reproduced with permission from Elsevier (*Lancet* 2001;**357**:1551–64).

tables demonstrate how complex information can be presented in a compact way using a two-dimensional comparison table that compares treatments in columns and countries in rows, and includes subgroup comparisons using additional rows. Such tables are invaluable as they obviate the need for complex text and enable the reader to fully appreciate where the treatment differences make the greatest impact.

Using tables instead of text

Table 3 is an example of a table taken from the methods section of a clinical trial. It contains categorization of the venous segments, which enables the reader to review their categorization easily. The accompanying text, being less wordy than if it was incorporated into the text, is easier to read. The authors use their categorization of the venous segments in their definition of type of reflux, as follows.

Table 3. Insonated venous segments [5].

Superficial venous system	Deep venous system
Saphenofemoral junction	Common or superficial femoral vein
Long saphenous vein (above knee)	Popliteal vein (above knee)
Long saphenous vein (below knee)	Popliteal vein (below knee)
Saphenopopliteal junction	
Short saphenous vein	
Calf-perforating veins	

Reproduced with permission from Elsevier (*Lancet* 2004;**363**:1854–9).

'Venous reflux' was identified as either:

- superficial (arising in any superficial segment)
- mixed superficial and segmental deep (one or two of the three insonated deep segments)
- mixed superficial and total deep (all three deep segments)

This defines the main subgroups that will be used in the analysis of this trial. However, this might not be considered a good use of a table in a journal manuscript where the number of tables is restricted; in this situation, tables should be used for detailed results of the study.

Reasons to include a figure in addition to, or instead of, a table

If there is one main outcome measurement for all patients included in the trial then it might be more helpful to show the results for this outcome in detail through a figure, rather than a table. For instance, the authors might include a dot plot or survival curve, according to the nature of the data collected. The IMAGES (Intravenous Magnesium Efficacy in Stroke) study (from which **Table 1** and **Figure 1** were extracted) reported the main outcome measure on all trial patients by including the following sentence: "When analyzed as time to event, the hazard ratio for death during the study was 1.18 (95% CI 0.97, 1.42, $P = 0.098$)"; they presented the corresponding survival curve shown in **Figure 2** [3].

Inclusion of this figure gives appropriate emphasis on the main outcome for all patients, as well as allowing extra detail to be observed (such as cumulative proportions of death at any time point and any changes in pattern by length of follow-up).

Figure 2. Kaplan–Meier plot of cumulative mortality [3].

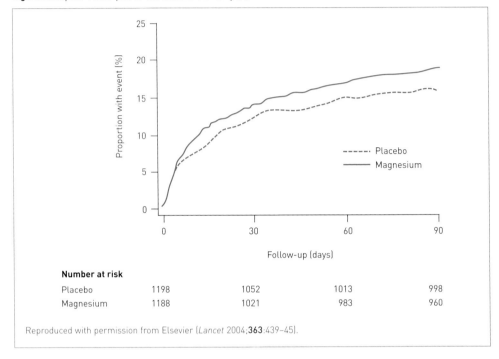

Reproduced with permission from Elsevier (*Lancet* 2004;**363**:439–45).

This IMAGES paper included a:

- trial profile
- baseline table
- figure/table reporting primary and secondary endpoints (our **Figure 1**)
- figure showing the primary endpoint in detail (our **Figure 2**)
- table reporting cause of death (our **Table 1**)
- figure/table reporting subgroup analyses (similar format to our **Figure 1**)
- table of adverse events (similar format to our **Table 1**)

This gives a comprehensive guide to the pertinent results that are needed.

When should table construction begin in a trial?

'Ghost', 'dummy', or 'template' tables are often drafted by a trial statistician according to the statistical analysis plan, and approved or amended by the principal investigators. Such tables provide layout, headings, and footnotes, but the fields remain empty of any data. Often, the appropriate time to construct such tables is at the beginning of the trial when case report forms are being designed to capture the data. Each piece of information should link to a data entry field(s). In a large clinical trial, it is often necessary to undertake interim analyses of the results, to be confident that it is appropriate to continue randomizing patients between the treatment arms. A large number of tables are usually constructed at this time – more than can be reported within the main published report.

Once the interim report has been constructed and reviewed, it is useful to take the opportunity to decide on the content and format of the tables for public presentations of the results and for the final publication; this enables the final report to be produced speedily once the datasets are cleaned and locked up. Remember that few people are privy to the interim results (only those on the data monitoring board) – this is a key reason for discussing the layout with empty tables. It also ensures that the focus of the results is decided upon without reference to the actual results obtained, which maintains objectivity. For instance, the focus is appropriately retained on the chosen main outcome measures and adverse effects, whilst also reporting the named additional outcome measures and any prespecified subgroup analyses.

Once the final report is produced, the computer-generated statistical output should be checked. It should also be carefully reviewed for errant calculations and to ensure that figures are displaying correct information. Consistency across different presentations of data and different methods of analysis can also be checked, for instance between a survival plot and the corresponding hazard ratio, comparing the odds ratios over a specified time period with hazard ratios, or comparing hazard ratios with mean survival times in the two groups.

Journal guidelines

Journals often specify the maximum number of tables and figures that can be incorporated in a manuscript. If they do not state this explicitly then you still need to ensure that the number is in accordance with other papers published in that journal. A general rule of thumb is to include no more than one table or figure per 1,000 words of text [6]. Many guidelines apply to most mainstream journals, whether or not they are stated explicitly. When submitting the paper to a journal, tables should be typed in double spacing, each on a separate page with a self-explanatory title. They should be placed at the end of the manuscript with their approximate locations indicated in the text [7]. Journals have different policies on whether it is necessary to explain abbreviations used in a footnote when they have previously been used in the text.

The CONSORT (Consolidated Standards of Reporting Trials) guidelines for reporting of clinical trials state that the number of participants (denominator) in each group included in each analysis must be reported, as well as whether the analysis was by 'intention-to-treat' (see **Chapter 22**) [1]. The guidelines also suggest that the results should be stated in absolute numbers when feasible (eg, 10/20, not 50%), although giving both can be considered good practice. For each primary and secondary outcome, the report should quote a summary of results for each group, and the estimated effect size and its precision (eg, 95% CI as in **Table 1**).

Authors must address multiplicity by reporting any other analyses performed, including subgroup analyses and adjusted analyses, indicating those that were prespecified and those that were exploratory (see **Chapters 23**, **25**, and **29**). All important adverse events or side-effects in each intervention group also need to be reported. International journals such as *The Lancet* require that all contributors abide by such guidelines.

Detailed advice on constructing a table

Once you are ready to construct a table, there are a number of guidelines to help produce the best format.

Overview
Purpose
Decide on the purpose of the table and what information should be included within it. For clinical trials, this is generally a comparison between two treatment groups, and the table will contain summary statistics for each treatment, as well as information directly comparing the two treatments.

Table size
Smaller tables can draw readers in more clearly to the main issue you want to get across, although a single row table might be best incorporated in the text. In a journal with a double-column page, a single-column table should not exceed 60 characters (and equivalent spaces) and a full-width table should not exceed 120 characters [6].

Unnecessary information
The best tables contain information that will be useful to the reader. Avoid repeating information in figures or text, other than the key outcomes. Balance the merits of giving the readers additional information with the possibility that the readers will feel overwhelmed if faced with too much information. This is often the case in tables of clinical characteristics.

Layout

Consider the layout of the table and anything that might make it easier to read – eg, subheadings, blank lines, or use of parentheses around 95% CIs or around percentages.

Totals

It might be desirable to include a row of totals, and sometimes subtotals – eg, when giving several different causes of death (**Table 1**). When two treatment arms are being compared, with information for each in a separate column, it is usually unhelpful to include a totals column to combine information from both trial arms. Consider adding a column combining treatment groups only if you have two similar treatments arms that can usefully be considered in combination, for comparison with the placebo group or another treatment group.

Titles and footnotes
Title/headings

The title should be a concise description of the information contained within the table. Row headings and column headings should describe what lies within them – where longer descriptions are necessary, supplementary information can be given in a footnote. If most/all columns contain the same type of information, details of this should be included in the table title or in a footnote, rather than in individual row headings (eg, footnote: "data are given as mean [standard deviation] unless stated otherwise").

Explanatory information

Remember that tables need to fully explain what is being compared. For instance, if quoting odds ratios, hazard ratios, or relative risks, state what outcome the ratios represent and which groups are being compared. The reader might need to look at row, column, and title headings to find all of this information.

Follow-up/outcomes

Provide the time to follow-up in the title of the table unless the trial has only one time line (ie, all patients were followed to 12 months). When outcomes that are not as final as death are included, it is important to specify whether the table reflects:

- the first outcome a patient suffers (as in a survival analysis)
- the worst outcome a patient suffers (hierarchical reporting)
- all outcomes separately (includes double counting if a patient suffers more than one event)

The specific method of reporting can be placed in the methods section of the text.

Adjustments

If analyses are adjusted, remember to specify what characteristics have been adjusted for. Clinical trials often report unadjusted results, unless stated otherwise in the protocol, which should then specify one or two things to adjust for or stratify by. For instance, the results might be stratified by recruitment center, or by patient characteristics used in stratified randomization.

Units

Make sure the units are quoted in the column or row headings, and ensure that all units are in accordance with the journal policy.

Reported numbers

Indicate the total numbers of patients that are being reported on – this could be included within the title row, if the same numbers are used for all analyses; otherwise, this information might need to be incorporated within the body of the table, perhaps to reflect different amounts of missing data for different outcome or predictor variables.

Analysis method

State whether the analysis is by intention-to-treat or per-protocol analysis, or any other method. If the analysis method is not mentioned in the table then it must be stated in the text.

Rounding

Any totals given should be calculated from the data before rounding. If data are rounded in the table, the publication should state that differences might occur between sums of component items and totals because of rounding.

Footnotes/references

Use footnotes for important information that does not fit elsewhere. References cited only in tables (or in legends to figures) should be numbered in accordance with a sequence established by the first identification in the text of that particular table (or illustration) [8].

Presenting numeric data in text and within fields of tables

The term 'field' refers to the cells where the numbers (or occasionally text information) are put within the table. Remember that the requirement to give units of measurement and to indicate the number of patients used in results (often reported in row or column headings of a table) also applies to data given within the text of the results section.

Significant figures (decimal places)

Use an appropriate number of decimal places so as not to give a false impression of precision (eg, if a percentage is out of <100 patients then no decimal places are needed). Perhaps use two decimal places for most things (unless there is little variation other than in the third decimal places and this is significant). The number of decimal places could depend on the number of patients in the study or the precision of the results – eg, if the CI is a few units wide then you would certainly not need more than one decimal place in the estimate. It is important to standardize the number of significant figures or decimal places in all values in a table or in all figures of a similar type.

P-values

Report *P*-values to two decimal places if $P > 0.05$, or as $P < 0.0001$ if appropriate, or else generally use two significant figure (except perhaps if around $P = 0.05$ to emphasize which side of $P = 0.05$ it falls). Remember that *P*-values are always positive; if the computer output reports the *P*-value as 0.0000, this implies that $P < 0.00005$ and it should be reported as $P < 0.0001$ [9]. Avoid the use of the abbreviation 'NS' for nonsignificant – it is always preferable to quote an exact *P*-value. This is particularly important if the *P*-value is only slightly greater than $P = 0.05$, to denote a trend in the treatment effect.

Descriptive statistics

For psychometric scales, indicate whether small numbers indicate healthier or more unwell patients. Percentages, ratios, averages, etc. might be helpful in a table for ease of comparison between columns – as well as reporting the ratio of numbers, where applicable (eg, report '5/10' for five cases out of 10, as required by CONSORT guidelines [1]). Standard deviations or other measures of spread should generally be quoted in baseline descriptive statistics.

Negative values

Avoid reporting negative values for comparisons where possible, eg, rather than saying there was an increase by –20%, state there was a decrease by 20%. An exception to this is within a table with a column for effect sizes for different outcomes or predictor variables; some may show increases, and some may show decreases.

Confidence intervals

Results that compare the treatment arms should generally be quoted with 95% CIs, as should any other results, too. Whilst remembering that statistical significance can be deduced from the CI on a comparison measure (odds ratio, difference, etc.), *P*-values may nevertheless be quoted in addition, depending on the preference of the authors, provided the table does not become too unwieldy as a result.

Specific information for fields of tables

Asterisks

P-values can sometimes be quoted using asterisks to indicate levels of significance, eg, in a larger table where quoting the P-values themselves would lead to a cumbersome table. The normal convention is to use * for $P < 0.05$, ** for $P < 0.01$, and *** for $P < 0.001$, for those values achieving statistical significance [9].

Blank cells

Always fill in blank cells, with zeros if appropriate, or with a note to say why the data is not available. If you use the abbreviation 'NA', state whether this refers to 'not available' or 'not applicable' [8]. If a large number of fields contain zeros or no information, this can be considered a waste of space and you need to consider restructuring the table or including the information in a different way (eg, combine some rows together).

Note on deducing statistical significance from confidence intervals

To deduce significance from a CI on a 'statistic of comparison', look to see whether the CI contains values that indicate there is no difference between the groups being compared. For example, does a 95% CI on an odds ratio, hazard ratio, or relative risk contain the value 1.0 within the range given? If so, then the results are consistent with there being no statistically significant difference between the two groups and we can deduce that *P* will be *greater* than 0.05. If the entire 95% CI is above (or below) 1.0 then there is evidence that there is a significant difference between treatment groups with respect to this outcome measure and *P* will be *less* than 0.05. Similarly, if a 95% CI for an estimated absolute difference in outcomes between treatments contains the value 0 (ie, the lower limit is negative and the upper limit is positive) then $P > 0.05$; otherwise, if the CI contains only positive or only negative values then $P < 0.05$ (see **Chapter 18**).

Finally, it is important is to make sure that:

- all the key results are contained within the report
- written interpretations are consistent with the tables
- repetition between tables and text is minimal

Conclusion

Tables are an effective way of presenting numeric data concisely, and are useful for presenting both the baseline characteristics of patients in each treatment group and the detailed results from a clinical trial. Tables should not be too large or complex to avoid overwhelming the reader, nor should they be too short, where the information might have been better incorporated within a few lines of text. Careful consideration is needed about what tables and figures to incorporate within a report and subsequent manuscripts, paying attention to the best way of presenting different types of information, as well as the maximum number allowed by journal editors. Tables need to be labeled sensibly, in such a way that the reader can understand the information contained within the table without reference to the text. Good tables, along with relevant figures (see the next chapter), allow trial construction to be clearly understood and results to stand out in a reader's mind.

References

1. Moher D, Schulz KF, Altman DG. The CONSORT statement: revised recommendations for improving the quality of reports of parallel-group randomised trials. *Lancet* 2001;**357**:1191–4.
2. Day RA. *How to Write and Publish a Scientific Paper.* Cambridge: Cambridge University Press, 1998:61–9.
3. Muir KW, Lees KR, Ford I, et al. Magnesium for acute stroke (Intravenous Magnesium Efficacy in Stroke trial): randomised controlled trial. *Lancet* 2004;**363**:439–45.
4. Villar J, Ba'aqeel H, Piaggio G, et al. WHO antenatal care randomised trial for the evaluation of a new model of routine antenatal care. *Lancet* 2001;**357**:1551–64.
5. Barwell JR, Davies CE, Deacon J, et al. Comparison of surgery and compression with compression alone in chronic venous ulceration (ESCHAR study): randomised controlled trial. *Lancet* 2004;**363**:1854–9.
6. Huth EJ. *Writing and Publishing in Medicine*. Philadelphia: Lippincott Williams & Wilkins, 1999:139–50.
7. *Psychology and Psychotherapy: Theory, Research and Practice*. Notes for Contributors. Available from: www.bps.org.uk/publications/jHP_6.cfm. Accessed May 5, 2005.
8. Wong, I. Editing tables of data. Queensland: Technical editor's eyrie. Available from: www.jeanweber.com/howto/ed-table.htm. Accessed May 5, 2005.
9. Altman DG, Bland JM. Presentation of numerical data. *BMJ* 1996;**312**:572.

Chapter 36

Use of Figures

Zoe Fox, Anil K Taneja, James F Lymp,
Duolao Wang, and Ameet Bakhai

Graphical representation of clinical data is used to provide visual information on the distributions or relationships of outcome variables, as well as illustrating the treatment effects observed in a study. Figures can illustrate the efficacy or safety of different treatments and provide a graphical comparison of those treatments among specific groups of patients. Publications benefit from graphical representations if they are easily interpretable and correctly applied. In this chapter, we discuss the various types of graphical representations that would be appropriate for different kinds of data. The advantages and disadvantages of specific graphical representations with a practical view are also illustrated.

Introduction

A graph or figure is a visual illustration of data, where data consist of observations of one or more variables. Data can be thought of as:

- categorical (qualitative)
- numeric (quantitative)

Categorical data are split into the following three groups:

- binary (containing two categories)
- nominal (more than two categories with no ordering)
- ordinal (more than two categories with inherent ordering)

Numeric data are more complicated and can be categorized as:

- discrete numeric (takes a whole number in a given range)
- continuous (taking any value, not necessarily an integer)
- censored (continuous data that can only be measured in a certain range)
- other data, such as rates or percentages

Graphs are usually produced post-analysis to provide the reader with a visual understanding of the global picture regarding the treatment effect. However, it is also important to visualize the data prior to its analysis [1,2]. Displaying the data beforehand enables one to see how it is distributed, in addition to spotting any outliers, unexpected values, or errors. This provides a prior global interpretation and allows for any corrections that might be required before performing the final analysis. A number of different figures can be employed for visual inspection of the data, but only well-documented, appropriate figures will illustrate the patterns sufficiently.

Basic characteristics of a graph

A useful graph displays both the magnitude and the frequency of individual data points from the distribution under consideration [3]. A graph should contain a title, and x and y axes with their respective labels. The x-axis is the horizontal axis and usually corresponds to the independent variable; the y-axis is the vertical axis and tends to relate to the dependent variable. Graphs should be clear and have short, informative titles describing the data that are displayed.

A useful graph will contain appropriately labeled axes and clearly presented information. The final graph should summarize the data by itself, without the

Figure 1. The percentage of patients who experienced protocol-defined virological failure in each treatment arm of the MaxCmin₁ study.

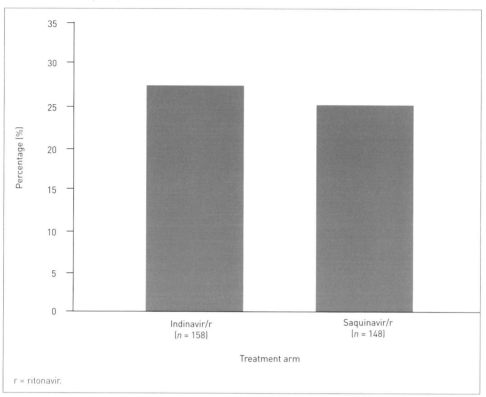

r = ritonavir.

need to refer to the text for further information. The scale of the axes needs to be included, and the maximum and minimum values should be specified. A legend and footnote can also be added to a graph to increase clarity. Overcrowding figures with details should be avoided to eliminate any confusion in understanding the graphical information.

Example: MaxCmin₁ trial

In this chapter, we will illustrate data from the MaxCmin₁ clinical trial using appropriate graphs. MaxCmin₁ was a randomized clinical trial set up to compare the safety and efficacy of ritonavir-boosted indinavir (IDV/r) versus ritonavir-boosted saquinavir (SAQ/r) in HIV-1-positive patients [4]. Out of the 306 patients who initiated their randomized regimen, 80 experienced protocol-defined virological failure (43 patients [27.2%] in the IDV/r arm and 37 patients [25.0%] in the SAQ/r arm) (**Figure 1**). In this basic graph, the two treatment arms appear on the *x*-axis and the outcome information (the percentage) is summarized on the *y*-axis.

Table 1. Number of patients (%) with protocol-defined virological failure in both treatment arms of the MaxCmin₁ study.

Reason failed	Indinavir/r n = 158	Saquinavir/r n = 148
Virologically	33 (20.9)	25 (16.9)
Lost to follow-up	8 (5.1)	8 (5.4)
Withdrew consent	1 (0.6)	3 (2.0)
Died	1 (0.6)	1 (0.7)
Total	43 (27.2)	37 (25.0)

r = ritonavir.

Commonly used graphs in clinical research

The choice of graph that will best fit the data depends on the distribution of the data (categorical or continuous) and the number of variables under consideration. Since categorical data consist of unique categories (eg, male/female) where each category is usually observed more than once, and continuous data contain distinct values (eg, height in cm) where each specific value appears infrequently, we use different methods for displaying each type of data. The most commonly used graphs to display single discrete numeric variables or categorical data are bar charts, pie charts, dot plots, and stem-and-leaf plots. Continuous data are usually displayed using histograms, dot plots, box plots, scatter plots, and line graphs, although continuous data are sometimes grouped in order to use graphical methods for categorical data. These graphs are described in detail in the following sections.

Bar charts

Bar charts can only be produced when the variable of interest is categorical or discrete numeric. They frequently occur in publications because they are visually very strong, useful for comparing more than one group, and easy to produce and interpret. Bar charts are produced by calculating the number of observations in each category; these observations are then translated into frequencies (or percentages), where the length of each bar is proportional to the frequency of observations in that category. Labels can be added to each bar to show the total number of patients contributing to that category. The bars on the bar chart are typically separated by gaps to indicate that the data are discreet.

In the MaxCmin₁ study, protocol-defined virological failure was broken down into true virological failures, patients who were lost to follow-up, patients who withdrew consent, and those who died (**Table 1**). These data can be presented in two ways using a bar chart:

Figure 2. A bar chart to show the distribution of protocol-defined virological failures by treatment arm in the MaxCmin₁ study.

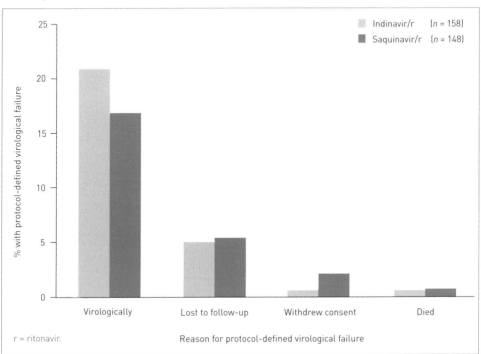

r = ritonavir.

- by looking at the percentage of all patients who have each type of virological failure in both treatment arms (**Figure 2**)
- by presenting this data as a segmented column chart to show the distribution of protocol-defined virological failures within each treatment arm (**Figure 3**)

Note that the column totals of a segmented bar chart add up to 100%. This reflects failure reasons for the patients who failed, but does not show the proportion of patients who failed in each treatment arm.

Care should be taken with bar charts because data can be presented in a number of different ways according to the message you want to depict. In addition, columns can be reordered to emphasize a specific effect, causing data to be misinterpreted more easily.

Pie charts
A pie chart is a circular diagram that is split into sections (slices), one slice for each category. Pie charts are produced using similar methods to bar charts. They

Figure 3. A segmented column chart to show the distribution of protocol-defined virological failures within each treatment arm in the MaxCmin$_1$ study.

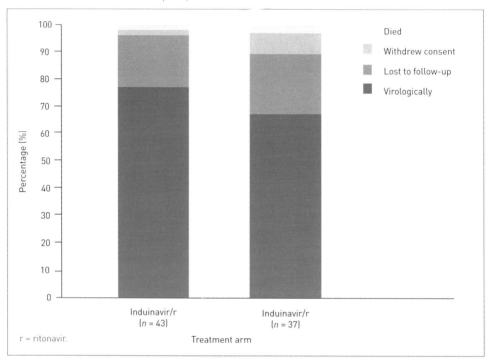

are visually appealing, but are less informative than bar charts because they focus on percentages. They lack data on the total number of frequencies in each category, although these can be added as labels if they do not confuse the interpretation. Pie charts are generally less desirable than bar charts because the data shown are proportional to the square of the frequency (ie, as area of a circle), rather than to the frequency itself, and thus any differences are over-represented. Also patients can only be counted once in a pie chart.

Figure 4 shows the same data as **Figure 3** for the IDV/r arm, but they are displayed using a pie chart rather than a bar chart. Although it is possible to produce two pie charts, one for the IDV/r arm and one for the SAQ/r arm, it is easier to compare data from these two treatment arms in a bar chart than a pie chart.

Dot plots
In a dot plot, each observation is represented by a single dot along a horizontal or vertical line. In the MaxCmin$_1$ study, it is possible to crudely compare the effects of the two regimens on immunological markers by producing a dot plot of the

Figure 4. A pie chart to show the distribution of protocol-defined virological failures for the indinavir/ritonavir arm of the MaxCmin$_1$ study (n = 158).

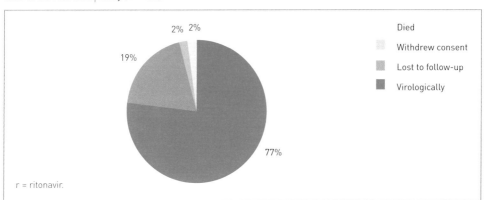

change in CD4 cell count from baseline to the end of 48 weeks of follow-up (**Figure 5**).

Dot plots can be used for both discrete and continuous data, but continuous data tend to be grouped, otherwise it can be cumbersome to plot the data and the plot becomes messy and hard to understand. These plots can contain a line that is perpendicular to the data points to show the median value and, similarly, lines can be included to represent the interquartile range (IQR). Multiple dot plots can be drawn alongside each other to allow comparisons to be made between groups.

Stem and leaf plots

A stem and leaf plot is a hybrid between a graph and a table. It is used for numeric data. This type of graph is usually drawn with a vertical stem and horizontal leaves. The vertical stem consists of the first few digits of the values arranged in numerical order, while the horizontal leaves are represented by the last digit(s) of each of the ordered values. Note that each of the digits in the leaves represents one data point. The resulting stem and leaf plot looks similar to a rotated histogram.

The advantages over a histogram are that:

- Stem and leaf plots are easy to draw by hand.
- Individual data values can be read from the graph, including the range, median, and IQR.
- They are useful for small datasets.

Figure 5. Dot plots to show the change in CD4 cell counts from baseline to the end of 48 weeks' follow-up for patients in the MaxCmin$_1$ study.

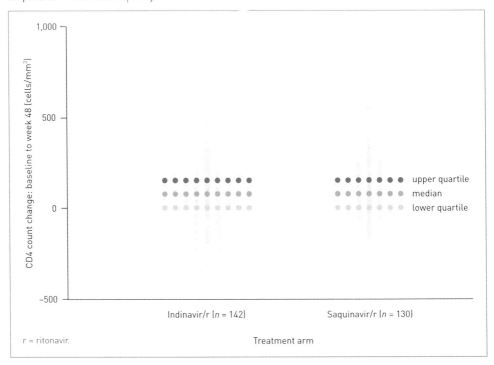

However, the median and IQR can be difficult to calculate if the dataset contains a large amount of data.

If we take a look at the baseline age of patients who initiated SAQ/r in the MaxCmin$_1$ study, a stem and leaf plot can be drawn as shown in **Figure 6**. With a little effort, you can see that the age range is 19–71 years, the median baseline age is 39 years, and the IQR is 34–48 years. Unfortunately, stem and leaf plots are not visually appealing and are therefore not used that frequently in medical literature.

Box plots for showing central location and outliers

A box plot, or box and whisker plot, is a diagrammatic representation of continuous data. It provides a visual means of exploring the skewness of the data and allows comparisons to be made between two or more groups. However, it only illustrates the median, IQR, and range, rather than all of the data individually. A basic box plot consists of a rectangle (the box) with arrows (the whiskers) extending out from the top and bottom. A box plot contains a '+' or horizontal line within the box to indicate the median. The bottom of the box corresponds to the lower

Figure 6. A stem and leaf plot to show the baseline age (years) for patients who initiated ritonavir-boosted saquinavir in the MaxCmin₁ study.

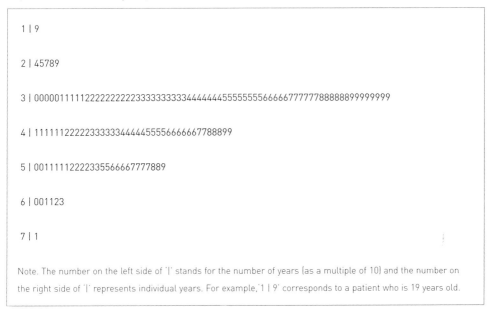

```
1 | 9

2 | 45789

3 | 000001111122222222222333333333334444444555555555666667777778888889999999999

4 | 11111122222333333444445555666666667788899

5 | 00111112222335566667777889

6 | 001123

7 | 1
```

Note. The number on the left side of '|' stands for the number of years (as a multiple of 10) and the number on the right side of '|' represents individual years. For example,'1 | 9' corresponds to a patient who is 19 years old.

quartile and the top to the upper quartile, while the whiskers terminate at the most extreme values in the dataset (including outliers).

If the data are not skewed then the plot will be perfectly symmetrical – the median will lie in the center of the box and both whiskers will extend for the same distance on either side. If the data are positively skewed then the median will be displaced to the bottom of the box, and if they are negatively skewed then the median will lie towards the top. There will also be an influence on the length of the whiskers.

For data that contain wide variation between observations it is more advisable to use a truncated box plot (**Figure 7**). In a truncated box plot, the whiskers extend out a specific statistical distance from the box (to the 5th and 95th percentiles, say) or to a point no further from the box than the IQR; all other observations (the outliers) are presented as dots beyond the whiskers. Different groups can be visually compared by aligning the box plots for each dataset, as long as they have been produced on the same scale. When more than one group is compared then the relative position of the horizontal line indicates the difference between medians. The relative height of the boxes indicates the difference in variation, and the relative overall height of the plots shows the difference between the ranges.

Figure 7. A truncated box and whisker plot to show the CD4 count at the end of 48 weeks' follow-up for patients in the MaxCmin$_1$ study.

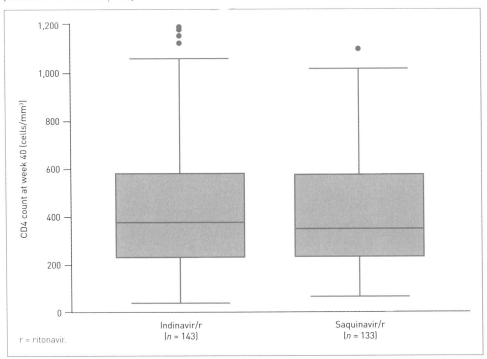

From **Figure 7**, you can see that there are no substantial differences in the CD4 count levels between the two treatment arms at week 48. The median measurements of both box plots are displaced to the bottom of the box, revealing a positive skew of the CD4 count data. This is emphasized by the shorter lower whisker and by the presence of outliers above the limits of the upper whiskers. Box plots can also be presented horizontally rather than vertically. They are simple to produce and useful for identifying outliers.

Histograms

Histograms look like bar charts (**Figure 8**). They are constructed in a similar fashion, but are used for continuous data rather than discrete numeric or categorical data. In order to create a histogram, data need to be separated into categories or bins where all the categories normally have equal width. The width of each bar relates to a range of values for that variable, and the area of the bar is proportional to the frequency of observations in that range. After defining the categories, the construction of a histogram is essentially the same as that of a bar chart.

Figure 8. Histograms showing how the distribution of CD4 counts at week 48 in the MaxCmin$_1$ study change according to the number of categories (bins).

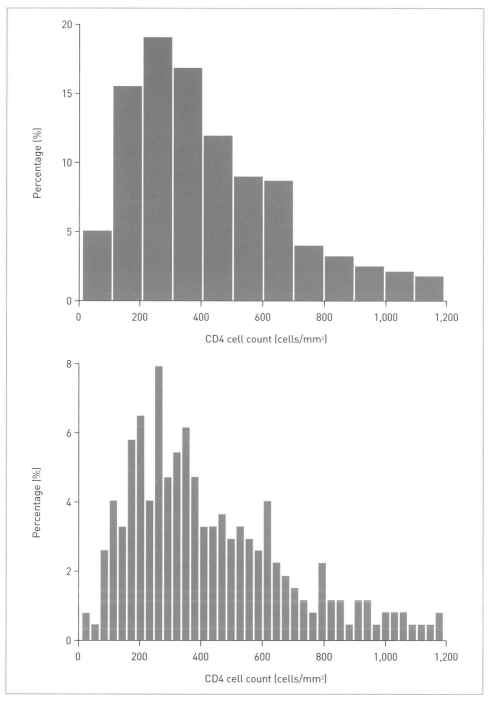

Both histograms and bar charts display the frequency density, except that histograms typically do not have spaces between the categories because the data are continuous. The appearance of a histogram is affected by how the categories are defined. An increase in the number of categories reduces the possible number of observations within the category. The number and width of the categories (bins) should be chosen according to clinically meaningful intervals. If this is not possible then they should be selected on a trial and error basis, with an overall aim of illustrating variations in the data. As a rough guide, 5–20 categories should be selected, depending on the number of observations in the dataset. This can result in a loss of information if the width of the categories is too wide; with too narrow categories, however, the graph will consist of the raw numbers (**Figure 8**). Note that most major statistical software packages do a reasonably good job of automatically selecting appropriate category widths.

Histograms are visually strong and useful for evaluating the spread and skew of the data, but are associated with some disadvantages. Firstly, it is difficult to compare two groups using a histogram; secondly, a histogram tells you how many values lie within a certain range, but without revealing the exact measurements.

Scatter plots

A scatter plot is a simple plot used to display the relationship between two continuous variables. One variable is termed the 'x' and the other the 'y'. Both variables are plotted against each other, the x variable along the *x*-axis and the y variable along the *y*-axis. The relationship between them can be expressed with the use of a regression line, which is usually calculated by a software package.

A scatter graph can be used to investigate whether there was a relationship between CD4 levels at baseline and week 48 in the MaxCmin$_1$ study (**Figure 9**). As we would expect, the trend line shows a highly significant relationship between the two variables (Spearman rank correlation coefficient = 0.83, $P < 0.0001$). On the other hand, a flat trend line does not imply that there is no relationship between the two variables under consideration. A weak relationship might exist, or the trend line might be misleading if its gradient and positioning are the result of a few influential points. For nonlinear relationships, other lines such as smoothing splines or lowess curves can be used, which try to funnel the points.

Line graphs

A line graph is a plot of numeric data where consecutive values are connected by a line (**Figure 10**). They can show repeated measures on a single individual to illustrate how a certain parameter, say the pharmacokinetic (PK) concentration of a drug, changes over time after it has been administered. In this case, the *x*-axis would correspond to the time and the *y*-axis would reflect the PK concentration.

Figure 9. A scatter plot showing the relationship between CD4 cell counts at baseline and at week 48 in the MaxCmin₁ study (n = 272).

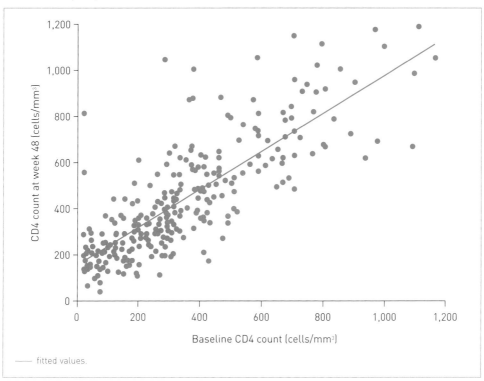

Line graphs can be used to depict fluctuating data containing peaks and troughs and are good for identifying trends. They are also used to show how the mean or median measurement of a marker fluctuates over time by treatment group.

Figure 10 shows the mean systolic blood pressure (SBP) at seven different time points for 2,028 patients followed over 36 months in an anonymous study. The dots correspond to the mean SBP at each visit and error bars have been added to show ± one standard error. This graph shows that SBP was consistently lower in group A compared to group B after randomization.

Kaplan–Meier plots are a type of line graph that are used to show how the percentage of patients who are event-free changes over time (see **Chapter 21**). Another example of a line plot is the receiver operating characteristic curve, which is a plot of the true-positive rate (sensitivity) versus the true-negative rate (1 – specificity) of a diagnostic test.

Figure 10. A line graph showing how mean systolic blood pressure (SBP) changes after randomization by treatment (bar stands for ± one standard error) (*n* = 2028).

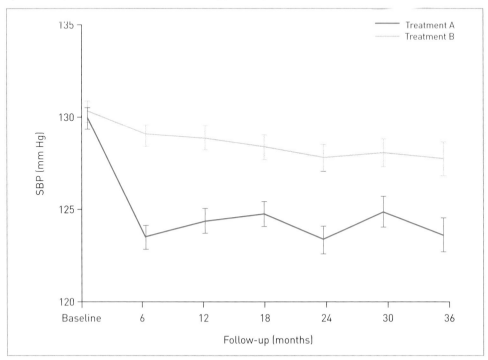

Caution should be employed regarding scales. When the length of time between observations is not uniform and the *x*-axis is not scaled accordingly then the graph might not reflect the data accurately. Similarly, if two line graphs are compared then they must be on the same scale, otherwise visual comparisons will be meaningless.

Spaghetti plots

If we consider the simple situation where we have separate line graphs showing the PK profile for each individual in a study, these lines could be combined in a single graph, sometimes called a spaghetti plot (**Figure 11**). Spaghetti plots are just several line graphs that have been overlaid. These plots are useful for PK data because they allow an assessment of the patterns of drug absorption and elimination, and also allow you to examine the between-subject variation. If individual lines are not all in the same direction or do not peak to the same degree then patients are exhibiting different responses to the drug, and further examination will be warranted to investigate the reasons for this.

Figure 11. A spaghetti plot showing individual pharmacokinetic concentration profiles in a study.

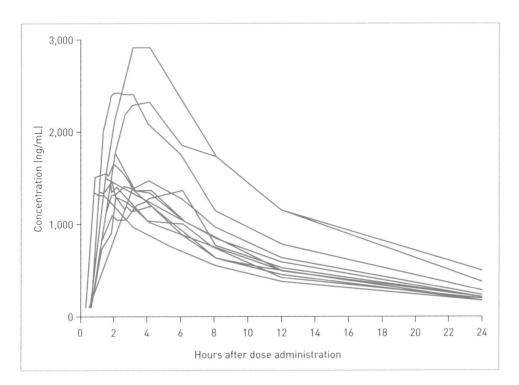

Forest plots

A forest plot displays point estimates and the corresponding confidence intervals (CIs) for multiple groups. Forest plots are most commonly used to present subgroups within a trial or the results of multiple studies as part of a meta-analysis, which is a formal method of comparing the results of several trials using the same intervention (see **Chapter 38**). Point estimates are usually obtained from simple or extended regression models such as logistic regression. In a systematic review of randomized controlled trials investigating the effects of corticosteroids on mortality in individuals with brain trauma, 13 trials were combined in a meta-analysis and the odds ratios of each study were presented using a forest plot (**Figure 12**) [5].

In this graph, the size of the marker represents the size of the corresponding study and the central vertical line represents no difference between the treatment and control arms. In meta-analyses, forest plots typically include a diamond at the base of the graph representing the combined estimate, or pooled intervention effect, from all of the studies. The center of the diamond corresponds to the pooled point estimate, and its horizontal tips represent the CIs based on the formal

Figure 12. A forest plot showing the overall and individual odds ratios for each study.

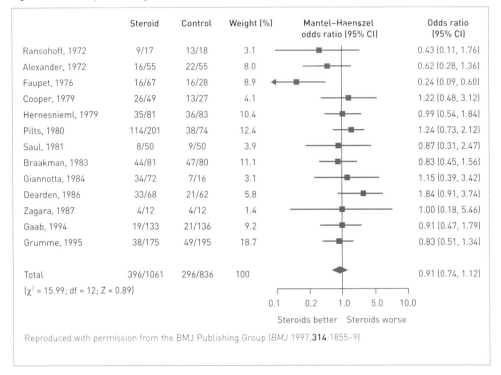

	Steroid	Control	Weight (%)	Mantel–Haenszel odds ratio (95% CI)	Odds ratio (95% CI)
Ransohoff, 1972	9/17	13/18	3.1		0.43 (0.11, 1.76)
Alexander, 1972	16/55	22/55	8.0		0.62 (0.28, 1.36)
Faupet, 1976	16/67	16/28	8.9		0.24 (0.09, 0.60)
Cooper, 1979	26/49	13/27	4.1		1.22 (0.48, 3.12)
Hernesnieml, 1979	35/81	36/83	10.4		0.99 (0.54, 1.84)
Pilts, 1980	114/201	38/74	12.4		1.24 (0.73, 2.12)
Saul, 1981	8/50	9/50	3.9		0.87 (0.31, 2.47)
Braakman, 1983	44/81	47/80	11.1		0.83 (0.45, 1.56)
Giannotta, 1984	34/72	7/16	3.1		1.15 (0.39, 3.42)
Dearden, 1986	33/68	21/62	5.8		1.84 (0.91, 3.74)
Zagara, 1987	4/12	4/12	1.4		1.00 (0.18, 5.46)
Gaab, 1994	19/133	21/136	9.2		0.91 (0.47, 1.79)
Grumme, 1995	38/175	49/195	18.7		0.83 (0.51, 1.34)
Total	396/1061	296/836	100		0.91 (0.74, 1.12)

$(\chi^2 = 15.99; df = 12; Z = 0.89)$

0.1   0.2   1.0   5.0   10.0

Steroids better   Steroids worse

Reproduced with permission from the BMJ Publishing Group (*BMJ* 1997;**314**:1855–9).

meta-analysis. While it is common to use 95% CIs for each trial and for the overall pooled effect, some researchers prefer to use wider CIs (often 99%) for the pooled estimate on the grounds that evidence regarding treatment benefit should be more convincing when combining the results of multiple studies. CIs for the pooled estimate are much narrower than for the individual studies because more patients contribute to the overall estimate, and consequently it is more precise.

Forest plots allow us to review at a glance a large collection of data testing the same relationship. They allow visual assessment of heterogeneity between groups by comparing the results of each study to see whether there is a single underlying effect, or a distribution of effects. If the results of the studies differ greatly, and the CIs for all of the studies do not overlap, then it might not be appropriate to combine the results. Although there is no statistical solution to this, heterogeneity between studies should not be seen simply as a problem for meta-analysis – it also provides an opportunity for examining why treatment effects differ in different circumstances [6].

Table 2. Summary of graphs used to display categorical and continuous data.

Graph	Features	Categorical data	Numeric data
Bar chart	• Frequency proportional to length of bar • Visually very strong, easy to interpret • Bars separated by gaps to indicate discrete data	Yes	No
Pie chart	• Percentages represent square of frequency • Differences between groups over-represented • Less informative than bar charts	Yes	No
Dot plot	• Each observation represented by a dot • Continuous data tend to be grouped • Can be used to display median value and IQR	No	Yes
Stem and leaf plot	• Each digit in a leaf represents a data point • Looks similar to a rotated histogram • Very easy to draw by hand if there are small amounts of data	No	Yes
Box plot	• Displays skew of data • Illustrates median, IQR, and range • Truncated box plot used to spot outliers	No	Yes
Histogram	• Continuous data usually displayed in categories of equal width • Bars do not have spaces between them • Area of bar is proportional to frequency	No	Yes
Scatter plot	• Displays relationship between two continuous variables, x and y, using a regression line • Influential points can mislead interpretation of line	No	Yes
Line graph	• All consecutive data are connected by a line • Can be used to depict fluctuating trends, median, and mean. • Overlaid line graphs can create a spaghetti plot	No	Yes
Forest plot	• Used to display point estimates and their confidence intervals for multiple groups • In meta-analyses, a diamond at the base of the graph represents the pooled intervention effect • Allows visual assessment of heterogeneity between groups	Yes	Yes
Funnel plot	• Used to compare treatment effects of individual studies in a meta-analysis • Plots study precision against corresponding treatment effect • Good for examining publication bias, but not fully robust	Yes	Yes
Graphs for three variables	• Mosaic displays represent multiway contingency tables • Icons supplement bar charts and pie charts, particularly with small sample size • Surface plots display quantitative data in three dimensions	Yes	Yes

IQR = interquartile range.

Funnel plots

A funnel plot can also be used to compare the treatment effects of individual studies in a meta-analysis. It is essentially a plot of the study precision against the corresponding treatment effect (see **Chapter 38** for more). Funnel plots are good for examining publication bias [7], but are not fully robust. In a review of 198 published meta-analyses, the shape of the funnel was determined by an arbitrary choice of the method to construct the plot. When different definitions of precision and/or effect measure were used, the conclusion about the shape of the funnel changed in 86% of cases [8].

Graphs for three variables

Other, less common, graphs that are used to display three dimensions include *mosaic displays*, *icons*, and *surface plots*. In brief, a mosaic display uses the strengths of a bar chart to represent multiway contingency tables [9]. Icons are a potential supplement to bar charts or pie charts, particularly when the sample size is small [10]. Surface plots are useful for displaying quantitative data in three dimensions, ie, there are x, y, and z axes for plotting points and the graph must be printed in a three dimensional representation [11].

Conclusion

Graphical representation facilitates the evaluation and comparison of outcome variables among different groups, and enables an appropriate choice of statistical methods. In this chapter, we have explored a variety of graphs that are commonly used in clinical reports (see **Table 2** for a summary). The choice of graph is determined by the purpose of the exercise and the type of data to present. In a trial report, all of the graphs should be appropriately labeled and contain sufficient information without needing to refer back to the text. Sometimes more than one graph is required, giving importance to simplicity.

References

1. Petrie A, Sabin C. *Medical Statistics at a Glance*. Oxford: Blackwell Publishing, 2000.
2. Kirkwood BR, Sterne JAC. *Essential Medical Statistics*. Oxford: Blackwell Publishing, 2003.
3. Norleans MX. *Statistical Methods for Clinical Trials*. New York: Marcel Dekker, 2000.
4. Dragsted UB, Gerstoft J, Pedersen C, et al. Randomized trial to evaluate indinavir/ritonavir versus saquinavir/ritonavir in human immunodeficiency virus type 1-infected patients: the MaxCmin$_1$ trial. *J Infect Dis* 2003;**188**:635–42.
5. Alderson P, Roberts I. Corticosteroids in acute traumatic brain injury: systematic review of randomised controlled trials. *BMJ* 1997;**314**:1855–9.

6. Bailey KR. Inter-study differences: how should they influence the interpretation and analysis of results? *Stat Med* 1987;**6**:351–60.

7. Egger M, Davey Smith G, Schneider M, et al. Bias in meta-analysis detected by a simple, graphical test. *BMJ* 1997;**315**:629–34.

8. Tang JL, Liu JL. Misleading funnel plot for detection of bias in meta-analysis. *J Clin Epidemiol* 2000;**53**:477–84.

9. Friendly M. Mosaic displays for multi-way contingency tables. *J Am Stat Assoc* 1994;**89**:190–200.

10. Elting LS, Martin CG, Cantor SB, et al. Influence of data display formats on physician investigators' decision to stop clinical trials: prospective trial with repeated measures. *BMJ* 1999;**318**:1527–31.

11. Phillips M, Cataneo RN, Greenberg J, et al. Breath markers of oxidative stress in patients with unstable angina. *Heart Dis* 2003;**5**:95–9.

Chapter 37

Critical Appraisal of a Report

Ameet Bakhai, Jaymin Shah, and Duolao Wang

The number of clinical trials being published in peer-reviewed journals continues to increase. While formal guidance is available on how to submit and systematically score such reports, in terms of their data, design, and presentation [1–3], there are few recommendations about how to interpret clinical trials [4]. Our perception of the results of trials may be influenced by expert peer presentations, media coverage, investment banking reports, and Internet debate, all of which can give opposing opinions. Therefore, healthcare professionals need to develop the ability to quickly and effectively evaluate the results of a clinical trial for themselves. In this chapter, we provide 10 key questions to assist in the evaluation of clinical trials, using a somewhat unconventional but critical approach to gauge a report in more depth.

Table 1. The quality of evidence as defined by the US Public Health Task Force Guide to clinical preventive services [15].

Quality of evidence	Type of study
I	Properly designed randomized controlled trial
II.1	Evidence obtained from well-designed controlled trials without randomization
II.2	Evidence obtained from well-designed cohort or case-control studies
II.3	Evidence obtained from multiple time series/observational studies, with or without intervention. Dramatic results in uncontrolled experiments (such as the results of the introduction of penicillin treatments in the 1940s) could also be regarded as this type of evidence
III	Opinions of respected authorities, based on clinical experience, descriptive studies, case reports, or reports of expert committees

1. Where was the report published?

Studies published in high-profile journals are likely to be widely read, evaluated, and debated. One formal measure of the influence of a journal is its impact factor. The impact factor is based on how often articles from that journal are referenced by subsequent publications in the 2 years following publication, and the impact factor of the journals in which the paper is referenced. The theory is that work of extraordinary merit will be referenced often. Thus, there is considerable competition to publish work in high-profile journals. It is generally believed that work published in such journals will have been carefully vetted for bias and major errors in methodology and design by both the editors and the reviewers invited to evaluate the paper by the journal. The reviewers – who are invariably experts in the subject being considered – provide excellent input and feedback to authors to improve their work where needed, or reject work of low quality, and thus promote a self-perpetuating mechanism for raising the standard of the articles published in these journals. The journal *Circulation* (impact factor 15) receives about 600 articles a month, but publishes less than 60 each month.

While clinical trials are the most scrutinized and valued reports in terms of clinical evidence, most journals will also publish reviews, hypotheses, and studies with small numbers of subjects if the work is novel or controversial; therefore, not all space is devoted to randomized trials. **Table 1** demonstrates the importance placed on randomized trials as the best source of evidence for the evaluation of the efficacy of therapies. A letter in the *BMJ* noted that the impact factor of top journals dropped as they began to publish more articles such as research letters, since the calculation process does not fully account for these types of article [5]. Therefore, the impact factor alone should not be used to assess the usefulness of an article published in a particular journal.

Furthermore, Pocock et al. reported that publication in a well-respected journal does not always correlate with ideal study design. They reviewed 45 reports published in the *BMJ*, the *New England Journal of Medicine*, and *The Lancet*. They found that the interpretation of large amounts of data was complicated by a common failure to specify in advance the intended size of a trial or statistical stopping rules for interim analyses, leading to a tendency to exaggerate treatment differences [6]. This problem is not unexpected: the reviewers assessing the study report might be experts in the disease area but they are not necessarily statistical experts, or experts in trial design.

2. How relevant is the question being asked by the study?

The introductory paragraph of a study report should state the exact question being asked. The reader then has to decide on the importance and relevance of the research question to the way he/she conducts his/her daily practice:

- Will the answer to the question alter the way in which patients are managed?
- Does the question relate to a substantial proportion of their routine practice or to a minority of patients?
- Has standard treatment changed since the beginning of the trial, so that the trial results are less relevant to current day practice?

An example of problems that can arise in prolonged trials was seen in a substudy of the very large ALLHAT (Anti-hypertensive and Lipid-lowering Treatment to Prevent Heart Attack Trial) study. In ALLHAT, patients with well-controlled hypertension, moderate dyslipidemia, and an additional cardiovascular risk factor were randomized to receive either pravastatin (40 mg daily) or "usual care" [7]. The aim of the study was to show that the addition of a statin to usual care would reduce all-cause mortality (the primary outcome measure) and/or coronary heart disease mortality (the secondary outcome measure).

A total of 10,355 patients were randomized to this substudy and followed for up to 8 years, but the substudy failed to show a significant difference in primary or secondary outcome measures. One of the possible explanations for this somewhat disappointing result was that the usual care in most practices included statin therapy for secondary prevention, and 26% of patients in the usual care arm were on a statin at the end of the trial. Such a significant treatment crossover was unlikely to have been expected at the beginning of the study, demonstrating how practice patterns can change faster than a trial can be completed and published.

3. Did patient selection particularly influence the results?

If, after scanning the abstract, you decide to interrogate the paper further, it is useful to focus on patient selection criteria before proceeding to the results. No trial can be properly evaluated without a detailed understanding of the study population, but authors often fail to adequately define and account for the types of subjects finally recruited to a study. The team designing the trial has to find the proper balance between restricting eligibility in order to obtain a relatively uniform group of subjects and minimizing exclusion criteria so as to make the results relevant to more patients. Many trials keep a screening register or log of study-eligible patients, as well as a log of those patients finally randomized. Both of these figures should be reported in the study manuscript. The ratio of patients screened to those recruited can often suggest whether the inclusion/exclusion criteria were broad enough to capture a large proportion of all patients with the disease.

Consider the AWESOME (Angina With Extremely Serious Operative Mortality Evaluation) clinical trial, which was designed to compare long-term survival in patients with medically refractory myocardial ischemia and a high risk of adverse outcomes with either a surgical revascularization (coronary artery bypass grafting) or a percutaneous intervention strategy, including stents [8,9]. This trial screened 22,662 patients, but randomized only 454, suggesting that the study focused on only a very specific subgroup of patients with coronary artery disease. Therefore, the results of this study are relevant to only a small cohort of all ischemic patients, and cannot be easily extrapolated to daily practice.

4. What do the recruitment rate and timing of publication tell us?

It is interesting to note when patients were recruited and when the study completed enrollment. If recruitment rates were much slower than the expected presentation rate of similar patients in normal practice, one might discuss the following points:

- Were the entry criteria too narrow, making recruitment difficult?
- Was the treatment protocol overly complicated, discouraging recruitment?
- Were the financial incentives for patient recruitment important? Financial incentives are usually unnecessary if the study addresses an issue that is important to both patients and clinicians.
- Were the correct centers chosen to recruit for this study, or was the subject of little interest to recruiting centers?
- Was recruitment slowed by an interim amendment to the protocol requested by the data and safety monitoring board, suggesting safety or statistical concerns at an early stage of the study?

The answers to some of these questions – such as the types of recruiting centers, the numbers recruited by each center, and whether the project was commercially funded – are often found in the appendices or notes. Issues such as commercial funding are also worth knowing since such studies tend to have higher recruitment rates than non-commercially funded projects.

The time between the end of follow-up and the time of publication can also be of interest. Most high-impact journals publish items 6–12 months after acceptance, unless fast tracked. Fast-tracked sections are available in some journals for trials addressing very topical or key issues, or for a major breakthrough. Editors of these sections aim to review and publish a report in as little as 2 months.

On the other hand, studies with results that are difficult to interpret, or with negative results, might be submitted or accepted for publication much later than positive, high-profile studies. The delay could be due to many suggestions from the reviewers – asking for additional work to improve the publication before acceptance – or to a number of previous journals considering and then rejecting the paper, each consideration taking 4–8 weeks, since authors are restricted to submitting the article to only one journal at a time. A journal might provide reviewers' comments on a web site, which can provide additional insights about the reasons for a lag in publication time, such as requests for additional patient numbers or reanalysis using other statistical methods.

5. Are the observed treatment differences due to systematic error (bias) or confounding?

In a clinical trial, the observed treatment effect regarding the safety and efficacy of a new drug can appear to be clinically and statistically significant and yet might be due to the result of systematic error or bias within the study [10]. Even the most careful measurement and elegant statistical analysis can not salvage a biased clinical trial, although learning about the mechanism of the bias might in itself be of scientific merit. The most common types of bias in clinical research are those related to subject selection and outcome measurement. A reader should therefore review a report with a question about whether such bias might have been prevented during the design and conduction. For example, did the patients in the trial get recruited in a clinical setting unrepresentative of the wider patient population – eg, patients only recruited in one country with highly developed medical services? This would then cause a geographical bias such that the results might not be reproducible in a different national setting. In addition, exclusion of subjects from statistical analysis because of noncompliance or missing data could bias an estimate of the true benefit of a treatment, particularly if more patients were removed from analysis in one group than the other. In randomized trials, outcomes should be compared among groups based on the original treatment assignment rather than based on the treatment received, as results from strategies other than intention-to-treat analysis are subject to potential bias.

Confounding is another factor that can contribute to the observed treatment difference in an outcome variable. Confounding occurs when a baseline characteristic (or variable) of patients is associated with the outcome but unevenly distributed between treatment groups. As a result, the observed treatment difference from the unadjusted (univariate) analysis can be explained by the imbalanced distribution of this variable. When reading a report, the most useful way to detect possible confounding factors is to examine the distribution of baseline characteristics by treatment group, to assess if the treatment groups are comparable.

6. Are negative trials worth reading in detail?

A negative clinical trial is one in which the observed differences are not large enough to satisfy a specified significance level (usually a $P < 0.05$ threshold), so the results are declared to be statistically nonsignificant. The tendency to defer publication of a negative trial creates so-called publication bias, with more positive-result studies being published. Studies that have yielded disappointing or negative results are less likely to be presented at scientific meetings, published promptly, or published in high-impact journals.

This reporting bias can imply that medical treatments are more useful than they really are. Despite evidence identifying investigators as the main cause of publication bias, investigators continue to claim that editorial bias is the main reason for nonpublication of negative or null results, and that this is why they do not submit negative findings. However, a study examining publication decisions for reports of controlled trials in *JAMA* found little evidence of a positive publication bias in that journal [11].

Thus, leading editors have an interest in publishing well-conducted negative or neutral trials. For the reader, it now becomes important to know not only which therapies benefit the management of certain diseases, but also those that do not. An example of a negative trial changing practice was the GUSTO-IV (Global Use of Strategies to Open Occluded Coronary Arteries) study [12]. This trial showed that abciximab therapy did not confer benefit on patients with acute coronary syndromes not needing urgent coronary investigations. Prior to this study, abciximab had been shown to be beneficial for almost all acute coronary syndrome populations, but GUSTO-IV showed that there was an increase in bleeding complications with this treatment without significant clinical benefit, prompting physicians to weigh the risk–benefit ratio more carefully. Therefore, there are lessons to be learnt from negative/neutral trials.

7. Was the study negative because it was inadequately powered?

With increased publication of trials with negative or neutral results, it is important to be clear whether the trial was negative due to errors in sample-size calculations or whether the new treatment strategy really was no different to the standard treatment. A trial should be large enough to detect a worthwhile effect as statistically significant if it exists, or to give confidence in the notion that the new treatment is no better than the control treatment.

Calculation of sample size is based on the expected difference in the primary outcome measure between the two groups being assessed, and the baseline event rate expected in the standard therapy group. The expected difference should also be worthwhile in real practice. For example, a 1% reduction in event rates is a useful difference to pursue if the event rate with standard therapy is around 5%–10%, but would be less meaningful if the event rate with standard therapy is 40%.

Underpowered studies are common because expectations are over-ambitious and additional patients might need to be recruited, but the funding to extend the study might not be available. Underpowered studies can lead to a Type II or beta error, ie, the erroneous conclusion that an intervention has no effect when the trial size is inadequate to allow a comparison. In contrast, a Type I or alpha error is the conclusion that a difference is significant when in fact it is due to chance. By convention, the threshold for considering a result as significant is set higher than for considering a study to be nonsignificant, therefore favoring traditional therapies over new therapies that lack established side-effect profiles [13].

8. Were the outcome measures reported appropriately?

A study's outcome measures need to be clearly defined. Standardized measurement criteria for outcomes are needed for the results to have clinical relevance. If multiple outcome measures are being collected, a precise statement should explain how these measures are to be prioritized and reported relative to the study objectives.

For example, one patient might have many adverse events during a study. The final statistical results for the study can then be based on a count of all the events, the patient's first event, or the worst event the patient suffered. The latter is important because some outcomes, eg, death, are more important than others, eg, an increase in the dose/number of medicines used to control symptoms. If all events are being measured, care must be taken to understand this, otherwise it can lead to a misunderstanding that generally the trial had high rates of adverse events.

When reviewing the results, it is important to ensure there are no hidden detrimental effects or other outcomes that might outweigh the benefits of the intervention under investigation. For example, authors often present the rates of death and then a combined rate of death or myocardial infarction (MI). If there is a 2% decrease in the death rate for the new treatment but only a 1% decrease for the combined endpoint, then it is important to consider the fact that there were more MIs with the new treatment. This is not necessarily at odds with the new treatment being beneficial, since if substantially fewer patients die then the patients living longer might have an increase in nonfatal complications, such as MI.

More commonly the situation is reversed in studies, with disease-specific outcomes being improved, but with (albeit nonsignificant) mortality rates for patients in the new treatment arm increasing. In meta-analyses combining the results of many such trials, two outcomes (such as death and relief of symptoms) can go in opposite directions, making the value of such therapies doubtful. It is also important that side-effects and their frequencies are presented – such as bleeding, weight gain, or drug interactions. These measures can easily sabotage an otherwise beneficial treatment.

Another way to tip results in favor of a new therapy is to only present the results from patients who were fully compliant with the new treatment protocol (per protocol analysis). However, excluding information from patients withdrawing from the study, perhaps because of side-effects, can favor the therapy that is more likely to cause side-effects. This is because the remaining patients are often younger and healthier, and they are able to continue taking medications despite mild side-effects, unlike more elderly patients or those with coexisting illnesses.

If the new therapy caused more side-effects, then in a per protocol-based analysis that group might have a somewhat healthier profile and hence less adverse outcomes from the disease process. The ideal report would include all patients in the analysis after they are randomized, regardless of what happens later (intention-to-treat analysis) – such as not being prescribed the treatment, being switched to the other treatment group, or only being partially compliant with the treatment.

Table 2. Items that should be included in reports of randomized trials [1]. Adapted from Reference [2].

Item	Comment
Heading	
Subheading	
Descriptor	
Title	Identify the study as a randomized trial
Abstract	Use a structured format
Introduction	State the prospectively defined hypothesis, clinical objectives, and planned subgroup analyses
Methods	
Protocol	Describe: • The planned study population, together with inclusion or exclusion criteria • Planned interventions and their timing • Primary and secondary outcome measure(s) and the minimum important difference(s), and indicate how the target sample size was projected • The rationale and methods for statistical analyses, detailing the main comparative analyses and whether they were completed on an intention-to-treat basis • Prospectively defined stopping rules (if warranted)
Assignment	Describe: • The unit of randomization (eg, individual, cluster, geographic) • The method used to generate the allocation schedule • The method of allocation concealment and the timing of assignment • The method to separate the generator from the executor of assignment
Masking (blinding)	Describe: • The mechanism (eg, capsules, tablets) • Similarity of the treatment characteristics (eg, appearance, taste) • Control of the allocation schedule (ie, the location of code during trial and when broken) • The evidence for successful blinding among the participants, the person doing the intervention, the outcome assessors, and the data analysts
Results	
Participant flow	Provide a trial profile summarizing the participant flow, numbers, and timing and follow-up of randomization assignment, interventions, and measurements for each randomized group
Analysis	State the estimated effect of intervention on primary and secondary outcome measures, including a point estimate and a measure of precision (confidence interval)
Discussion	State the results in absolute numbers when feasible (eg, 10/20, not 50%) Present summary data and appropriate descriptive and interferential statistics in sufficient detail to permit alternative analyses and replication Describe prognostic variables by treatment group and any attempt to adjust for them Describe deviations from the planned study protocol together with the reasons State specific interpretations of study findings, including sources of bias and imprecision (internal validity) and discussion of external validity, including appropriate quantitative measures when possible State general interpretations of the data in light of the totality of the available evidence

9. What are the implications of the study results and discussion?

In the discussion section of the article, readers should expect to find a balanced interpretation of the results, taking into account any previous work. A guide to the format of a submission of a clinical trial is shown in **Table 2**. The biological plausibility of the results should be addressed, along with the impact on current medical practice. Although the authors will offer their interpretation of the data, the reader must draw their own conclusions about the importance and impact of the results compared with conventional treatment strategies. A significant report may lead to changes in guidelines, but this usually requires either a very large definitive study or at least two large independent trials supporting the same conclusion.

The conclusions of the publication might be biased or restricted in commercially funded studies. Major journals have guidelines for the disclosure of industry's role in a clinical trial. These guidelines require the authors to disclose full details of their role (and the sponsors) in a study. Some journals insist that the responsible author sign a statement indicating that he or she accepts full responsibility for the conduct of the trial, has had full access to the data, and has control of the decision to publish, independent of the commercial sponsors funding the work [14].

10. What were the limitations of the study?

Having decided to read the full study manuscript, it is essential to appreciate the limitations of a study. Indeed, most discussions with peers about a recent trial report are won by the person who understands the flaws of a study, in addition to the positive implications. The authors of a study are usually aware of most of their study's limitations, but often they will only write about those that can be defended. While these are valid tactics, the best investigators will discuss all the limitations and recommend how future studies should be conducted to overcome these. Some limitations are inherent to most studies – such as the phenomenon that most participants in a trial are generally healthier as a result of exclusion criteria – and so the ability of study results to be generalized should also be discussed. A balanced discussion suggests the mark of careful and considerate clinical scientists and researchers, and lends the overall report more credibility.

Conclusion

Inevitably, there is far more information being published then can be read and committed to memory. It is therefore natural to restrict our focus to titles relevant to our own work. For these titles, we scan the abstract and decide whether to read the full paper. Mental notes can then be made about the number of patients enrolled, the duration of follow-up, and the dose of the new therapy being tested. With a little more effort, a few more points can also be easily gleaned, allowing a more considered evaluation of the significance of a clinical trial report, which in turn might make the results more memorable.

References

1. Altman DG, Schulz KF, Moher D, et al. The revised CONSORT statement for reporting randomized trials: explanation and elaboration. *Ann Intern Med* 2001;**134**:663–94.

2. Moher D, Schulz KF, Altman DG, et al. The CONSORT statement: Revised recommendations for improving the quality of reports of parallel-group randomized trials. *JAMA* 2001;**285**:1987–91.

3. Greenhalgh T. Assessing the methodological quality of published papers. *BMJ* 1997;**315**:305–8.

4. Critical Appraisal Skills Programme Website, Learning and Development Public Health Resource Unit. Available from http://www.phru.nhs.uk/casp/casp.htm. Accessed March 23, 2005.

5. Joseph KS. Quality of impact factors of general medical journals. *BMJ* 2003;**326**:283.

6. Pocock SJ, Hughes MD, Lee RJ. Statistical problems in the reporting of clinical trials. A survey of three medical journals. *N Engl J Med* 1987;**317**:426–32.

7. The Antihypertensive and Lipid-Lowering Treatment to Prevent Heart Attack Trial (ALLHAT-LLT). Major outcomes in moderately hypercholesterolemic, hypertensive patients randomized to pravastatin vs. usual care. *JAMA* 2002;**288**:2998–3007.

8. Morrison DA, Sethi G, Sacks J, et al. Percutaneous coronary intervention versus coronary artery bypass graft surgery for patients with medically refractory myocardial ischemia and risk factors for adverse outcomes with bypass: a multicenter, randomized trial. Investigators of the Department of Veterans Affairs Cooperative Study #385, the Angina With Extremely Serious Operative Mortality Evaluation (AWESOME). *J Am Coll Cardiol* 2001;**38**:143–9.

9. Morrison DA, Sethi G, Sacks J, et al. Percutaneous coronary intervention versus coronary bypass graft surgery for patients with medically refractory myocardial ischemia and risk factors for adverse outcomes with bypass. The VA AWESOME multicenter registry: Comparison with the randomized clinical trial. *J Am Coll Cardiol* 2002;**39**:266–73.

10. Pocock SJ. *Clinical Trials: A Practical Approach*. Chichester: John Wiley & Sons, 1983.

11. Olson CM, Rennie D, Cook D, et al. Publication bias in editorial decision making. *JAMA* 2002;**287**:2825–8.

12. Simoons ML on behalf of the GUSTO Investigators. Effect of glycoprotein IIb/IIIa receptor blocker abciximab on outcome in patients with acute coronary syndromes without early coronary revascularisation: the GUSTO IV-ACS randomised trial. *Lancet* 2001;**357**:1915–24.

13. Wang D, Bakhai A. Practical issues in trial design. Part 7: Choosing the right sample size for a randomized controlled trial. *Clinical Researcher* 2001;**1**(6):36–9.

14. International Committee of Medical Journal Editors. Uniform requirements for manuscripts submitted to biomedical journals. *Ann Intern Med* 1997;**126**:36–47.

15. Agency for Healthcare Research and Quality. Guide to clinical preventive services. 3rd edition. 2000–2003. Report of the US Preventive Services Task Force. Available from: http://www.ahrq.gov/clinic/cps3dix.htm. Accessed March 23, 2005.

Chapter 38

Meta-Analysis

Duolao Wang, Felicity Clemens,
and Ameet Bakhai

Data for the assessment of new therapies may initially come
from several modest-sized studies. It is not uncommon for
these data to be either contradictory or to vary regarding the
size of the treatment benefit. In situations like this, a meta-
analysis might be valuable. A meta-analysis is a systematic
method for combining the results of multiple similar studies
to allow more accurate conclusions to be drawn from a larger
pooled number of subjects. Although the complexity of the
methods used for a meta-analysis can be a limitation, a
well-conducted meta-analysis provides a powerful guide
to the benefits of a therapy and may pave the way for a large,
definitive trial. In this chapter, we discuss how the meta-
analysis technique is gaining increasing credibility and
attracting more scrutiny, making it useful for all researchers
and clinicians to appreciate the essence of this method.

What is a meta-analysis?

Gene Glass first used the term 'meta-analysis' in 1976 to refer to a philosophy, not a statistical technique. Glass suggested that reviewing the literature in itself was a research technique and should therefore be performed as systematically as more formal research. Since then, the term meta-analysis has meant literally an analysis of several individual analyses or studies, or an amalgamation of previously published and unpublished research on a specific intervention. To perform a meta-analysis, the results of two or more independent studies are combined in a meaningful way that still addresses the original clinical question. The output from a meta-analysis typically consists of an overall mean treatment difference, derived from a weighted average of the treatment difference from each study and a confidence interval. The weighting given to each study depends on its quality, precision, and size.

For example, we recently conducted a meta-analysis on the impact of beta-blockers on mortality in patients with heart failure. Twenty-two relevant studies were identified. While the largest single trial had 3,991 patients and the smallest had just 12 patients, the meta-analysis had a total of 10,480 patients [1]. **Table 1** displays the differences in the mortality rates of 14 of the individual studies that had at least one death in each treatment arm. The meta-analysis shows that beta-blockers reduce the odds of death by about one-third [1], an effect somewhat different from the results of many of the 14 studies.

What is the aim of a meta-analysis?

The aim of a meta-analysis is to estimate the treatment effect with the greatest possible power and precision [2–5]. By including the study populations of several trials, a real treatment difference can be detected more easily due to an increased sample size, and the precision of estimating that difference is improved. A well-conducted meta-analysis is time consuming and expensive, but it is still unlikely to be as expensive as conducting a new, larger trial.

What basic steps are involved in a meta-analysis?

There are five steps involved in a meta-analysis [4,6]:

Step 1: Formulation of the study question
The aim of the analysis should be specific and clear, for example:
"Do beta-blockers reduce mortality in patients with heart failure when used in addition to standard therapies?"

Table 1. Characteristics and results of 14 trials on the effect of beta-blockers on mortality in heart failure patients [1].

Primary author/ trial name	Design	Treatment (dose)	Mean age (years ± SD)	Follow-up (years)	All-cause mortality	
					Treated events/ total events	Control events/ total events
Anderson	RCT	Metoprolol (12.5 mg up to 50 mg twice daily)	51 ± 3	1.6	5/25 (20.0%)	6/25 (24.0%)
Engelmeier	RCT, double-blind	Metoprolol (6.25 mg up to 100 mg once daily over 4–6 weeks)	51 ± 8	0.8	1/9 (11.1%)	2/16 (12.5%)
MDC	RCT, double-blind	Metoprolol (10 mg up to 150 mg over 7 weeks)	49 ± 12	1.5	23/194 (11.8%)	21/189 (11.1%)
Fisher	RCT, double-blind	Metoprolol (6.25 mg up to 50 mg twice daily)	63 ± 10	0.5	1/25 (4.0%)	2/25 (8.0%)
CIBIS	RCT, double-blind	Bisoprolol (1.25 mg up to 5 mg once daily over 4 weeks)	60 ± 1	1.9	53/320 (16.6%)	67/321 (20.9%)
Bristow	RCT, double-blind	Bucindolol (12.5 mg, 50 mg and 200 mg)	56 ± 2	0.2	4/105 (3.8%)	2/34 (5.9%)
Krum	RCT, double-blind	Carvedilol (25 mg twice daily)	56 ± 2	0.3	3/33 (9.1%)	2/16 (12.5%)
PRECISE	RCT, double-blind	Carvedilol (25 mg up to 50 mg, twice daily)	61 ± 11	0.5	6/133 (4.5%)	11/145 (7.6%)
US Carvedilol	RCT, double-blind	Carvedilol (6.25 mg up to 25–50 mg twice daily over 2–10 weeks)	58 ± 12	0.5	22/696 (3.2%)	31/398 (7.8%)
Carvedilol efficacy[a]	RCT, double-blind	Carvedilol[b]			2/70 (2.9%)	2/35 (5.7%)
Colucci	RCT, double-blind	Carvedilol (12.5 mg up to 50 mg twice daily over 6 weeks)	55 ± 11	1	2/232 (0.9%)	5/134 (3.7%)
ANZHFG	RCT, double-blind	Carvedilol (3.125 mg up to 25 mg twice daily over 2–5 weeks)	67[c]	1.6	20/207 (9.7%)	26/208 (12.5%)
CIBIS II	RCT, double-blind	Bisoprolol (1.25 mg up to 10 mg over 5 weeks)	61[c]	1.3	156/1327 (11.8%)	228/1320 (17.3%)
MERIT-HF	RCT, double-blind	Metoprolol (12.5 mg up to 200 mg)	64 ± 9	1	145/1990 (7.3%)	217/2001 (10.9%)

[a]Carvedilol efficacy in severe heart failure. Data presented at the Cardiorenal Advisory Panel Meeting of the US Food and Drug Administration. Protocol 239 (May 2, 1996). [b]No dose is available for this study. [c]No SD is available for this study. ANZHFG = Australia–New Zealand Heart Failure Group; CIBIS = Cardiac Insufficiency Bisoprolol Study; CIBIS II = Cardiac Insufficiency Bisoprolol Study II; MDC = Metoprolol in Dilated Cardiomyopathy Trial; MERIT-HF = Metoprolol CR/XL (controlled release [AstraZeneca's Topol XL]) Randomized Intervention Trial in Heart Failure; PRECISE = Prospective Randomized Evaluation of Carvedilol in Symptoms and Exercise; RCT = randomized controlled trial; SD = standard deviation; US Carvedilol = US Carvedilol Heart Failure Study Group.

Table 2. Sources of information for meta-analyses.

• Search for peer-reviewed material in electronic medical databases, such as:
  – MEDLINE (including Pre-MEDLINE)
  – Embase
  – BIDS
  – ISI
  – The Cochrane Collaboration Library

• Review published books that are relevant to the subject or conference material from meetings devoted to the subject, such as abstract books
• Search specific Internet sites relevant to the disease, including national and international societies of specialists (for beta-blockers, the American College of Cardiology or the European Society of Cardiology web sites) and clearing houses of guidelines for the treatment of that disease/condition
• National or local registries and further unpublished studies can also contribute to the meta-analysis. For these, approach recognized experts and leading medical centers in the specific disease area
• Communicate with the research and clinical affairs departments of specialist pharmaceutical companies to gain published or unpublished study data

• Do a general search of Internet sites using medical search engines, such as OMNI, and general search engines such as:
  – www.Google.com
  – www.AltaVista.com
  – www.Yahoo.com

Step 2: Literature search

To answer the study question, it is important to capture as many relevant studies as possible. The methods used to gather information for a meta-analysis are shown in **Table 2**.

In the beta-blocker study we used a computerized bibliographic method to search the MEDLINE database from January 1998–January 2000 using keywords and phrases such as 'beta-blocker', 'clinical trials', and 'congestive heart failure'. We also searched reports of abstracts from conferences on cardiology and heart failure for the period of 1996–2000.

Step 3: Study selection

Only studies that have a similar design can be retained from all of the studies identified. While formal match-scoring systems (systems to evaluate how similar the studies are) exist and can allow us to control the contribution that a study makes to the meta-analysis, some simple criteria can be used to match the studies to be combined. These are as follows:

• trial design, eg, parallel versus crossover, randomized controlled trials (RCTs) versus non-RCTs
• included patient populations, eg, heart failure patients with or without coronary artery disease

- excluded patient populations, eg, heart failure patients over 65 years old or with renal disease
- treatment strategies, eg, beta-blockers versus placebo or diuretics
- primary outcomes, eg, mortality or hospital readmissions

In general, meta-analyses favor randomized double-blind trials, as biases are minimized or distributed evenly by the process of random allocation. More liberal inclusion criteria can make the studies broader (allowing retrospective or non-randomized studies) but the conclusions might be more subjective [5]. Ideally, the inclusion criteria must aim to address the main research question [6]. For example, a study looking at the treatment effect on quality of life should exclude trials that do not use quality of life as an outcome.

The researcher should also aim to identify negative or indifferent studies that might not have been published, or studies awaiting publication. Research registers can be consulted and well-known researchers can be contacted directly. Hospitals with an interest in the condition under examination might be aware of ongoing trials or unpublished data.

Publication bias

Publication bias is an immediate problem facing researchers conducting a thorough meta-analysis, since journals prefer to publish trials with significant positive findings rather than trials with negative or indifferent findings. The existence of publication bias can be inferred by constructing a funnel plot [7].

A funnel plot is a simple scatter plot of the treatment effects (such as odds ratios [ORs]) estimated from individual studies on the *x*-axis, against a measure of the precision of each study (such as sample size or standard error) on the *y*-axis. The name 'funnel plot' arises from the fact that estimation of the true treatment effect by each component study becomes more precise as the sample sizes of the component studies increase. Therefore, small studies will produce estimates of the effects that will scatter more widely at the bottom of the graph, and will converge for larger studies if these are well matched. In the absence of publication bias, the plot should resemble a symmetrical inverted funnel. A funnel plot for the data in **Table 1** is given in **Figure 1**; it shows no evidence of asymmetry or publication bias. For more about publication bias and funnel plots, please refer to references [4] and [7].

Step 4: Data extraction and quality assessment

Once the final set of studies is identified, the relevant information must be extracted from each study and an assessment of the quality of the available data must be made. Information on study design, patient characteristics, treatments,

Figure 1. Funnel plot of the data from the 14 trials displayed in Table 1. The plot resembles a symmetrical inverted funnel, suggesting no publication bias in this meta-analysis.

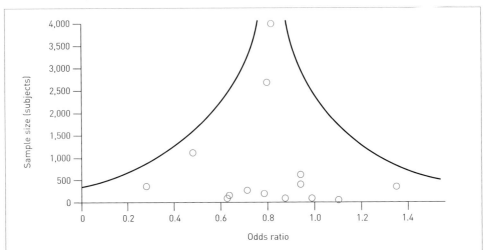

study duration, and primary and other outcomes should be extracted in a standard form to be used for further statistical analysis.

Step 5: Statistical analysis

The final step of a meta-analysis is to combine the information from the different studies by employing appropriate statistical methods to enable interpretation of the pooled effect. This combination might take place at the level of individual patient data or at the level of aggregate trial results and outcomes of interest. There are two basic data requirements for a meta-analysis of aggregate trial results:

- A common measure of treatment effect, such as OR, risk ratio, or mean difference, must be used to compare the different treatment strategies used in each study.
- The variance (or standard error) of the treatment effect must be calculated for each study.

In the beta-blocker study example, the measure of the chosen treatment effect was the OR for the mortality of patients on beta-blockers versus placebo, a commonly used statistic [8].

Table 3. A fixed-effects model (the Woolf method) for computing a pooled odds ratio (OR) estimate and its 95% CI based on 2×2 tables.

Data structure:

Suppose there are k studies, each having data in the form of a 2×2 table:

	Event		Total
	Yes	No	
Treatment A	a_i	b_i	$a_i + b_i$
Treatment B	c_i	d_i	$c_i + d_i$
Total	$a_i + c_i$	$b_i + d_i$	n_i

Assumptions:

ORs are identical and fixed across all studies, and differences in the ORs are only due to within-study variation

Computing steps:

(1) Calculate natural logarithm of the OR for the ith study:

$$\ln(OR) = \ln\left(\frac{a_i \times d_i}{b_i \times c_i}\right)$$

(2) Calculate the standard error (SE) of $\ln(OR)$:

$$SE_i = \sqrt{\frac{1}{a_i} + \frac{1}{b_i} + \frac{1}{c_i} + \frac{1}{d_i}}$$

(3) Compute the weighting for each study:

$$w_i = \frac{1}{SE_i^2}$$

(4) Calculate the pooled logarithm of the fixed-effects OR:

$$\ln(OR) = \frac{\sum_{i=1}^{k} w_i \ln(OR_i)}{\sum_{i=1}^{k} w_i}$$

(5) Calculate the standard error for $\ln(OR_c)$:

$$SE_c = \frac{1}{\sqrt{\sum_{i=1}^{k} w_i}}$$

(6) Do an antilogarithm conversion to obtain the estimate of the pooled OR:

$$OR_c = \exp(\ln(OR_c))$$

(7) Calculate the 95% CI for OR_c:

$$\exp(\ln(OR_c) \pm 1.96 SE_c)$$

Interpretation:

(1) OR_c represents the combined treatment effect

(2) The 95% CI ($\exp(\ln(OR_c) \pm 1.96 SE_c)$) gives the possible range of the true treatment effect. If the CI does not include the value I, then the average effect of treatment B is different from that of treatment A. If this is not the case, there is no evidence that the effects are different

---

What is the appropriate statistical method?

Two types of models are commonly used to conduct a meta-analysis; the *fixed-effects model* and the *random-effects model*. These are each used under different circumstances, but both create a combined estimate of treatment effect.

The fixed-effects model

The fixed-effects model assumes that the meta-analysis is trying to estimate one overall treatment effect for all the studies included in the analysis. This implies that the researcher believes that there is a common 'true' treatment effect underlying the studies and that the results of these studies will vary randomly about this true effect. This model can be used when considering studies that match closely in design and methodology. **Table 3** demonstrates the computing procedures of one of the fixed-effects models (the Woolf method) [9]. By applying this model to the data in **Table 1**, the results generated for the estimated pooled OR and its 95% CI

Figure 2. Meta-analysis of the effect of beta-blockers on mortality in heart failure patients.

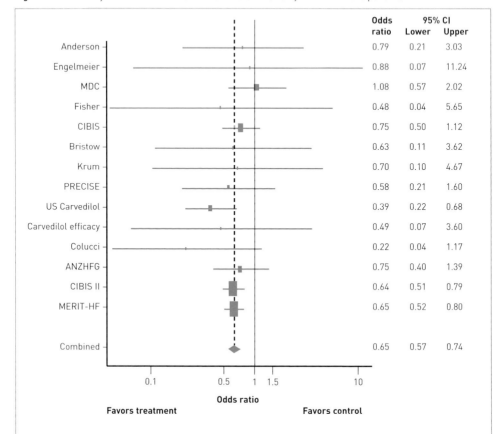

The figure shows the odds ratios (ORs) and their 95% confidence limits for 14 randomized trials studying the effect on mortality of beta-blockers compared with controls. The blocks represent the point estimates for each trial and the horizontal lines the 95% CIs. The size of each block is approximately proportional to the statistical weight of the trial in the meta-analysis. The diamond represents the pooled estimate and its 95% confidence interval. The ORs are displayed on a log scale so that the differences in the CIs can be easily seen. The solid vertical line represents no difference in the treatment effect between two treatments. The heterogeneity test statistic (Q) is 8.44, and, since $k - 1 = 13$, $Q < k - 1$, which suggests no evidence of heterogeneity amongst the trials (see Table 4).

are: $OR_F = 0.65, 95\%$ CI 0.57, 0.74. The results of the meta-analysis are also plotted in **Figure 2**, indicating that the use of beta-blockers, compared with placebo, reduced the odds of death by 35% with a range of 26%–43%.

The random-effects model

The random-effects model assumes that there is a different underlying effect for each study and takes this into account as an additional source of variation. This means that the studies included in the meta-analysis do not necessarily estimate the same treatment effect, since some features of a study's design, such as the

Table 4. A random-effects model (the DerSimonian–Laird method) for computing a pooled odds ratio (OR) estimate and its 95% CI based on 2 × 2 tables.

Data structure: Same as in **Table 1** **Assumptions:** ORs are different across studies. Differences in ORs are not only due to within-study variation but also to between-study variation **Computing steps:** (1) Calculate the heterogeneity test statistic, Q°: Null hypothesis: the k underlying ORs are equal Test statistic: $Q = \sum_{i=1}^{k} w_i (OR_i - OR_F)$ Definitions of w_i, OR_i, OR_F are the same as in **Table 3**. (2) Calculate the between-study variability: $$\tau = \max\left(0, \frac{Q - (k-1)}{\sum_{i=1}^{k} w_i - \left(\frac{\sum_{i=1}^{k} w_i^2}{\sum_{i=1}^{k} w_i}\right)}\right)$$ (3) Calculate the weighting for each study: $$w_i^* = \frac{1}{\dfrac{1}{w_i} + \tau}$$	(4) Calculate the pooled logarithm of the random-effects OR estimate: $$\ln(OR_R) = \frac{\sum_{i=1}^{k} w_i^* \ln(OR_i)}{\sum_{i=1}^{k} w_i^*}$$ (5) Calculate the standard error (SE) for $\ln(OR_R)$: $$SE_R = \frac{1}{\sqrt{\sum_{i=1}^{k} w_i^*}}$$ (6) Do an antilogarithm conversion to obtain an estimate of the pooled OR: $$OR_R = \exp(\ln(OR_R))$$ (7) Calculate the 95% CI for OR_R: $$\exp(\ln(OR_R) \pm 1.96SE_R)$$ **Interpretation:** (1) If $Q \geq k - 1$, then there is evidence of statistical heterogeneity, ie, the ORs are different across the studies[a]. Otherwise, ther is no evidence that the ORs are different (2) OR_R gives the combined treatment effect: $\exp(\ln(OR_R) \pm 1.96SE_R)$ gives the possible range of the true treatment effect and, if the 95% CI does not include the value 1, then the pooled effect of treatment B is different from that of treatment A

[a] For the formal statistical test, please refer to reference 3.

populations included, do not fully match the other studies. These different effects are amalgamated and the meta-analysis is used to estimate an overall effect. Therefore, a random-effects model gives more weight to smaller studies and its overall estimate has a wider confidence interval [2,3,5,9]. Some authors regard this approach to be conceptually problematic because one of the fundamental assumptions inherent in this model is that the studies included are a random sample from a hypothetical population of studies [3].

The procedures for using the DerSimonian–Laird random-effects model are described in **Table 4**, where they are applied to the data from **Table 1**. A test for heterogeneity (the difference in beta-blocker effect on mortality between studies) for this meta-analysis was performed. The value of the heterogeneity test statistic (Q) was 8.44, and, since $k - 1 = 13$, $Q < k - 1$, which indicates that the included studies are very similar (there is no evidence of statistically significant heterogeneity; see **Table 4**). The pooled estimate of the effect of beta-blocker treatment on mortality using the random-effects model is: $OR_R = 0.65$, 95% CI

Table 5. Meta-analysis of 10 hypothetical trials using the Woolf fixed-effects model and the DerSimonian–Laird random effects model.

Study	Treated events/ total events	Control events/ total events	Odds ratio (95% CI)	Fixed-effects model weighting	Random-effects model weighting
1	15/130	15/135	1.04 (0.49, 2.23)	6.65	2.21
2	21/400	17/135	0.38 (0.20, 0.75)	8.51	2.39
3	14/60	24/50	0.33 (0.15, 0.75)	5.77	2.11
4	6/40	18/40	0.22 (0.07, 0.63)	3.37	1.67
5	12/1010	35/760	0.25 (0.13, 0.48)	8.75	2.41
6	138/1400	175/765	0.37 (0.29, 0.47)	64.73	3.16
7	15/500	20/525	0.78 (0.40, 1.54)	8.28	2.37
8	6/110	2/105	2.97 (0.59, 15.06)	1.46	1.01
9	65/150	40/100	1.15 (0.69, 1.92)	14.53	2.7
10	5/70	2/35	1.27 (0.23, 6.90)	1.34	0.96
Combined OR (95% CI)				0.47 (0.39, 0.55)	0.55 (0.36, 0.85)

The heterogeneity test (Q) for the random-effects model analysis was 34.66, and, since $k - 1 = 9$, $Q > k - 1$, which indicates that the 10 studies are statistically heterogeneous. The fixed-effects model weights each study according to its sample size, so the largest trial has the most weight. On the other hand, the weightings generated by the random-effects model are less varied, giving relatively more weight to smaller studies, yielding a wider confidence interval for the pooled odds ratio than occurs with the fixed-effects model.
CI = confidence interval; OR = odds ratio.

0.57, 0.74. For the data in **Table 1**, the between-study variability is zero ($\tau = 0$; see **Table 4**), therefore these results are identical to those from the fixed-effects model.

Table 5 compares the meta-analysis of 10 hypothetically heterogeneous trials using the Woolf fixed-effects and DerSimonian–Laird random-effects models. Testing the random-effects model for heterogeneity gives $Q = 34.66$, and, since $k - 1 = 9$, $Q > k - 1$, which indicates that the 10 studies are statistically heterogeneous. The estimated between-study variability is 0.30 ($\tau = 0.30$). The results from the meta-analysis show that the random-effects model gives smaller studies more weight and yields a wider confidence interval for the pooled OR than occurs with the fixed-effects model.

There will only be a substantial difference in the pooled treatment effect computed by the two methods if there is considerable heterogeneity between the component studies. Whether the fixed- or random-effects model should be used for a specific meta-analysis depends on the presence of statistically significant heterogeneity (evaluated by formal heterogeneity testing). The random-effects model is usually recommended when statistically significant heterogeneity is present between study results. More importantly, the source of heterogeneity should be investigated to identify the types of clinical heterogeneity in terms of, eg, patient selection, baseline disease severity, dose schedules, and years of follow-up, that might explain all or part of the statistical heterogeneity [10]. In the absence of statistically significant heterogeneity, the fixed-effects model is advocated [4].

What key objectives are there when results are presented?

In any meta-analysis it is important that the account of the analysis is transparent and that the reasons for including and excluding various studies and other data are documented. Both the sources and the search strategy for this evidence need to be described and the criteria used to assess the quality of the included studies should be detailed. By doing this, any bias inadvertently caused by the researcher due to his/her method of study selection is transparent and the reader can appreciate the limitations of the evidence base, the efforts made to address these limitations, and how robust the inferences drawn from the results are. The results of a meta-analysis can be best presented in a graph like **Figure 2**.

What are the main concerns about meta-analysis?

Meta-analysis is a useful way of combining available evidence. The most common criticism is that the pooled estimate is not a meaningful measure and it is not applicable to 'real life' medical practice for a number of reasons [4]. These reasons include differences between studies, poor quality of some or all of the studies included, and a selection bias towards published studies. Essentially, the criticisms are that when the data come from several separate studies, adjustments might not account for the differences between the studies.

The second problem, right from the outset, is that in a meta-analysis it is impossible to know which studies are missing because they were never captured, even at the stage of screening for generally relevant studies. An inexpert search of the literature might not identify all relevant studies [4,6].

Thirdly, each of the studies included in the meta-analysis will have their own problems with internal validity [4,6]. The biases existing within each study will be passed on to the meta-analysis and they will affect its conclusions. It is therefore essential that study quality is considered when a preliminary literature search is performed.

Lastly, a meta-analysis is usually performed when the results of modest studies conflict or there is a large variability in the size of the treatment effect. If data from large trials with matching criteria were available, a meta-analysis would not be needed.

While meta-analyses are increasingly being performed in medical research, the analysis is only as good as the team performing the work. The art of this science is still developing in an attempt to overcome several limitations. A strong meta-analysis will pay careful attention to the inputs (ie, patients, endpoints, and trial design) and will be clear about the methods and assumptions used. Finally, individuals who are contemplating performing a meta-analysis are advised to work together with researchers and statisticians with experience in this field.

Conclusion

The results of a meta-analysis can provide a significant weight of evidence and, although the complexity of the method is a limitation, this analysis allows clinical questions to be addressed in the absence of data from a large, definitive randomized trial. Where evidence for the benefit of a new treatment over standard therapy conflicts between modest-sized studies or there is variation in the size of the benefit, a meta-analysis gives a more accurate measure of the true effect of the therapy or intervention. Meta-analyses are therefore here to stay, and are being performed in many specialties other than healthcare. There is therefore an increasing need for researchers to be able to appreciate the place of meta-analyses and the results they generate, bearing in mind their complexities.

References

1. Shibata MC, Flather MD, Wang D. Systematic review of the impact of beta-blockers on mortality and hospital admissions in heart failure. *Eur J Heart Fail* 2001;**3**:351–7.
2. Chalmers TC. Meta-analysis in clinical medicine. *Trans Am Clin Climatol Assoc* 1987;**99**:144–50.
3. DerSimonian R, Laird NM. Meta-analysis in clinical trials. *Control Clin Trials* 1986;**7**:177–86.
4. Egger M, Davey Smith G, Altman D, editors. *Systematic Reviews In Health Care: Meta-Analysis In Context*. London: BMJ Publishing Group, 2001.

5. Everitt BS, Pickles A. *Statistical Aspects of the Design and Analysis of Clinical Trials*. London: Imperial College Press, 1999.

6. L'Abbe KA, Detsky AS, O'Rourke K. Meta-analysis in clinical research. *Ann Intern Med* 1987;**107**:224–33.

7. Egger M, Davey Smith G, Schneider M, et al. Bias in meta-analysis detected by a simple, graphical test. *BMJ* 1997;**315**:629–34.

8. Bakhai A, Wang D. Practical issues in trial design. Part 5: Relative risk ratios and odds ratios. *Clinical Researcher* 2001;**1**(8):34–6.

9. Fleiss JL. The statistical basis of meta-analysis. *Stat Methods Med Res* 1993;**2**:121–45.

10 Thompson SG. Why sources of heterogeneity in meta-analysis should be investigated. *BMJ* 1994;**309**:1351–5.

Glossary

ANOVA (analysis of variance)

A statistical method for comparing several means by comparing variances. It concerns a normally distributed outcome (response) variable and a single categorical (predictor) variable representing treatments or groups. ANOVA is a special case of a linear regression model by which group means can be easily compared.

Bias

Systematic errors associated with the inadequacies in the design, conduct, or analysis of a trial on the part of any of the participants of that trial (patients, medical personnel, trial coordinators, or researchers), or in publication of the results, that make the estimate of a treatment effect deviate from its true value. Systematic errors are difficult to detect and cannot be analyzed statistically, but can be reduced by using randomization, treatment concealment, blinding, and standardized study procedures.

Confidence intervals

A range of values within which the 'true' population parameter (eg, mean, proportion, treatment effect) is likely to lie. Usually 95% confidence intervals are quoted which implies there is 95% confidence in the statement that the 'true' population parameter will lie somewhere between the lower and upper limits.

Confounding

A situation in which a variable (or factor) is related to both the study variable and the outcome so that the effect of the study variable on the outcome is distorted. For example, if a study found that coffee consumption (study variable) is associated with the risk of lung cancer (outcome), the confounding factor would be cigarette smoking, since coffee drinking is often performed with the use of cigarettes, which is the true risk factor for lung cancer. Thus we can say that the apparent association of coffee drinking with lung cancer is due to confounding by cigarette smoking (confounding factor). In clinical trials, confounding occurs when a baseline characteristic (or variable) of patients is associated with the outcome but unevenly distributed between treatment groups. As a result, the observed treatment difference from the unadjusted (univariate) analysis can be explained by the imbalanced distribution of this variable.

Correlation coefficient (r)

A measure of the linear association between two continuous variables. The correlation coefficient varies between –1.0 and +1.0. The closer it is to 0, the weaker the association. When both variables go in the same direction (eg, height and weight) r has a positive value between 0 and 1.0 depending on the strength of the relationship. When the variables go in opposite directions (eg, left ventricular function and life-span) r has a negative value between 0 and –1.0, depending on the strength of this inverse relationship.

Covariates

Generally used as an alternative name for explanatory variables in the regression analysis but more specifically referring to variables that are not of primary interest in an investigation. Covariates are often measured at baseline in clinical trials because it is believed that they are likely to affect the outcome variable and consequently need to be included to estimate the adjusted treatment effect.

Descriptive/inferential statistics

Descriptive statistics are used to summarize and describe data collected in a study. To summarize a quantitative (continuous) variable, measures of central location (ie, mean, median, mode) and spread (eg, range and standard deviation) are often used, whereas frequency distributions and percentages (proportions) are usually used to summarize a qualitative variable. Inferential statistics are used to make inferences or judgments about a larger population based on the data collected from a small sample drawn from the population. A key component of inferential statistics is hypothesis testing. Examples of inferential statistical methods are the t-test and regression analysis.

Endpoint

A clearly defined outcome associated with an individual subject in clinical research. Outcomes may be based on safety, efficacy, or other study objectives (eg, pharmacokinetic parameters). An endpoint can be quantitative (eg, systolic blood pressure, cell count), qualitative (eg, death, severity of disease), or time-to-event (eg, time to first hospitalization from randomization).

Hazard ratio

In survival analysis, the hazard (rate) represents an instantaneous event rate (incidence rate) at a certain time for an individual who has not experienced an event at that time. A hazard ratio compares two hazards of having an event between two groups. If the hazard ratio is 2.0, then the hazard of having an event in one group is twice the hazard of having an event in the other group. The computation of the hazard ratio assumes that the ratio is consistent over time (proportional hazards assumption).

Hypothesis testing or significance testing

A statistical procedure for assessing whether an observed treatment difference was due to random error (chance) by calculating a P-value using the observed sample statistics such as mean, standard deviation, etc. The P-value is the probability that the observed data or more extreme data would have occurred if the null hypothesis (ie, no true difference) were true. If the calculated P-value is a small value (eg, <0.05), the null hypothesis is then rejected and we say that there is a statistically significant difference.

Intention-to-treat analysis

A method of data analysis based on the intention to treat a subject (ie, the treatment regimen a patient was assigned at randomization) rather than the actual treatment regimen he received. As a consequence, subjects allocated to a treatment group are followed up, assessed, and analyzed as members of that group regardless of their compliance to that therapy or the protocol, irrespective of whether they later crossed over to another treatment group, or whether they discontinued treatment.

Kaplan–Meier estimate and survival curve

A survival curve shows an estimate of the fraction of patients who survive over the follow-up period of the study without an event of interest (eg, death). The Kaplan–Meier estimate is a simple way of computing the survival curve, taking into account patients who were lost to follow-up or any other reasons for incomplete results (known as censored observations). It usually provides a staircase graph of the fraction of patients remaining free of event over time.

Meta-analysis

The systematic review and evaluation of the evidence from two or more independent studies asking the same clinical question to yield an overall answer to the question.

Normal distribution

A bell-shaped symmetric distribution for a continuous variable with the highest frequency at a mean value and the lowest frequency further away from this mean value. A normal distribution can be completely described by two parameters: mean (μ) and variance (σ^2). In the special case of $\mu = 0$ and $\sigma^2 = 1$, it is called the standard normal distribution.

Number needed to treat (NNT)

This term is often used to describe how many patients would need to be given a treatment to prevent one event. It is determined from the absolute difference between one treatment and another. For example, in a randomized study, a group receiving treatment A had a death rate of 12.5% and a group on treatment B had a death rate of 15.0% in groups matched for size and length of follow-up. Comparing the two treatments there was an absolute risk reduction of 15% – 12.5% = 2.5% for treatment A. From this we can derive that the NNT (= 1/0.025) is 40. This means 40 patients need to be given treatment A rather than treatment B to prevent one additional death.

Odds ratio (OR) and risk ratio (RR)

These terms compare the probability of having an event between two groups exposed to a risk factor or treatment. The risk ratio (RR) is the ratio of the probability of occurrence of an event between two groups. The odds ratio (OR) is the ratio of patients with and without an event in each group. For example, if the number of deaths in the treatment and control arms (both of sample size 100) of a randomized study are 50 and 25 respectively, the RR = (50/100) / (25/100) = 2. The treatment group has a 2-fold relative risk of dying compared with the control group. The OR = (50/50) / (25/75) = 3, indicating that the odds of death in the treatment arm is 3-fold that of the control arm.

Per-protocol analysis

A method of analysis in which only the subset of subjects who complied sufficiently with the protocol are included. Protocol compliance includes exposure to treatment, availability of measurements, correct eligibility, and absence of any other major protocol violations. This approach contrasts with the more conservative and widely accepted 'intention-to-treat' analysis.

Power

The probability of rejecting the null hypothesis (eg, no treatment difference) when it is false. It is the basis of procedures for calculating the sample size required to detect an expected treatment effect of a particular magnitude.

Random error

An unpredictable deviation of an observed value from a true value resulting from sampling variability. It is a reflection of the fact that the sample is smaller than the population; for larger samples, the random error is smaller, as opposed to systematic errors (bias) that keep adding up because they all go in the same direction.

Regression analyses

Methods of explaining or predicting outcome variables using information from explanatory variables. Regression analyses are often used in clinical trials to estimate the adjusted treatment effect taking into account differences in baseline characteristics, and in epidemiological studies to identify prognostic factors while controlling for potential confounders. Commonly used regression models include linear, logistic, and Cox regression methods.

Risk factor

A risk factor can be defined as anything in the environment, personal characteristics, or events that make it more or less likely one might develop a given disease, reach an adverse event, or experience a change in health status. For example, raised cholesterol is a risk factor for heart attacks.

Standard error

A measure of the random variability of a statistic (eg, mean, proportion, treatment effect) indicating how far the statistic is likely to be from its true value. For example, standard error of the mean (SEM) indicates uncertainty of a single sample mean ($\overline{X}$) as an estimate of the population mean (μ). A smaller SEM implies a more reliable estimate of the population mean. Standard error can be used to calculate a confidence interval of an estimated population parameter. The smaller the standard error, the narrower the confidence interval, and the more precise the point estimate of the population parameter.

Treatment effect

An effect attributed to a treatment in a clinical trial, often measured as the difference in a summary measure of an outcome variable between treatment groups. Commonly expressed as a difference in means for a continuous outcome, a risk difference, risk ratio, or odds ratio for a binary outcome, and a hazard ratio for a time-to-event outcome.

Univariate/multivariate analysis

The term variate refers to the term variable. A univariate analysis examines the association between a single variable and an outcome variable (correctly called a bivariate analysis), for example, age and occurrence of stroke. In a multivariate analysis, associations between many variables are examined simultaneously. In particular, multivariate regression analysis can be used to assess the relative importance and contribution of each predictor variable to the outcome variable. For example, a multivariate logistic regression can be undertaken to identify the most important prognostic factors among several risk factors (eg, age, sex, systolic blood pressure, and cholesterol level) that predict the occurrence of stroke.

Abbreviations

3TC	lamivudine
ACE	angiotensin-converting enzyme
ALLHAT	Anti-hypertensive and Lipid-Lowering Treatment to Prevent Heart Attack Trial
ANCOVA	analysis of covariance
ANOVA	analysis of variance
ANZHFG	Australia-New Zealand Heart Failure Group
APC	activated protein C
AUC	area under the curve
AWESOME	Angina With Extremely Serious Operative Mortality Evaluation
BBB	bundle branch block
BHAT	Beta-blocker Heart Attack Trial
bpm	beats per minute
Ca	calcium
CABG	coronary artery bypass graft
CAD	coronary artery disease
CAL	chronic airways limitation
CANDLE	Candersartan versus Losartan Efficacy
CAP	community-acquired pneumonia
CARET	Beta-Carotene and Retional Efficacy Trial
CAST	Cardiac Arrhythmia Suppression Trial
CEC	clinical events committee
CESAR	Conventional Ventilation or Extra Corporeal Membrane Oxygenation for Severe Adult Respiratory Failure
CF	cystic fibrosis
CF-WISE	Withdrawal of Inhaled Steroids Evaluation Study in Patients with Cystic Fibrosis
CHARM	Candesartan in Heart failure – Assessment of Reduction in Mortality and morbidity
CHF	chronic heart failure
CI	confidence interval
CIBIS	Cardiac Insufficiency Bisoprolol Study
CIBIS II	Cardiac Insufficiency Bisoprolol Study II
CONSORT	Consolidated Standards of Reporting Trials
CRASH	Corticosteroid Randomization After Significant Head Injury
CRF	case record form
CRT	cluster randomized trial
CURE	Clopidogrel in Unstable Angina to Prevent Recurrent Events
D4T	stavudine

DBP	diastolic blood pressure
DDI	didanosine
DSMB	data and safety monitoring board
DMSC	data and safety monitoring committee
ECG	electrocardiogram
EF	error factor
EFV	efavirenz
EUCTD	EU Clinical Trials Directive
FDA	Food and Drug Administration
FEV_1	forced expiratory volume in 1 second
GISSI	Gruppo Italiano per lo Studio della Streptochinasi nell'Infarto Miocardico
GRACE	Global Registry of Acute Coronary Events
GUSTO-IV	Global Use of Strategies to Open Occluded Coronary Arteries
HAART	highly active anti-retroviral therapy
HOPE	Heart Outcomes Prevention Evaluation
hosp	hospitalization
HRT	hormone replacement therapy
ICC	intra-cluster correlation coefficient
ICH	The International Conference on Harmonisation of Technical Requirements for Registration of Pharmaceuticals for Human Use
ICH-GCP	The International Conference on Harmonisation guidelines for Good Clinical Practice
ICS	inhaled corticosteroids
IDV	indinavir
IMAGES	Intravenous Magnesium Efficacy in Stroke
IMS	intravenous magnesium sulfate
IMP	investigational medicinal product
IQR	interquartile range
IRB	institutional review board
ISIS-2	Second International Study of Infarct Survival
ISIS-4	Fourth International Study of Infarct Survival
ITT	intention-to-treat
KM	Kaplan–Meier
LLQ	lower limit of quantitation
LOCF	last observation carried forward
MAGPIE	Magnesium Sulphate or Placebo for Women with Pre-Eclampsia
MAR	missing at random
MCAR	missing completely at random

MDC	Metoprolol in Dilated Cardiomyopathy Trial
MERIT-HF	Metoprolol CR/XL (controlled release [AstraZeneca's Topol XL]) Randomized Intervention Trial in Heart Failure
MHRA	Medicines and Healthcare Products Regulatory Agency
MI	myocardial infarction
MNAR	missing not at random
NA	not applicable
NFV	nelfinavir
NYHA	New York Heart Association
OC	oral captopril
OM	oral mononitrate
OR	odds ratio
ORACLE	Broad Spectrum Antibiotics for Preterm, Prelabour Rupture of Fetal Membranes
OSIRIS	Open Study of Infants at High Risk of or with Respiratory Insufficiency – the Role of Surfactant
P	*P*-value
P	phosphorus
PBC	primary biliary cirrhosis
PCI	percutaneous coronary intervention
PCI-CURE	Percutaneous Coronary Intervention and Clopidogrel in Unstable Angina to Prevent Recurrent Ischemic Events
PD	pharmacodynamic
PI	principal investigator
PK	pharmacokinetic
PP	per-protocol
PRAIS-UK	Prospective Registry of Acute Ischemic Syndromes in the United Kingdom
PRECISE	Prospective Randomized Evaluation of Carvedilol in Symptoms and Exercise
PROMIS-UK	Prospective Registry of Outcomes and Management in Acute Ischemic Syndromes in the United Kingdom
PUFA	polyunsaturated fatty acids
QALYs	quality-adjusted life-years
r	ritonavir
RALES	Randomized Aldactone Evaluation Study
RCT	randomized controlled trial
RITA	Randomized Intervention Trial of Angina
RITA 3	Noninvasive Versus Invasive (Angiography) in Patients with Unstable Angina or Non-Q Wave Infarct
RR	risk ratio/relative risk

SAQ	saquinavir
SBP	systolic blood pressure
SD	standard deviation
SE	standard error
SEM	standard error of the mean
SMO	site management organization
Syst-Eur	Systolic-Hypertension-Europe
TARGET	Do Tirofiban and ReoPro Give Similar Efficacy Outcomes Trial
TB	tuberculosis
TMC	Tacrolimus Versus Microemulsified Cyclosporin in Liver Transplantation
US Carvedilol	US Carvedilol Heart Failure Study Group
ZDV	zidovudine

Index

Note: Page numbers in *italics* refer to tables or boxed material. Page numbers in **bold** refer to figures. *vs* indicates a comparison.